The Bacterial L-Forms

MICROBIOLOGY SERIES

Series Editors
ALLEN I. LASKIN
Sommerset, New Jersey

RICHARD I. MATELES
Stauffer Chemical Company
Westport, Connecticut

Volume 1   Bacterial Membranes and Walls
edited by Loretta Leive

Volume 2   Eucaryotic Microbes as Model Developmental Systems
edited by Danton H. O'Day and Paul A. Horgen

Volume 3   Microorganisms and Minerals
edited by Eugene D. Weinberg

Volume 4   Bacterial Transport
edited by Barry P. Rosen

Volume 5   Microbial Testers: Probing Carcinogenesis
edited by I. Cecil Felkner

Volume 6   Virus Infections: Modern Concepts and Status
edited by Lloyd C. Olson

Volume 7   Methods in Environmental Virology
edited by Charles P. Gerba and Sagar M. Goyal

Volume 8   Microtubules in Microorganisms
edited by Piero Cappucinelli and N. Ronald Morris

Volume 9   Handbook of Indigenous Fermented Foods
edited by Keith H. Steinkraus

Volume 10   Unusual Microorganisms: Gram-Negative Fastidious Species
edited by Edward J. Bottone

Volume 11 Laboratory Manual for Medical Microbiology
edited by The Faculty of the Department of Microbiology, Schools of Medicine and Dentistry, State University of New York at Buffalo

Volume 12 Infectious Diarrheal Disease: Current Concepts and Laboratory Procedures
edited by Paul D. Ellner

Volume 13 Microbial Degradation of Organic Compounds
edited by David T. Gibson

Volume 14 The Silage Fermentation
by Michael K. Woolford

Volume 15 The Mycobacteria: A Sourcebook *(in two parts)*
edited by George P. Kubica and Lawrence G. Wayne

Volume 16 Nonfermentative Gram-Negative Rods: Laboratory Identification and Clinical Aspects
edited by Gerald L. Gilardi

Volume 17 The Bacterial L-Forms
edited by Sarabelle Madoff

Other Volumes in Preparation

The Bacterial L-Forms

edited by

Sarabelle Madoff

Departments of Medicine and Bacteriology
Massachusetts General Hospital
Boston, Massachusetts

MARCEL DEKKER, INC.   New York and Basel

Library of Congress Cataloging-in-Publication Data
Main entry under title:

The Bacterial L-forms.

(Microbiology series ; v. 17)
Includes index.
1. L-form bacteria. I. Madoff, Sarabelle. II. Series
QR73.B33   1986   616'.014   85-31145
ISBN 0-8247-7480-9

COPYRIGHT © 1986 by MARCEL DEKKER, INC.   ALL RIGHTS RESERVED

Neither this book nor any part may be reproduced or transmitted in any form or by any means, electronic or mechanical, including photocopying, microfilming, and recording, or by any information storage and retrieval system, without permission in writing from the publisher.

MARCEL DEKKER, INC.
270 Madison Avenue, New York, New York 10016

Current printing [last digit]:
10 9 8 7 6 5 4 3 2 1

PRINTED IN THE UNITED STATES OF AMERICA

Dedicated to the Memory of
Dr. Louis Dienes
Scientist, Teacher, and Friend

Foreword

The bacterial L-forms have been subjects of laboratory research for a half-century, engaging the fascinated concern of microbiologists, pathologists, immunologists and, in recent years, molecular biologists and geneticists. This book attests to the sheer volume of work accomplished in the past 50 years; the extensive bibliographies following each chapter provide a glimpse into the huge literature that has accumulated from laboratories all around the world.

A lot has been learned about L-forms, to be sure. A casual reader might leaf through the book quickly and conclude that all the facts must now be in hand, and that he needed only time enough to settle down for a fairly long read, with complete comprehension of these peculiar organisms as the reward. But a closer reading tells otherwise. These are among the strangest creatures in nature, and virtually everything that is known about them gives rise to new and more puzzling questions. Fifty years out, the research on L-forms is still in its earliest stage, with what seems like everything in the world still awaiting to be discovered.

The authors make plain their own puzzlement, but also their long devotion to their subject. There is something ineluctably attractive about L-forms. Despite the many technical difficulties they impose on an investigator, including their finicky habits of life and their tendency to behave unpredictably, it is easy to get hooked on them.

It may be permissible, in an introduction, to say something about these microorganisms that would be unsuitable in any of the scientific chapters. I think that what I have to say would win head-nodding agreement from most of the authors, maybe all. It is this: L-forms are charming creatures. Once you have seen their fantastic colonies, especially when illuminated under a Dienes-stained coverslip, they become absolutely irresistible. They are, to use a word rarely employed in scientific discourse (except by the chemists for crystals in the old days), beautiful, nothing less.

The things that have been learned about them so far, and the questions being raised for the future, are of the most down-to-earth, practical importance. There is a shared hunch that they may turn out to be significant pathogens in certain chronic human diseases, perhaps including genitourinary disorders, even rheumatoid arthritis (my own hunch). The molecular biologists might look forward to a lifetime of puzzlement over the profound genetic alterations set in play when an ordinary bacterium changes to its L-form, and then back again.

The experimental pathologists may be nearly ready for the development of totally new models of infectious disease. And the evolutionary biologists, wondering over the origins of endosymbiotic organelles in eukaryotic cells, may find in L-forms the beginnings of theory. Not to mention the expanding community of mycoplasmologists, who still need to straighten out the lineage of their favorite organisms, and who should have L-forms somewhere on their minds.

All of these and more are excellent reasons for going to work on L-forms and writing up grant proposals. But the real reason, the one that sooner or later compels attention and makes it impossible *not* to work on L-forms, is that they are, in themselves, so enchanting.

Lewis Thomas
Memorial Sloan-Kettering Cancer Center
New York, New York

Preface

Historically, the bacterial L-forms have been studied primarily for their intrinsic scientific merit. The fact that a bacterium under certain conditions can enter into a wall-less state, that it can survive in this state, and that it can ultimately revert to its usual bacterial form (or lose the ability to revert), is in itself remarkable. This phenomenon cannot be insignificant in the life of bacteria.

It is the intent of this book to present the current state of knowledge of the L-forms of bacteria. In the past, interest was centered around cultural techniques, morphologic transformations, and to a lesser degree, metabolism and physiology of the L-forms. It is now clear that there are still many gaps in our understanding of these cell wall-deficient organisms. However, we have come a long way. In recent years, the L-forms have come to be recognized not only as bacterial curiosities, but as invaluable tools in many new and innovative areas of microbial research. With the recent advances in molecular biology, the bacterial L-forms are being used as special models for bacterial function at the molecular level. Molecular genetic studies may be greatly enhanced by the use of the L-forms. They can be used to study the biosynthesis of bacterial membranes, the mechanisms of antibiotic effects on bacteria and their membranes, ribosomal functions, the replication of DNA and plasmid-related effects, and many other aspects of bacterial physiology at the genetic level.

It is important to recognize the diversity of these studies. Reports from many scientific disciplines that have benefited from the study of bacterial L-forms are included in this volume, from fundamental studies of ultrastructure, morphology, and reproduction to the broader areas of the physical, biochemical, and genetic aspects of bacterial variation. Considerations of host defense mechanisms and other antigenic factors and of susceptibility to antimicrobial agents are included. The study of these complex and divergent disciplines can be expected to yield valuable information as to the role of the L-forms in the biology of bacteria and their participation and significance in infectious disease processes.

In addition, the fascinating problem of possible phylogenetic relationships among bacteria, the L-forms, and the mycoplasmas is discussed. Present concepts of evolutionary pathways in bacteria should receive considerable impetus through attention to the many varieties of cell wall-deficient microorganisms.

The principal groups of bacteria that have been studied extensively have been accorded separate chapters. Of necessity, many others have had to be omitted because of limitations of space. However, throughout the volume, extensive references to all manner of bacterial L-forms are included.

Seventeen investigators are represented in this volume; each has contributed the most recent information on the state of current research in his or her own particular area of interest and expertise. A considerable amount of previously unpublished data is included, as is a comprehensive review of our current concepts of the role of the bacterial L-forms in disease, a matter of vital interest to every worker in the field. Thus this volume is intended not only for the microbiologist concerned with cell wall-deficient organisms, but for other interested microbiologists, and for cell biologists, molecular biologists, membrane biochemists, and geneticists, as well as for clinicians and immunopathologists in the infectious diseases.

I wish to express my sincere appreciation to the authors for their contributions and for the time, effort, and interest expressed in the realization of this book. I am grateful also for the helpful suggestions of Dr. J. R. King, Dr. P. F. Smith, and Dr. R. M. Cole. I wish to thank Kenneth Demsky for secretarial assistance. Thanks are due to my daughter Eve and to the other members of my family for providing support, encouragement, and humor. For assistance with the final preparation of this volume, I am grateful to the staff of Marcel Dekker, Inc.

Sarabelle Madoff

Contents

Foreword (Lewis Thomas)		*v*
Preface		*vii*
Contributors		*xi*

1	Introduction to the Bacterial L-Forms *Sarabelle Madoff*	1
2	Origins and Evolution of Wall-Less Prokaryotes *Harold Neimark*	21
3	L-Forms of Group D *Streptococcus* *James R. King*	43
4	Macromolecular Synthesis, Survival, and Cytotoxicity of an L-Form of *Streptococcus pyogenes* *Charles Panos*	59
5	L-Forms of *Bacillus* *Richard W. Gilpin and Frank E. Young*	99
6	β-Lactam-Induced *Proteus* L-Forms *Jean-Marie Ghuysen, Martine Nguyen-Disteche, and André Rousset*	127
7	*Brucella* L-Forms—Their Occurrence and Characteristics *Betty A. Hatten and Janine Schmitt-Slomska*	163
8	L-Forms of *Neisseria* *John W. Lawson*	185
9	L-Forms of *Pseudomonas aeruginosa* *John Z. Montgomerie*	195

10	Biology of Cell Wall-Defective Forms of *Nocardia* Blaine L. Beaman	203
11	L-Forms as Models for the Study of Antibiotic Activities Janine Schmitt-Slomska	229
12	Immunology of Bacterial L-Forms Raymond J. Lynn	263
13	Interaction of Cell Wall-Defective Bacteria with Host Defenses Zell A. McGee	277
14	L-Forms and Bacterial Variants in Infectious Disease Processes William N. Pachas	287

Index   *319*

Contributors

Blaine L. Beaman, Department of Medical Microbiology and Immunology, University of California School of Medicine, Davis, California

Jean-Marie Ghuysen, Department of Microbiology, University of Liège, Liège, Belgium

Richard W. Gilpin,* Department of Microbiology and Immunology, The Medical College of Pennsylvania, Philadelphia, Pennsylvania

Betty A. Hatten, Department of Clinical Laboratory Sciences, Oklahoma University Health Sciences Center, Oklahoma City, Oklahoma

James R. King, Division of Anti-Infective Drug Products, Center for Drugs and Biologics, Food and Drug Administration, Rockville, Maryland

John W. Lawson,† Department of Microbiology, Clemson University, Clemson, South Carolina

Raymond J. Lynn, Department of Microbiology, University of South Dakota, School of Medicine, Vermillion, South Dakota

Zell A. McGee, Department of Medicine, Center for Infectious Diseases, University of Utah School of Medicine, Salt Lake City, Utah

Sarabelle Madoff, Departments of Medicine and Bacteriology, Massachusetts General Hospital, Boston, Massachusetts

John Z. Montgomerie, Infectious Disease Division, University of Southern California School of Medicine, Los Angeles, California

---

*Present affiliation: Department of Biochemistry, Jefferson Medical College, Thomas Jefferson University, Philadelphia, Pennsylvania

†Present affiliation: Department of Medical Microbiology, University of Birmingham, Birmingham, United Kingdom

Harold Neimark, College of Medicine, State University of New York, Brooklyn, New York

Martine Nguyen-Disteche, Department of Microbiology, University of Liège, Liège, Belgium

William N. Pachas, Department of Medicine, Spaulding Rehabilitation Hospital and Harvard Medical School, Boston, Massachusetts

Charles Panos, Department of Microbiology, Jefferson Medical College, Thomas Jefferson University, Philadelphia, Pennsylvania

André Rousset,[*] Department of Bacteriology, University of Strasbourg, Strasbourg, France

Janine Schmitt-Slomska, U.65 INSERM: National Institute of Health and Medical Research, Department of Microbiology, Faculty of Medicine, Nimes, France

Frank E. Young,[†] Department of Microbiology, University of Rochester School of Medicine and Dentistry, Rochester, New York

---

[*]*Present affiliation*: Department of Bacteriology, University of Dijon, Dijon, France
[†]*Present affiliation*: Office of the Commissioner, U.S. Food and Drug Administration, Washington, District of Columbia

1
Introduction to the Bacterial L-Forms

SARABELLE MADOFF
Departments of Medicine and Bacteriology, Massachusetts General Hospital, Boston, Massachusetts

I. Historical Aspects	2
II. Terminology and Definitions	2
III. Induction of L-Forms	5
IV. Morphology and Ultrastructure	6
V. Reproduction and Reversion	9
VI. Reversion of L-Forms and Identification of Revertants	9
VII. Genetic Factors	12
VIII. Evolutionary Aspects	13
IX. Occurrence and Pathogenicity	14
X. Future Investigations	15
References	15

It is the very strangeness of nature that makes science engrossing.
Lewis Thomas

The purpose of this introductory chapter is to present a brief overview of the biology of the bacterial L-forms and to place within this framework the work of the many investigators contributing to this volume. The diversity of the research in this field is so broad in scope that an attempt to correlate these studies seems indicated. Salient points are included to present the current knowledge in the field and to interrelate the many pathways of study undertaken by the different laboratories.

I. HISTORICAL ASPECTS

The history of the L-forms is by now well known. Fifty years ago the efforts of Klieneberger and Dienes ushered in a new era in the world of microbiology. Klieneberger isolated tiny colonies resembling the organisms of bovine pleuropneumonia (now known as *Mycoplasma mycoides*) from a culture of *Streptobacillus moniliformis*. These seemed to be growing in symbiosis with the bacillus and were named L_1 (L for Lister Institute) [1]. Dienes acknowledged the resemblance of the colonies to mycoplasma but he challenged the concept of symbiosis when he studied the development of the L_1 from the streptobacillus and demonstrated its return to the bacillary form [2]. He succeeded in isolating L-form colonies from other bacterial species showing spontaneous transformation and established that bacteria could continue to multiply in the absence of the rigid cell wall [3]. This discovery opened the way to a new understanding of bacterial morphology and reproductive processes and stimulated other investigators to study these phenomena. (For an early review, see Dienes and Weinberger [4].

Two other observations played a critical role in the progress made in this field. One was the discovery by Pierce that penicillin could induce the transformation of the streptobacillus to the L-form [5], an observation that was confirmed in many other bacterial species [4,6-8]. The second notable advance was the recognition by Sharp that osmotic protection, as offered by increased salt concentration of the medium, was necessary for the development and growth of L-forms from Group A streptococci [9,10]. Sucrose and other osmotic stabilizers were found to be effective with other bacterial species [11]. The requirement of some species for animal serum in the medium had already been recognized [4]. It was also found that exposure of the bacteria to the effects of bacteriostatic chemicals, to amino acids, to lysozyme and other muralytic enzymes, to phage, and to hyperimmune sera could also result in L-form induction and growth [12-14]. Thanks to these important advances, it has been possible to study L-forms from many diverse bacterial species (Table 1) [15,21].

II. TERMINOLOGY AND DEFINITIONS

Although the terms "L-forms" and "L-phase variants" have been used interchangeably, the term "L-forms" is preferred by most workers in the field. The terms "L-phase" and "L-phase variants" tend to be misleading because they imply that an "L-phase" is a natural state that is universal to all bacteria. In truth it is known that L-forms have been produced only from certain strains of some bacterial species (for a complete discussion of L-form terminology, see McGee et al. [16] and Dienes [17]).

Table 1 Bacterial Genera from Which L-forms Have Been Derived

Agrobacterium	*Erysipelothrix*	*Salmonella*
Bacillus	*Escherichia*	*Sarcina*
Bacteriodes	*Flavobacterium*	*Serratia*
Bartonella	*Haemophilus*	*Shigella*
Bordetella	*Listeria*	*Staphylococcus*
Brucella	*Neisseria*	*Streptobacillus*
Clostridium	*Proteus*	*Streptococcus*
Corynebacterium	*Pseudomonas*	*Vibrio*

Source: Madoff [21]. Copyright by Springer-Verlag (1981).

Controversy notwithstanding, the essential nature of the bacterial L-forms remains clear and indisputable. An L-form may be defined as a special type of growth derived or induced from a bacterium following suppression of the rigid cell wall. The classical bacterial forms are replaced by soft spherical granular forms and large bodies which penetrate the agar medium and produce colonies that resemble those of the mycoplasma (Fig. 1). L-form colonies can be propagated indefinitely in the presence of the inducing agent in appropriate media. Alternatively, when the inducing agent is removed, an L-form may either revert to the parent bacterium or it may have become stabilized for growth as an L-form and no longer be capable of reversion.

Spheroplasts and protoplasts are spherical structures originating from bacteria following partial (spheroplasts) or complete (protoplasts) removal of the cell wall by enzymatic digestion in a hyperosmolar environment [18]. Under certain conditions either spheroplasts or protoplasts may initiate L-type growth when transferred to L-form media providing the proper osmotic support. Thus, "spheroplast L-forms" and "protoplast L-forms" are descriptive for L-forms differing in properties relating to the presence or absence of cell wall constituents. (For a complete discussion, see Chapter 6.)

"Cell wall-deficient bacteria" is a term used to describe a variety of bacterial forms showing abnormal morphology and/or requiring osmotic protection for their growth. Such bacterial variants have been isolated from clinical specimens and have been variously described as "atypical," "transitional," or "aberrant" [16]. Fortunately these terms are being discarded in favor of "cell wall-deficient bacteria." Henceforth these bacterial forms would better be described in terms of morphological, serological, and biochemical properties, and, if possible, by genetic analysis. In this way, unusual isolates will be characterized, the terminology will be simplified and the literature will be rendered more comprehensible.

"Revertant bacteria" (bacteria recovered from the L-forms) most often retain the essential characteristics of the parent strain. One major difference is the

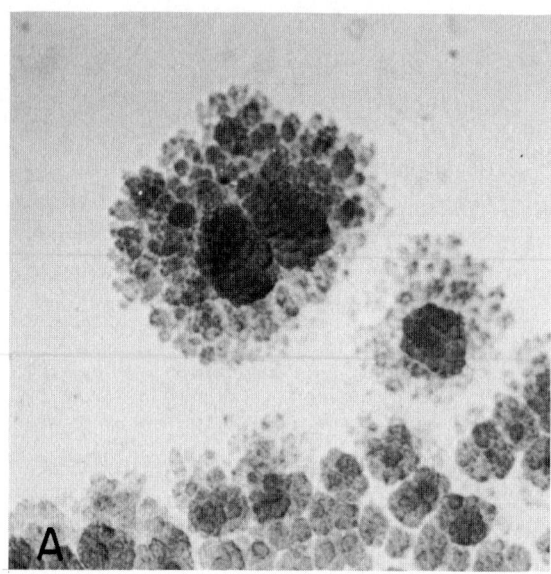

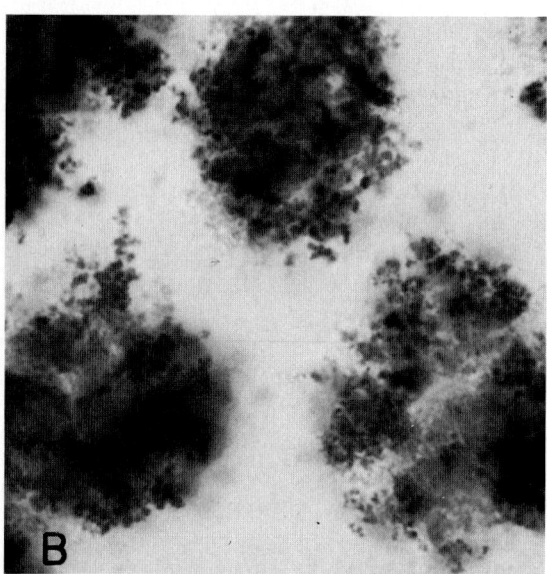

Figure 1 Dienes-stained preparations on agar. *(A)* L-forms of *Neisseria gonorrhoeae* (magnification ×65). *(B)* L-forms of *Streptococcus pyogenes* (magnification ×110). (*Source*: Madoff [21]. Copyright by Springer Verlag, 1981.)

greater tendency of revertant bacteria to again produce L-forms. Other significant alterations noted in revertant bacteria include changes in cell composition, in structure and function, in the production of enzymes and toxins, in antigenic factors, and in sensitivity to antibiotics. The dynamics of L-transformation are operative not only during conversion and adaptation to growth, but also during the process of reversion, and it is important to consider whether the changes observed represent alterations of phenotype or of genotype. (For discussions, see Chap. 3-6, inclusive.)

At this point it is necessary to emphasize the diversity of the L-forms. It is well known to all investigators that L-forms probably represent a polyglot mixture of considerable variability. L-forms produced in a given situation, at different times, or from different organisms cannot be equated to one another. The properties of L-forms may be greatly influenced by physical, environmental, and biological factors. Even those derived from the same organism, but in different hands or by different methods, may show marked differences. Thus, given the present state of our knowledge of the L-forms, a description of a particular L-form culture in terms of morphology and ultrastructure alone is insufficient. Investigators should include other pertinent data, such as the origin of the parent, the method of induction, requirements for osmotic protection, tendency for reversion, extent of wall defectiveness, and some comparative information on the physiological and biochemical properties of the parent bacterium, the derived L-forms, and the revertant forms. Only thus will the essential information regarding a specific L-form culture be made available.

III. INDUCTION OF L-FORMS

The induction and maintenance of the L-forms of various bacterial species are described in the respective chapters. Selective procedures have been provided by Madoff in a previous publication [21]. Therefore, only a few general principles will be mentioned here. It is understood that it is unwise to lay down specific rules for any organism; the key to success is trial and error.

In general, L-forms are induced by exposing the bacteria to an inducing agent on a suitable medium. Important requirements of the medium include the proper consistency of the agar gel, the presence of animal serum, and the correct osmolarity. The penicillins are the most effective inducing agents. Other antibiotics that interfere with cell wall synthesis, such as cycloserine, ristocetin, bacitracin, vancomycin, and the cephalosporins, have also been used. High concentrations of amino acids, notably glycine and phenylalanine and other agents such as lysostaphin and the peptidases, have also been utilized in L-form production.

L-forms can be induced by lytic enzymes that digest the murein of the cell wall of bacteria. When bacteria are treated with lysozyme in a hyperosmolar medium, protoplasts or spheroplasts are formed; either of these, when released, may produce L-forms when transferred to media of appropriate osmolarity (Fig. 2) [21,22]. Gooder and Maxted, as early as 1961, produced L-forms of Group A streptococcus using a phage-associated muralytic enzyme found in a Group C phage lysate [23]. This method proved successful with many other strains of streptococcus.

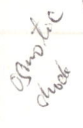

Most gram-negative bacteria can be converted to L-forms on media of the normal physiological osmolarity. Most gram-positive bacteria and some gram-negative species require increased osmotic protection for L-form growth. (For discussions of osmotic stress and L-form lysis, see Chap. 3 and 13.) Sodium chloride is the commonly used osmotic stabilizer; sucrose plus Mg^{2+} can be more effective for some strains. The combination of sucrose and sodium chloride has also been successful. Polyvinylpyrrolidone (PVP) was found to be an important osmotic stabilizer. Other agents include neutral salts, oleic acid, spermine, and sodium succinate, to mention only a few.

Modifications in inducing agent and/or environmental conditions may be decisive for the success of an experiment. For example, in induction studies with the pneumococcus, the definitive factor was the use of penicillin within an extremely narrow range of concentration [24]. In *Neisseria* species, the selection of particular lots of PVP and dialysis thereof were found to be critical in the frequency of L-form induction [25] (see Chap. 8). Induction studies with bacteria exposed to differing experimental conditions may result in L-forms of dissimilar physiological properties. Some strains of bacteria have been impervious to all tested methods of induction.

Following exposure of the bacteria to the inducing agent, it may take from several hours to several days for L-colonies to appear in the cultures. When penicillin is used in a gradient, the L-colonies may be detected by the naked eye or with the hand lens in the zone of bacterial inhibition. Microscopic identification of the colonies as L-forms is made by the stained agar technique of Dienes in the manner used for mycoplasma [26,27]. As with mycoplasmas, serial passage in subcultures is obtained by the well known "push block" technique [28]. Growth in broth may be initiated with agar blocks also, but, in contrast to mycoplasmas, a long period of adaptation may be necessary to obtain an adequate concentration of viable organisms. Likewise, growth in chemically defined media is not easily obtained, but a few species have been adapted to grow in such media [29,30].

IV. MORPHOLOGY AND ULTRASTRUCTURE

The reader is referred to the chapters dealing with specific organisms for descriptions of morphology at the ultrastructural level; however, a few general principles will be stated here. As Hijmans and Clasener aptly wrote [31], "The

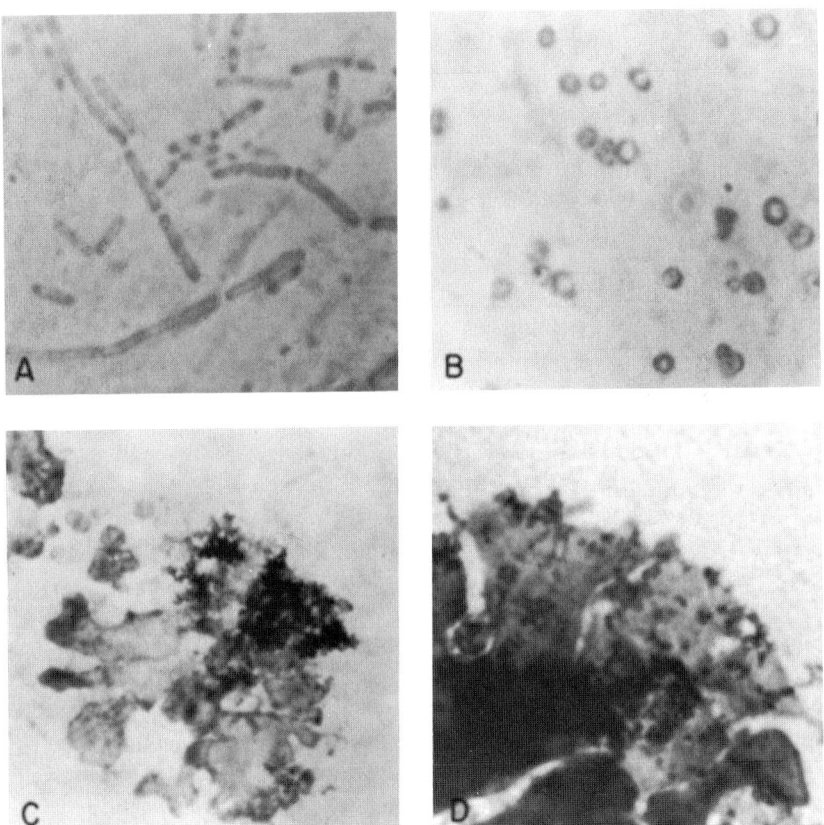

Figure 2 Induction of L-forms of *Bacillus* spp. by treatment with lysozyme. Dienes-stained preparations (magnification × 2250). *(A)* Organisms grown 2 hr in broth medium. *(B)* Following incubation for 2 hr, in the presence of lysozyme, protoplasts are formed, then transferred to hypertonic L-form agar medium. *(C)* Protoplasts enlarge to large bodies with granular elements developing into L-form colony. *(D)* Detail of periphery of mature L-form colony. (*Source*: Madoff [21]. Copyright by Springer-Verlag, 1981.)

major part of our knowledge of the morphological phenomena connected with the growth of L-forms is based on the diligent observations and descriptions of Louis Dienes" [32-34]. According to Dienes, the large bodies serve as a link between the bacteria and the L-forms. The initial step in induction is the enlargement of the bacterial cell. In some instances the large bodies fragment, releasing typical bacterial forms. Alternatively, small L-form bodies develop within or at the periphery of the large bodies. These are spherical, fragile, and plastic, and as they multiply, they penetrate the agar medium forming an L-colony. As seen microscopically, an L-colony resembles a mycoplasma colony in that the center portion is embedded in the agar; the peripheral growth on the surface is less dense and is composed of aggregates of large bodies. The familiar "fried-egg appearance" is the usual result. Compared with mycoplasma the L-colonies usually have a coarser structure and can be considerably larger than mycoplasma colonies. Configuration of the colonies is variable; species differences as well as methods of induction, conditions of the medium, and passage history may be important factors [4,12,21,26].

Partial loss of cell wall by the bacteria usually produces the readily revertible "B-type" spheroplast L-forms, whereas the complete loss of cell wall yields the "stable" or difficult-to-revert "A-type" protoplast L-forms. Ultrastructural studies have illustrated the complete absence of bacterial cell wall in A-type L-colonies. Streptococci, staphylococci, corynebacteria, and some other gram-positive bacteria tend to produce A-type colonies exclusively [35]. By electron microscopy, B-type L-colonies show remnants of cell wall that are similar to that of the parent bacteria but lack the rigidity. Layers of altered mucopeptide are often visible [34,36]. Enterobacteriaceae and other gram-negative species such as proteus may produce B-type L-colonies predominantly. However, it is important to note that both protoplast L-forms (A-type) and spheroplast L-forms (B-type), or either, may be produced under special conditions and that either can become stabilized to the extent that they no longer revert to bacterial form [19,33,37,38] (see Chap. 6). Thus it appears that the presence (or absence) of cell wall constituents is not the only essential property in the revertibility of the L-forms. Numerous examples of this unexplained paradox appear in the literature. In *Neisseria* [39] and in *Hemophilus influenzae* [40,41], L-forms that were revertible under certain conditions showed only the presence of cytoplasmic membrane by electron microscope. In thin sections of *Bacillus* sp., no trace of cell wall could be seen; in some, multilayered structures surround the membrane [42] (see Chap. 5). In *Nocardia* spp. both A- and B-type colonies are seen, with considerable variation among both types. A comprehensive survey of the comparative ultrastructure of some bacterial L-forms has been presented by Cole [36].

L-forms of a strain of *Escherichia coli* show the presence of laminate structures and microtubules [43]. These bear a resemblance to core structures observed in *Streptococcus faecalis* [44], *Pseudomonas aeruginosa* [45], and *Nocardia* sp. (see Chap. 10 for illustration). The nature and function of these tubular structures have not yet been established.

V. REPRODUCTION AND REVERSION

L-forms of diverse bacterial species are surprisingly similar in morphology and reproductive processes. Although "elementary bodies" as small as 200-300 nm are seen, the size of the smallest units capable of cell division remains uncertain [36]. Mechanisms of cell replication, as in mycoplasma, appear to vary from binary or asymmetric division to budding or segmentation of the small dense bodies from large spherical forms. In *Proteus* L-forms, the sequential enlargement of protoplasmic bodies followed by the release of new granular forms [34] was described by Dienes and Bullivant and by Cole [36]. In L-forms of *H. influenzae*, small dense bodies are seen at the periphery of large cells as condensations apparently capable of detachment as budding forms [40]. Green et al. have proposed a reproductive cycle for the L-forms of *S. faecalis* [46]. Small L-form bodies divide by binary fission and budding and develop within mature "mother" forms. During reversion, mesosome-like structures are formed in a similar manner, as described by Landman et al. in *Bacillus subtilis* [47]. Wyrick and Gooder studied the reversion of L-forms of *Streptococcus faecium* with ferretin-labeling [48]. Reversion arises through excretion of cell wall material around the L-forms. Portions of cell wall associated with cell membrane form a "scaffolding" to recreate the complete bacterial cell wall. Significant contributions to the study of L-form replication and reversion are to be found in Chaps. 3-11.

In summary, L-form processes indicate that if there are orderly mechanisms in the life cycle of L-forms they are not entirely clear. It is not yet known how the genome segregates in the formation of the new and viable L-form elements [36]. Many factors appear to be involved in the processes of reversion to the bacterial state. Evidence for the loss of revertibility points to genetic alterations of the stable L-forms.

VI. REVERSION OF L-FORMS AND IDENTIFICATION OF REVERTANTS

As stated above, L-cultures are referred to as "stable" when the ability to revert to the parent bacterium is lost. In some species, when the cultures have become stabilized, reversion can no longer be effected under any known conditions. For others, special techniques have been devised. Reversion of *B. subtilis* has been effected by changes in the physical environment, e.g., by increasing the agar concentration or by the use of gelatin in the media [49]. Similar techniques

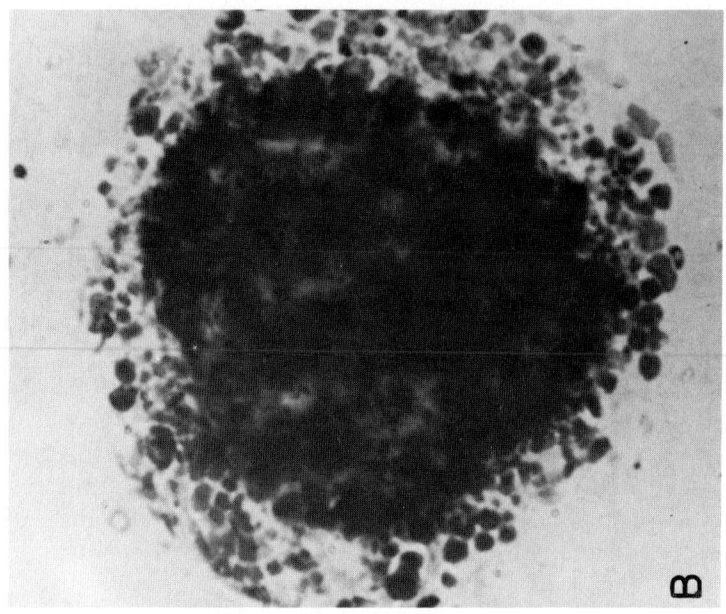
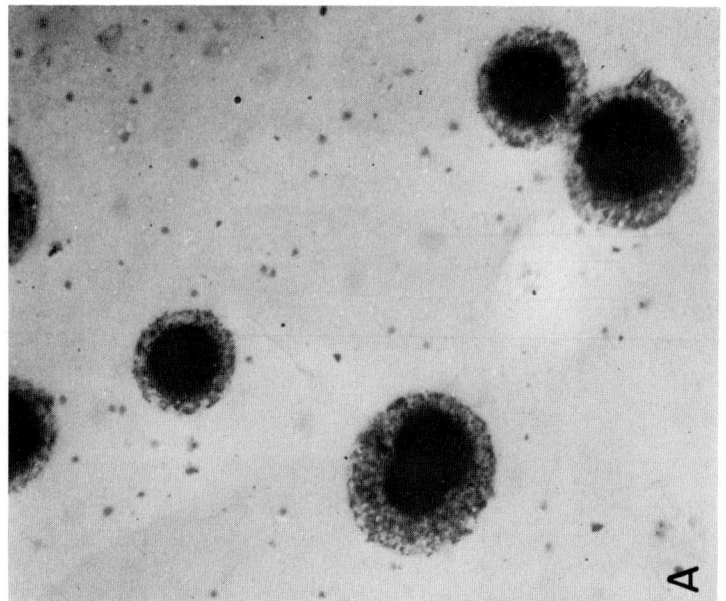

Figure 3 *(A)* L-forms of *Haemophilus influenzae*, 96 hr incubation. L-colonies show deep granular growth at the center and a periphery of large body surface growth (magnification ×250). *(B)* L-colony in subculture in the presence of *Neisseria perflava* factor(s) after 10 days' incubation (magnification ×4500).

BACTERIAL L-FORMS

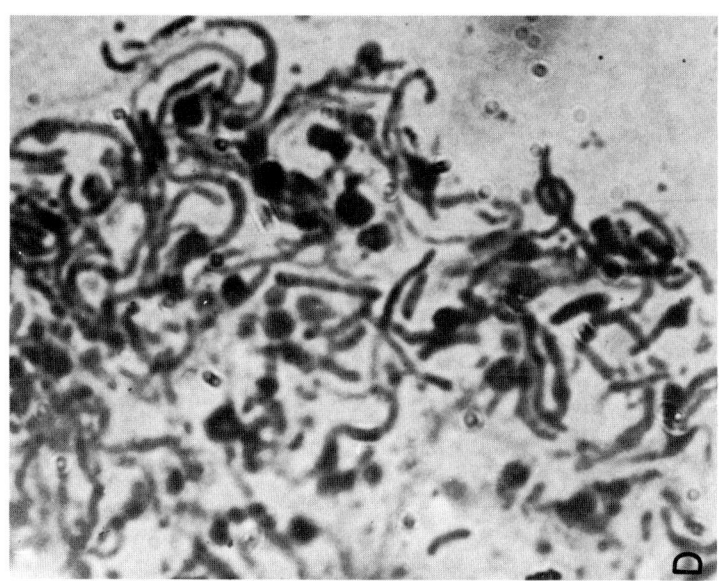

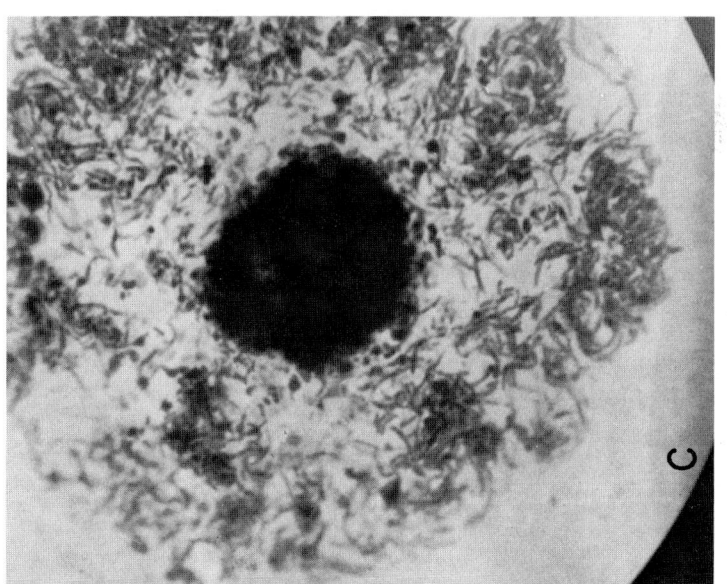

(C) Reverting L-colony of *Haemophilis influenzae* shows central L-type granular growth. Surface growth consists of large bodies and swollen, filamentous forms (magnification ×100). *(D)* Enlargement of periphery of revertant colony showing pleomorphic and filamentous reverting bacterial forms (magnification ×4500). (*Source*: Madoff [41]. Copyright by Springer International, 1979.)

using gelatin were employed successfully with streptococcus L-forms [50]. In rare instances, reversion of L-forms has been influenced by the presence of factors produced by other bacteria or fungi [51]. Landman and Halle induced reversion of *B. subtilis* L-forms by the use of *B. subtilis* cell wall material as a primer of cell wall regeneration [52]. In *H. influenzae,* growth and reversion of L-forms were found to be enhanced by a low-molecular-weight peptide produced by a strain of *Neisseria perflava* discovered as a contaminant in the culture (Fig. 3) [41]. Observations such as these deserve further investigation.

The identification of a stable, nonreverting L-form from an unknown source may be extremely difficult. Modified biochemical tests useful for the parent bacteria may aid in the characterization of L-form isolates [53,54]. Serological testing may provide additional useful information [55,56]. However, as noted in Chapter 12 by Lynn, some antigenic components presented by the L-forms may differ from those offered by the intact bacteria. Comparison of membrane proteins appears to offer a reliable method for comparing L-forms and bacteria [36,57]. An interesting suggestion is made by Martin et al. that the presence of penicillin binding protein patterns in stable L-forms, as observed in proteus, may prove useful in the identification of the bacterial parent of an unknown L-form [58]. The early molecular genetic studies of DNA base composition and DNA hybridization provided a significant breakthrough in comparative genetic studies of bacteria, their derived L-forms, and mycoplasma [59]. With the application of the newer more sensitive techniques of DNA hybridization, there is considerable optimism that this difficult problem, the study of the genetic relatedness among these microorganisms, may be greatly clarified in the future.

VII. GENETIC FACTORS

Genetic differences among bacteria in a population may be decisive in the production of L-forms. In one classic experiment by Hijmans and Dienes, only one of 20 streptococcus colonies was shown to produce progeny capable of L-transformation [60]. The finding of spontaneous L-form colonies in a strain of *Erysipelothrix rhusiopathiae* suggested that variant bacteria or mutants may appear in the normal bacterial population under certain conditions such as aging of the cultures [61]. Biochemical studies support the hypothesis of genetic determinants in the conversion to the L-form. Stable L-forms of *Streptococcus pyogenes* were found to be defective in important stages of cell wall synthesis [62,63]. The physiology of the cytoplasmic membranes was radically altered when the cultures became adapted to survive in normal physiologic medium [64]. Gregory and Gooder noted the loss of enzyme function in *S. faecium* L-forms at the membrane stage of peptidoglycan synthesis [65]. Pachas and Schor suggested that penicillin had a mutagenic affect on *Proteus* L-forms, resulting in both structural and functional changes [66]. Differences in antibiotic sensitivity patterns in L-forms and their revertant bacteria are highly suggestive of genetic modifications [67] (for discussion, see Chap. 11). Stable L-forms of a phytopathogenic bacterium (genus *Erwinia*) have been produced by ultraviolet irradiation with apparent mutagenic affect [68].

There is still a paucity of studies at the molecular level. However, in a unique study, Hoyer and King demonstrated the loss of a portion of the chromosomal DNA in a stable L-form of *S. faecalis* [69]. Landman suggested the use of L-forms as important genetic models for studies of transformation, transduction, and phage infection [70]. In a significant study, Wyrick et al. used DNA-mediated transformation to transfer the characteristics of the stable L-form state to recipient intact cells of *B. subtilis* [71]. In Chapter 5 Gilpin and Young review the important pioneer work that has been done in the area of genetic transformation with L-forms of *Bacillus* sp. They discuss evidence for the proposal that the stable L-form phenotype of *B. subtilis* represents a genetic mutant.

Future studies by molecular biologists and geneticists should do much to explore the role of the L-forms as a factor of genetic change in bacteria. Furthermore, since genetic manipulation of the L-forms is now possible, their use as models in DNA technology is a new area for future research.

L-forms induced on media of high osmolar value have been adapted to grow on media of normal osmolarity. Significant alterations, indicating either selection or mutation, have resulted from such adaptation. Studies with adapted L-forms of a *Streptococcus pyogenes* suggest that a mutational effect may have occurred. In contrast to the original L-form cultures, the altered L-forms were shown to have a marked pathogenic affect in vivo [64] (for comprehensive discussion, see Chap. 4). Observations with L-forms of streptococcus MG may be significant with respect to possible mutagenic effects [72]. Following long-term cultivation and gradual step-wise adaptation to medium of normal osmolarity, altered colonies emerged that markedly resembled mycoplasma colonies. When tested serologically, they reacted specifically with *Acholeplasma laidlawii* by growth inhibition and fluorescent antibody tests. Infinite care in repeated trials was taken to rule out the possibility of contamination with the mycoplasma. Similar studies of adaptation were performed with an L-culture of *Corynebacterium* spp. [73]. These findings are in no way bizarre, but an extension of numerous previous observations on bacterial and L-form variation [19,20,33,74], and they raise interesting questions regarding possible genetic mutations and evolutionary pathways in the life of bacteria.

VIII. EVOLUTIONARY ASPECTS

The study of phylogenetic relationships between classical bacteria and cell wall-defective microorganisms represents a major interest in this volume. In Chapter 2

Neimark has provided an elegant and comprehensive review of the subject and has presented the evidence for the derivation of mycoplasma from the bacteria. His own pioneer work has demonstrated definite evolutionary relationships between selected strains of streptococcus and acholeplasma; the L-forms were not included in these studies. Dienes and many others, however, referred repeatedly to the biologic similarities between L-forms and mycoplasma and ventured the opinion that evolutionary processes in bacteria may have led to the emergence of mycoplasma through the mediation of the L-forms [33,34,75]. The view that the L-forms may participate in a significant manner in bacterial evolution needs to be studied at the molecular level.

IX. OCCURRENCE AND PATHOGENICITY

The little-known aspects of the occurrence and pathogenicity of the L-forms in disease are reviewed in Chapter 14. In animal experimentation the L-forms have failed to show pathogenicity unless reversion to the bacteria occurred in vivo. On the other hand, L-forms of certain bacteria retain the pathogenic potential of the parent bacteria. For example, toxin production is retained by the L-forms of clostridia [76] and *Corynebacterium diphtheriae* [77]. Neuraminidase is produced by L-forms of *Vibrio cholerae* [78]. The L-forms of *Staphylococcus aureus* retain the ability to produce coagulase [79], and the L-forms of *Streptococcus pyogenes* are able to produce both M protein and streptolysin [80].

Certain factors in persisting and recurrent infections may predispose to the production of wall-defective organisms [81]. The L-forms have a survival advantage over bacteria under certain conditions that are not conducive to the growth of bacteria. Exposure to antibiotics, to cellular enzymes, and to host defense mechanisms may constitute important factors for the persistence of cell wall-defective organisms in certain disease processes. Thus, patients with long-term infections of the urinary tract including those with pyelonephritis, or patients with septicemia, meningitis, or endocarditis of long duration who have failed to demonstrate normal bacterial isolates, may provide fruitful sources for experimental cultivation of clinical material. Domingue et al. have recently presented some significant results supporting this view [82].

It may be of interest here that human serum with complement kills certain L-forms but is without effect on the parent bacteria. (For discussion of host defense mechanisms, see Chap. 13.)

In summary, the L-forms may not be primary pathogens, but the indications for their potential pathogenicity deserve further exploration. Future research should considerably expand our knowledge of the importance of these organisms in disease.

X. FUTURE INVESTIGATIONS

The study of the bacterial L-forms in disease cries out for investigation(s) with new experimental models and techniques.

Studies with bacterial L-forms have already had a profound influence on the way in which we view bacteria [83]. They have contributed significantly to our knowledge of the structure, function, and genetic composition of the bacterial cell. The modern microbiologist can profit from a knowledge of the bacterial L-forms. Future investigators should pursue the presence of the L-forms in the natural environment of bacteria, plants, insects, and invertebrates with the ultimate view of establishing their role in the life of bacteria and in clinical infections. Bacteria are exposed to traumatic influences exerted by environmental changes, host-dependent interactions, and biologic interdependency with other microorganisms. In this context, evolutionary trends and pathologic conditions may be the result of genetic modification of bacteria mediated by changes in their cell wall. To the molecular biologist, the existence of the L-forms of bacteria as a means of preserving the species is a fascinating aspect of the living organism [83]. Do the bacterial L-forms represent the genetic response of the viable organism to selective pressures of the environment? Indeed, readers of Steven Jay Gould may find in the stable L-form state another example of what he has termed "punctuated equilibrium"—the appearance of a new and different subspecies of a well-known biologic (bacterial) entity [84].

REFERENCES

1. Klieneberger, E. (1935). The natural occurrence of pleuropneumonialike organisms in apparent symbosis with *Streptobacillus moniliformis* and other bacteria. *J. Pathol. Bacteriol.* 40:93–105.
2. Dienes, L. (1939). "L" organism of Klieneberger and *Streptobacillus moniliformis*. *J. Infect. Dis.* 65:24–42.
3. Dienes, L. (1939). L type variant forms in cultures of various bacteria. *Proc. Soc. Exp. Biol. Med.* 42:773–778.
4. Dienes, L. and Weinberger, H. J. (1951). The L-forms of bacteria. *Bacteriol. Rev.* 15:245–288.
5. Pierce, C. H. (1942). *Streptobacillus moniliformis*, its associated L_1 form and other pleuropneumonia-like organisms. *J. Bacteriol.* 43:780.
6. Dienes, L. (1947). Isolation of pleuropneumonia-like organisms from *H. influenzae* with the aid of penicillin. *Proc. Soc. Exp. Biol. Med.* 64:166–168.
7. Dienes, L. (1948). The isolation of L type cultures from *Bacteroides* with the aid of penicillin and their reversion into the usual bacilli. *J. Bacteriol.* 56:445–456.
8. Dienes, L., Weinberger, H. J., and Madoff, S. (1950). The transformation of typhoid bacilli into L forms under various conditions. *J. Bacteriol.* 59:755–764.

9. Sharp, J. T. (1954). L Colonies from hemolytic streptococci: New technic in the study of L-forms of bacteria. *Proc. Soc. Exp. Biol. Med. 87*: 94–97.
10. Dienes, L. and Sharp, J. T. (1956). The role of high electrolyte concentration in the production and growth of L-forms of bacteria. *J. Bacteriol. 71*: 208–213.
11. Lederberg, J. and St. Clair, J. (1958). Protoplasts and L-type growth of *Escherichia coli*. *J. Bacteriol. 75*:143–160.
12. Madoff, S., Burke, M. E., and Dienes, L. (1967). Induction and identification of L-forms of bacteria. *Ann. N.Y. Acad. Sci. 143*:755–759.
13. Hijmans, W., van Boven, C. P. A., and Clasener, H. A. L. (1969). Fundamental biology of the L-phase of bacteria in *The Mycoplasmatales and the L-phase of Bacteria* (L. Hayflick, ed.), Appleton-Century-Crofts, New York, pp. 67–143.
14. Madoff, S. and Pachas, W. N. (1970). Mycoplasma and the L-forms of bacteria in *Rapid Diagnostic Methods in Medical Microbiology* (C. D. Graber, ed.), Williams and Wilkins, Baltimore, pp. 195–217.
15. Hijmans, W. and Clasener, H. A. L. (1971). A survey of the L-forms of bacteria in *Mycoplasma and the L-forms of bacteria* (S. Madoff, ed.), Gordon and Breach, New York.
16. McGee, Z. A., Whittler, R. G., Gooder, H., and Charache, P. (1971). Wall-defective microbial variants: Terminology and experimental design. *J. Infect. Dis. 123*:433–438.
17. Dienes, L. (1973). Nomenclature of bacterial L-forms and cell wall-defective bacteria. *J. Infect. Dis. 127*:476–477.
18. Brenner, S., Dark, F. A., Gerhardt, P., Jeynes, M. H., Kandler, O., Kellenberger, E., Klieneberger-Nobel, E., McQuillen, K., Rubio-Huertos, M., Salton, M. R. J., Strange, R. E., Tomcsik, J., and Weibull, C. (1958). Bacterial protoplasts. *Nature 181*:1713–1715.
19. Dienes, L. (1970). Permanent alterations of the L-forms of *Proteus* and *Salmonella* under various conditions. *J. Bacteriol. 104*:1369–1377.
20. Pachas, W. N. and Currid, V. R. (1974). L-form induction, morphology and development in two related strains of *Erysipelothrix rhusiopathiae*. *J. Bacteriol. 119*:476–482.
21. Madoff, S. (1981). The L-forms of bacteria in *The Prokaryotes: A Handbook on Habitats, Isolation and Identification of Bacteria* (M. P. Starr, H. Stolp, H. G. Truper, A. Balows and H. G. Schlegel, eds.), Springer-Verlag, Berlin, Heidelberg, pp. 2225–2237.
22. King, J. R. and Gooder, H. (1970). Induction of enterococcal L-forms by the action of lysozyme. *J. Bacteriol. 103*:686–691.
23. Gooder, H. and Maxted, W. R. (1961). External factors influencing structure and activities of *Streptococcus pyogenes* in *Microbial Reaction to Environment* (G. G. Neynell and H. Gooder, eds.), Cambridge University Press, Cambridge, pp. 151–173.
24. Madoff, S. and Dienes, L. (1958). L forms from pneumococci. *J. Bacteriol. 76*:245–250.

25. Bacigalupi, B. A. and Lawson, J. W. (1973). Defined physiological conditions for the induction of the L-form of *Neisseria gonorrhoeae*. *J. Bacteriol.* 116:778–784.
26. Madoff, S. (1960). Isolation and identification of PPLO. *Ann. N.Y. Acad. Sci.* 79:383–392.
27. Dienes, L. (1967). Permanent stained agar preparation of mycoplasma and L-forms of bacteria. *J. Bacteriol.* 93:689–692.
28. Madoff, S. and Pachas, W. N. (1976). Mycoplasma and the L-forms of bacteria in *Rapid Diagnostic Methods in Medical Microbiology* (C. D. Graber, ed.), Williams and Wilkins, Baltimore, pp. 195–217.
29. van Boven, C. P. A., Kastelein, M. J. W., and Hijmans, W. (1967). A chemically defined medium for the L-phase of group A Streptococci. *Ann. N.Y. Acad. Sci.* 143:749–754.
30. Gilpin, R. W., Young, F. E., and Chatterjee, A. N. (1973). Characterization of a stable L-form of *Bacillus subtilis*. *J. Bacteriol.* 113:486–499.
31. Hijmans, W. and Clasener, H. A. L. (1971). A survey of the L-forms of bacteria in *Mycoplasma and the L-forms of Bacteria* (S. Madoff, ed.), Gordon and Breach, New York, pp. 37–47.
32. Dienes, L. (1967). Morphology and reproductive process of L-forms of bacteria 1. streptococci and staphylococci. *J. Bacteriol.* 93:693–702.
33. Dienes, L. (1968). Morphology and reproductive processes of bacteria with defective cell wall in *Microbial Protoplasts, Spheroplasts and L-forms* (L. B. Guze, ed.), Williams and Wilkins, Baltimore, pp. 74–93.
34. Dienes, L. and Bullivant, S. (1968). Morphology and reproductive processes of the L-forms of bacteria. *J. Bacteriol.* 95:672–682.
35. Dienes, L., Madoff, S., and Bullivant, S. (1966). Study of L-forms as seen in thin sections with the electron microscope in *Current Research on Group A Streptococcus* (R. Caravano, Excerpta Medica Foundation, Amsterdam, pp. 342–345.
36. Cole, R. M. (1971). Some implications of the comparative ultrastructure of bacterial L-forms in *Mycoplasma and the L-forms of bacteria* (S. Madoff, ed.), Gordon and Breach, New York, pp. 49–83.
37. Martin, H. H. and Lehmann, R. (1970). Stable L-forms of *Proteus mirabilis* as spontaneous and induced mutants. *Proc. 10th Int. Congr. Microbiol.* p. 9 (Mexico City).
38. Louis, C. and Schmitt-Slomska, J. (1977). Effect of polymyxin B on the ultrastructure of the stable *Proteus mirabilis* L-forms in *Spheroplasts, Protoplasts and L-forms of Bacteria* (J. Roux, ed.), Ed. INSERM, vol. 64, Paris, pp. 197–210.
39. Lawson, J. W., and Bacigalupi, B. (1977). Induction and reversion of the L-forms of *Neisseria gonorrhoeae* in *Spheroplasts, Protoplasts and L-forms of Bacteria* (J. Roux, ed.), Ed. INSERM, vol. 64, Paris, pp. 96–106.
40. Madoff, S. (1977). L-forms of *Haemophilus influenzae*: Morphology and ultrastructure in *Spheroplasts, Protoplasts, and L-forms of Bacteria* (J. Roux, ed.), Ed. INSERM, vol. 64, Paris, pp. 15–26.

41. Madoff, S. (1979). L-forms of *Haemophilus influenza*: Growth and reversion as influenced by a strain of *Neisseria perflava. Curr. Microb.* 2:43–46.
42. Wyrick, P. B. and Rogers, H. J. (1973). Isolation and characterization of cell-wall defective variants of *Bacillus subtilis* and *Bacillus licheniformis. J. Bacteriol.* 116:456–465.
43. Eda, T., Kanda, Y., and Kimura, S. (1976). Membrane structures in stable L-forms of *Escherichia coli. J. Bacteriol.* 127:1564–1567.
44. Cohen, M., McCandless, R. G., Kalmanson, G. M., and Guze, L. B. (1968). Core-like structures in transitional and protoplast forms of *Streptococcus faecalis* in *Microbial Protoplasts, Spheroplasts and L-forms* (L. B. Guze, ed.), Williams and Wilkins, Baltimore, pp. 94–109.
45. Hubert, E. G., Potter, C. S., Hensley, T. J., Cohen, M., Kalmanson, G. M., and Guze, L. B. (1971). L-forms of *Pseudomonas aeruginosa. Infect. Immun.* 4:60–72.
46. Green, M. T., Heidger, P. M., and Domingue, G. Proposed reproductive cycle for a relatively stable L-phase variant of *Streptococcus faecalis. Infect. Immun.* 10:915–927.
47. Landman, O. E., Ryter, A., and Frehel, C. (1968). Gelatin-induced reversion of protoplasts of *Bacillus subtilis* to the bacillary form: Electronmicroscopic and physical study. *J. Bacteriol.* 96:2154–2170.
48. Wyrick, P. B. and Gooder, H. (1977). Reversion of *Streptococcus faecium* cell-wall defective variants to the intact bacterial state in *Spheroplasts, Protoplasts and L-forms* (J. Roux, ed.), Ed. INSERM, vol. 64, Paris, pp. 59–88.
49. Landman, O. E. and Forman, A. (1969). Gelatin-induced reversion of protoplasts of *Bacillus subtilis* to the bacillary form: Biosynthesis of macromolecules and wall during successive steps. *J. Bacteriol.* 99:576–589.
50. King, J. R. and Gooder, H. (1970). Reversion to the streptococcal state of enterococcal protoplasts, spheroplasts and L-forms. *J. Bacteriol.* 103:692–696.
51. Madoff, S. (1974). Influence of microbial factors on the reversion of L-forms of *Hemophilus influenzae* and streptococci. (Abstr) Annual Meeting ASM, G246.
52. Landman, O. E. and Halle, S. (1963). Enzymically and physically induced inheritance changes in *Bacillus subtilis. J. Mol. Biol.* 7:721–738.
53. Cohen, R. L., Wittler, R. G., and Faber, J. E. (1968). Modified biochemical tests for characterization of L-phase variants of bacteria. *Appl. Microbiol.* 16:1655–1662.
54. Asnani, P. J. and Gill, K. (1980). Biological properties of L-forms and their parent bacteria. *Acta Microbiologica Acad. Sci. Hung.* 27:131–134.
55. Lynn, R. J. and Haller, G. L. (1968). Bacterial L-forms as immunogenic agents in *Microbial Protoplasts, Spheroplasts and L-forms* (L. B. Guze, eds.), Williams and Wilkins, Baltimore, pp. 270–278.
56. Feinman, S. B., Prescott, B., and Cole, R. M. (1973). Serological reactions of glycolipids from streptococcal L-forms. *Infect. Immun.* 8:752–756.
57. King, J. R., Theodore, T. S., and Cole, R. M. (1969). Generic identification of L-forms by polyacrylamide gel electrophoretic comparison of extracts from parent strains and their derived L-forms. *J. Bacteriol.* 100:71–77.

58. Martin, H. H., Schilf, W., and Schiefer, H. G. (1980). Differentiation of mycoplasmatales from bacterial protoplast L-forms by assay for penicillin binding proteins. *Arch. Mikrobiol. 127*:297-299.
59. Somerson, N. L., Reich, P. R., Chanock, R. M., and Weissman, S. M. (1967). Genetic differentiation by nucleic acid homology III. Relationships among mycoplasma, L-forms and bacteria. *Ann. N.Y. Acad. Sci. 143*: 9-20.
60. Hijmans, W. and Dienes, L. (1955). Further observations on L-forms of *Alpha*-hemolytic Streptococci. *Proc. Soc. Exp. Biol. Med. 90*:672-675.
61. Pachas, W. N. and Currid, V. R. (1974). L-form induction, morphology and development in two related strains of *Erysipelothrix rhusiopathiae*. *J. Bacteriol. 119*:576-582.
62. Cohen, M. and Panos, C. (1966). Membrane lipid composition of *Streptococcus pyogenes* and derived L-form. *Biochemistry 5*:2385.
63. King, J. R., Prescott, B., and Caldes, G. (1970). Lack of murein in formamide-insoluble fraction from the stable L-form of *Streptococcus faecium* strain F 24. *J. Bacteriol. 102*:296-297.
64. Leon, O. and Panos, C. (1976). Adaptation of an osmotically fragile L-form of *Streptococcus pyogenes* to physiological osmotic conditions and its ability to destroy human heart cells in tissue culture. *Infect. Immun. 13*: 252-262.
65. Gregory, W. W. and Gooder, H. (1978). Inhibition of peptidoglycan biosynthesis as a postcytoplasmic reaction in a stable L-phase variant of *Streptococcus faecium*. *J. Bacteriol. 135*:900-910.
66. Pachas, W. W. and Schor, M. (1977). Some biologic and genetic characteristics of *Proteus* L-forms in *Spheroplasts, Protoplasts and L-forms of Bacteria* (J. Roux, ed.), Ed. INSERM, vol. 64, Paris, pp. 129-146.
67. Schmitt-Slomska, J. and Roux, J. (1977). Cell wall defective organisms as a model for the study of antibiotic activity in *Spheroplasts, Protoplasts and L-forms of Bacteria* (J. Roux, ed.), Ed. INSERM, vol. 64, Paris, pp. 185-196.
68. Cabezas de Herrera, E. and Garcia Jurado, O. (1977). Stable L-forms of *Erwinia cartovora* induced by ultraviolet irradiation in *Spheroplasts, Protoplasts and L-forms of Bacteria* (J. Roux, ed.), Ed. INSERM, vol. 64, Paris, pp. 107-118.
69. Hoyer, B. H. and King, J. R. (1969). Deoxyribonucleic acid sequence losses in a stable streptococcal L-form. *J. Bacteriol. 97*:1516-1517.
70. Landman, O. E. (1968). Protoplasts, spheroplasts and L-forms viewed as a genetic system in *Microbial Protoplasts, Spheroplasts and L-forms* (L. B. Guze, ed.), Williams and Wilkins, Baltimore, pp. 319-332.
71. Wyrick, P., McConnell, M., and Rogers, H. (1973). Genetic transfer of the stable L-form state to intact bacterial cells. *Nature 24*:505-507.
72. Madoff, S. (1976). Mycoplasma and L-forms: Occurrence in bacterial cultures. *Health Lab. Sci. 13*:159-166.
73. Pachas, W. N. and Schor, M. (1983). Diphtheroid L-form variants resembling *A. laidlawii* (Abstr). Annual Meeting ASM, p. 97.

74. Dienes, L. and Pachas, W. N. (1971). Observations suggesting the development of Streptococci from pleomorphic filamentous gram negative bacteria. *Yale J. Med. Microbiol.* *43*:337–350.
75. Smith, P. F. (1971). *The Biology of Mycoplasmas*, Academic, New York.
76. Scheibel, I. and Assandri, J. (1959). Isolation of toxigenic L-phase variants from *Cl. tetani. Acta Pathol. Microbiol. Scand. 46*:333–338.
77. Kanei, C., Uchida, T., and Yoneda, M. (1978). Isolation of the L-phase variant from toxigenic *Corynebacterium diphtheriae* C7 (B). *Infect. Immun. 20*:167–172.
78. Madoff, M., Annenberg, S. M., and Weinstein, L. (1961). Production of neuraminidase by L-forms of *Vibrio cholerae. Proc. Soc. Exp. Biol. Med. 107*:776–777.
79. Mattman, L. H., Tunstall, L. H., and Rossmore, H. W. (1961). Induction and characteristics of staphylococcal L-forms. *J. Microbiol. 7*:705–713.
80. Sharp, J. T., Hijmans, W., and Dienes, L. (1957). Examination of the L-forms of Group A streptococci for the group specific polysaccharide and M protein. *J. Exp. Med. 105*:153–159.
81. Kagan, G., Vulfovitch, Y., Gusman, B., and Raskova, R. (1977). Persistence and pathological effect of streptococcal L-forms in vivo in *Spheroplasts, Protoplasts and L-forms of Bacteria* (J. Roux, ed.), Ed. INSERM, vol. 64, Paris, pp. 247–258.
82. Domingue, G. J., ed. (1982). *Cell Wall-deficient Bacteria, Basic Principles and Clinical Significance*, Addison-Wesley, Reading, Massachusetts.
83. Pachas, W. N. and Madoff, S. (1978). Biological significance of bacterial L-forms in *Microbiology-1978* (D. Schlessinger, ed.), Am. Soc. Microbiol., Washington, D.C., pp. 412–415.
84. Gould, S. J. (1983). *Hen's Teeth and Horse's Toes*, W. W. Norton, New York, London.

2
Origins and Evolution of Wall-Less Prokaryotes

HAROLD NEIMARK
College of Medicine, State University of New York, Brooklyn, New York

I. Introduction	21
II. Categories of Wall-Less Prokaryotes	22
A. Mycoplasmas	22
B. Bacterial L-Forms	24
III. Origins of the Mycoplasmas	27
IV. Evolution of the Mycoplasmas	31
V. Concluding Remarks	35
References	36

I. INTRODUCTION

The surface of a bacterial cell determines the result of many interactions between the bacterium and its environment, and surface structures have long been a major theme of study in bacteriology [1-5]. Bacteria that lack the important envelope component, the cell wall, occur with some frequency in nature and the existence of these wall-less prokaryotes appears to reflect a mechanism for responding to or circumventing environmental factors. Partial or total loss of cell wall components may have quite far-reaching effects beyond merely producing a wall-less cell because of the relation between genome segregation, cell division and wall growth [6-8]. Whether the loss of cell walls was a primary event or wall genes were lost concomitantly or as a consequence of other chromosomal alterations will be discussed later.

II. CATEGORIES OF WALL-LESS PROKARYOTES

Two general categories of wall-less prokaryotes customarily have been recognized: mycoplasmas (formerly called pleuropneumonia-like organisms, PPLO) and bacterial L-forms, the subject of this volume. For many years the relationship between these wall-less prokaryotes was unclear, largely because of the then prevalent difficulties in studying these bacteria (for an extensive and balanced review of this period, see Ref. 9). Although they share some characters resulting from the wall-less state (for example, the formation of similar "fried-egg" colonies), it is now clear that the differences between mycoplasmas and L-forms are considerable and fundamental. In addition, a third category of wall-less prokaryotic cellular forms will be discussed below.

A. Mycoplasmas

1. General Characteristics

Mycoplasmas are naturally occurring wall-less prokaryotes with the general characteristics and cellular organization of bacteria. However, in contrast to bacteria they are small in size (0.33-1.0 μm); indeed, they are the smallest known cells capable of autonomous replication. Mycoplasma cells are bounded only by a single lipoprotein membrane [10-13], but membranes of many mycoplasmas have been observed to be surrounded by an amorphous layer that in several instances has been identified as mucopolysaccharide [14].

In occurrence, mycoplasmas are not rare or unusual but rather are found either as pathogens or commensals in association with a wide variety of mammals, birds, insects, and plants [15]. At present count, nearly 80 distinct species have been described, with many of these being isolated within the last 5 years. These wall-less bacteria have been set apart from all other prokaryotes in the class Mollicutes, order Mycoplasmatales, and classified into the following genera: *Mycoplasma, Acholeplasma, Ureaplasma, Spiroplasma,* and *Anaeroplasma* (Table 1).

In addition to the mycoplasmas that have already been isolated, many other wall-less prokaryotes resembling mycoplasmas have been observed in insects and other invertebrates [16], amphibians, and plants, but have not been cultivated (reviewed in Ref. 17). Consequently, it appears that many more mycoplasmas remain to be cultivated and that only parts of the group have been characterized. It is now evident, then, that wall-less prokaryotes constitute a large class of biologically interesting microorganisms that are commonly and broadly distributed in nature.

2. Genome Sizes

Mycoplasmas also are distinguished from the majority of bacteria, including L-forms, by their small genomes [18] which fall into two separate size classes

Table 1 Properties of the Mycoplasmas

Genus	Current number of species	Genome		Cholesterol requirement	Characteristics	Habitat
		Size (megadaltons)	G + C content (%)			
Mycoplasma	>70	~500	23–40	+	Fermentative and nonfermentative; gliding motility in some	Animals
Ureaplasma	2	~500	27–30	+	Urease activity; hexokinase and lactate dehydrogenase absent	Animals
Acholeplasma	>8	~1000	29–35	–	FDP-activated lactate dehydrogenase	Animals, insects, plant surfaces
Spiroplasma	>3	~1000	26–29	+	Helical filaments; flexing motility	Insects, plants, (animals)
Anaeroplasma (uncertain affiliation)	2	Unknown	~29 ~40	+/–	Obligate anaerobes	Rumen of cattle and sheep

[19,21] that cluster around 470 megadaltons (Mdal) (range, ~440–540 Mdal; mycoplasmas and ureaplasmas) and 1000 Mdal (acheloplasmas and spiroplasmas), or approximately twice the size of the small chromosome species. The mycoplasmas comprising the small size class are unique in having chromosomes smaller than those of any free-living prokaryotes. Only the genomes of the obligately parasitic intracellular chlamydia (genome size 660 Mdal [22]), and the bacterial inclusion bodies found in certain protozoa (discussed below) even approach this small size. The 1000-Mdal class, although unusually small in size, is not unique since its values overlap the smallest sizes observed in a few walled bacteria, i.e., 990 Mdal and 1000 Mdal for the parasitic bacteria *Neisseria meningitidis* and *Hemophilus influenzae*, respectively [23]. This class also overlaps the lower range of Rickettsiae genomes which span from about 1000 Mdal upwards to 1490 Mdal [24,25]; only one member of this group, the agent of Trench fever, has been cultivated. The 1000-Mdal size class is not limited to parasitic bacteria, however, since the thermoacidophile *Thermoplasma acidophilum* [26] and *Methanobacterium thermoautotrophicum* [27] have genomes of about 1000 Mdal. Thermoplasma clearly is a wall-less prokaryote and originally was grouped with the mycoplasmas; however, it was considered to be of uncertain taxonomic affiliation [28]. It was suggested that thermoplasma might be a wall-defective variant of a thermoacidophilic bacterium [29] and lipid structure studies indicated that thermoplasma in fact is closely related to other thermoacidophilic, halophilic, and methanogenic bacteria [30]; subsequently, thermoplasma was confirmed to be an archaebacterium [31].

B. Bacterial L-Forms

Bacterial L-forms, by definition, arise directly from known bacterial species. L-forms can occur spontaneously in a few species but they can be induced from virtually all gram-positive and gram-negative bacteria under suitable conditions by treatment with one of several agents that interfere with cell wall formation, such as penicillin, lysozyme, high concentrations of certain amino acids (e.g., glycine), or specific antibody (see Chap. 1). The conversion to L-forms essentially is a population effect where many or most of the surviving cells in a culture convert; for gram-positive bacteria, including streptococcus and bacillus, suitable manipulation of treatment and medium conditions results in a mass conversion, in certain strains, to the L-form (see Chap. 5). Removal of the inducing agent usually results in reversion to the parental bacterial form. (The term "parent" will be used to denote the precursor of L-forms; the term "progenitor" or "antecedent" will be used to describe the bacterial precursors of mycoplasmas.) However, continued cultivation in the presence of inducing agents occasionally results in the development of stable L-forms.

Aside from the loss of their cell walls, L-forms in most cases appear to be little changed genetically from their bacterial parents and retain most of the parental biochemical characters. DNA-DNA hybridization studies (see Ref. 32 for a survey) between bacteria and their L-forms support this notion. An important exception is pathogenicity. Most pathogenic bacteria (except those where pathogenicity is due to exotoxin production or an extracellular virulence factor) lose pathogenicity when they convert to the L-form, and generally they regain pathogenicity on reversion to the walled form. In addition, Black and co-workers [29] pointed out that flagellated bacteria lose motility upon conversion to protoplasts and spheroplasts, even though these wall-deficient cells retain flagella; similarly, L-phase variants of flagellated bacteria also are invariably nonmotile but unfortunately, few observations on the fate of flagella following L-phase induction have been made. Black et al. [29] did examine the L9 L-phase of *Proteus mirabilis* and, using electronmicroscopy, were unable to observe flagella in negatively stained preparations. It should be noted that few genetic studies comparing bacteria and their stable L-forms have been carried out. One stable L-form of *Streptococcus faecalis* is known to have lost approximately 4-6% of its chromosome in the transition from its parent [33].

A third category of wall-less cellular elements derived from prokaryotes, albeit greatly altered in composition, can be considered if one accepts that plastids, the eukaryotic photosynthetic organelles, evolved from prokaryotes. The endosymbiont hypothesis for the origin of plastids proposes that these organelles descended from photosynthetic prokaryotes which were taken in as endosymbionts within host cells ("protoeukaryotic cells"), and these later developed into eukaryotes [34-36]. This category probably also contains the mitochondria of eukaryotes and perhaps as well the hydrogenosomes [37,38] of anaerobic trichomonads; however, the evidence for these cellular organelles is not as extensive as for chloroplasts and, in the case of mitochondria, is replete with puzzles.

An important question in evolutionary biology is how these organelles, which contain separate autonomously replicating genomes, evolved. Closely tied to the origin of eukaryotic organelles is the origin of eukaryotic cells themselves, one of the grand questions of evolutionary biology. It is generally accepted that eukaryotes evolved from prokaryotes or from a common ancestor shared with prokaryotes. Two alternate theories have been suggested to explain how organelles of prokaryotic ancestry reached their present nearly indispensable status in eukaryotic cells: (1) the endosymbiont theory, already mentioned, proposes that eukaryotic organelles are derived from different genetic lines of free-living prokaryotes that early in evolution entered into the progenitor of the eukaryotic cell [34]; (2) the alternate theory is that eukaryotes and their organelles evolved from one progenitor through differentiation, the so-called direct filiation theory (see Ref. 39 for a discussion).

An interesting hypothesis that combines some features of each theory and requires a role for a wall-less prokaryote in the formation of eukarotes has been proposed by Cavalier-Smith [40]. In brief, he postulated that the ancestor of all eukaryotes was an oxygen-evolving cyanobacterium that possessed cytochromes. A first step would have been loss of the cell wall to produce a cyanobacterial "L-form"; this membrane-bound cell then developed the functions of endocytosis and phagocytosis, which were proposed to be crucial for the rise of the eukaryotic cell. Whether one agrees with this hypothesis or not, it does raise valid questions that any theory must address, namely, how were cell walls lost, and how did a membrane-bound nucleus arise.

In the case of plastids, the similarities between the organelles and cyanobacteria have been documented extensively and the evidence that plastids evolved from cyanobacteria is very strong [35,41-43]; this is so whether one supports the theory that plastids arose from cyanobacteria through endosymbiosis or by direct filiation. However, the existence of an intermediate form that appears to be a bridge between plastids and cyanobacteria provides still more support for the endosymbiotic origin of plastids and may provide insight into the evolutionary process. *Cyanophora paradoxica* is a small biflagellate protist that contains intracellular cyanobacteria-like structures surrounded by a vacuolar membrane. Originally the inclusions, which have the characteristic cyanobacterial photosynthetic apparatus and a thin peptidoglycan cell wall, were thought to be a symbiotic cyanobacterium. However, the inclusion bodies have a very small chromosome [44] and are now called cyanelles. The genome of the cyanelle is only 117 Mdal [44], approximately one-tenth that of cyanobacteria, and resembles plastid DNA in size and structure [45]. This genome, which can code for only about 120 proteins of average molecular weight 50,000, presumably is too small to encode a sufficient number of proteins for the cyanelle to exist as a free-living organism. Now the cyanelle is considered to have descended from a cyanobacterium [46] which has been modified through loss of genetic material, allowing it to adjust to its host and live as an endosymbiont in an obligatory symbiotic relationship.

It is particularly relevant to the discussion here that the genome size of the cyanelle is very small—approximately one-fifth that of mycoplasma or ureaplasma genomes and even considerably more reduced in size relative to cyanobacterial genomes—yet cyanelles have retained the capacity to synthesize a thin peptidoglycan cell wall. There are numerous other examples where genome size presumably has been reduced and some degree of wall synthesis has been retained. As already mentioned, chlamydia, which also grow in vacuoles in the host cell cytoplasm, possess small genomes; *Chlamydia trachomatis*, in contrast to mycoplasmas [47], possesses penicillin-binding proteins [48] and has some wall structure but lacks detectable muramic acid [48]. Infectious, intracellular endosymbionts or parasites, apparently derived from bacteria, also appear to be widespread among protozoa, particularly ciliates [49]. The genome sizes of four of these symbiont particles, *lambda, mu, pi* [50], and *omicron* [51] have been determined and all are small (estimated from renaturation kinetics to range from about 400 to 600 Mdal); also each particle contains multiple genome copies. *Omicron*, a prokaryote found in the cytoplasm of *Euplotes aediculatus*, is reported to be gram-negative and its genome size appears to be approximately 640 Mdal [51]. If the small genome cyanelles do represent an intermediate stage in the formation of chloroplasts from cyanobacteria, then in at least some cases, complete loss of the cell wall did not occur until major reductions in genome size had first taken place. For many of the intracytoplasmic particles, insufficient information is available at present to determine whether they originally had small chromosomes [51] or whether they too have undergone genome size reduction.

In the case of mitochondria, endosymbiosis also is an attractive hypothesis. The search among contemporary bacteria for descendants of the prokaryotes that could have given rise to mitochondria has involved studies of metabolic characteristics and structural homologies of proteins and ribosomal RNAs [38,42,52,53]. Various investigators have recognized in making comparisons that selective pressures bearing on a prokaryote in an intracellular environment may be quite different [54] from those affecting an extracellular or free-living prokaryote. The finding of somewhat different genetic codes in mitochondria from yeast, wheat, and humans [54,55] has greatly complicated matters. In addition, the transfer of DNA segments between the genome and the mitochondrial genome has occurred and this process could have further obscured the origin of the organelle DNA [56]. Nevertheless, attractive evidence pointing to a group of bacteria that includes *Paracoccus denitrificans* and the purple nonsulfur photosynthetic bacteria (Rhodospirillaceae) has been developed [38,57,58]. These bacteria have the requisite mitochondrial-type respiratory chain and there are structural homologies between their cytochrome *c* and mitochondrial cytochrome *c* [53]. Also, some clues to possible prokaryotic antecedents may be obtained from comparisons of 5S ribosomal RNAs [59]. The wheat mitochondria 5S rRNA has been sequenced and it has most of the features of prokaryotic 5S rRNA [60]; interestingly, the helix V region of the mitochondria 5S rRNA is truncated as is the helix V region of mycoplasma 5S rRNAs [60] (discussed below).

III. ORIGINS OF THE MYCOPLASMAS

The origins of mycoplasmas, their relationship to one another, and their relationship to other prokaryotes came into question when it was recognized that virtually all bacteria can produce wall-deficient growth forms ("L-forms") that closely resemble the naturally occurring mycoplasmas [61]. Two opposing hypotheses have been offered to explain the relationship of mycoplasmas to other prokaryotes [62-64] : one hypothesis holds that mycoplasmas are a true biological class, all of whose members are phylogenetically related through common evolution; the other hypothesis holds that mycoplasmas are an artificial assemblage of wall-less prokaryotes derived from various bacteria. In terms of bacterial evolution, it was implicit in the former hypothesis that the extant mycoplasmas would be the surviving descendants of exceedingly primitive bacteria that existed before the development of a peptidoglycan-based cell wall [32].

Genetic heterogeneity is a major feature of the mycoplasmas and the group is made up of organisms with diverse morphological, antigenic, nutritional, and physiologic properties. As the principal physiological groupings of mycoplasmas were established, it became clear that the mycoplasmas were also heterogeneous [65] in such fundamental characters as metabolic pathways, DNA base composition, and even genome size (reviewed in Ref. 32). Particularly, the range of mycoplasma GC contents was so broad that the mycoplasmas could not be compatibly contained in a single genus [65,66]. To conform to the hypothesis that mycoplasmas are a true biological class, it would have been necessary to interpret the fundamental heterogeneity observed among mycoplasmas as reflecting the breadth of a very large biological group that had evolved to produce such diverse species. However, this hypothesis and its variations were difficult to support because one had to explain how the diverse mycoplasma biotypes came to parallel many of the very same biotypes found among walled bacteria. The discovery of additional mycoplasma biotypes, such as spiroplasmas and organisms possessing gliding motility, broadened and deepened the diversity of life forms that were encompassed within the group.

Fermentative mycoplasmas are a prominent segment of the mycoplasmas, and about half of the known isolates ferment glucose and accumulate acid endproducts. At least 16 fermentative organisms so far examined accumulate D- or L-lactic acid as a major product of glucose fermentation [32], and both homofermentative and heterofermentative mycoplasmas have been recognized. Several workers [67-69] pointed out that physiological and metabolic similarities exist between the fermentative mycoplasmas and lactic acid bacteria; both groups of organisms ferment glucose by the Embden-Meyerhof pathway and accumulate lactate, usually do not synthesize heme enzymes, and have a flavin-terminated respiratory system. Recent studies confirm the absence of cytochromes from several representative acholeplasmas and mycoplasmas [70]. When it was found that one large segment of the mycoplasmas, the sterol nonrequiring acholeplasmas, possess fructose diphosphate-activated lactate dehydrogenases that are strikingly similar to the unique lactate dehydrogenases found in streptococci [71-73], studies were carried out to determine whether these mycoplasmas are phylogenetically related to members of the genus *Streptococcus*.

Subsequently, we proved that acholeplasmas are phylogenetically closely related to streptococci and that they descended from streptococci [32,74]. The evidence was obtained largely from comparative enzyme studies and immunological studies, the latter utilizing highly specific antisera against purified glycolytic enzyme proteins [74,75].

Other close similarities, in addition to the structural homology shared by several of their glycolytic enzymes, can be found between acholeplasmas and streptococci. Shaw and Baddiley [76] showed that bacteria could be grouped on the basis of the structures of their glycolipids, resulting in a taxonomic scheme very similar to that obtained by traditional methods; Shaw [77] then pointed out that the lipid composition of those mycoplasmas that have been examined is akin to that of gram-positive bacteria. We noted [32] that information on mycoplasma lipids [77,78] is in accord with our findings, and that lipids from *Acholeplasma laidlawii* and other acholeplasmas closely resemble, or are identical, to those of streptococci [10]. Furthermore, at least two acholeplasmas, *A. laidlawii* and *Acholeplasma granularum*, accumulate free phospholipids with structures similar to that of the lipid anchor for glycerol teichoic acid in streptococci [79].

No immunological cross-reactions were obtained against any of several representative small genome mycoplasmas, indicating either that these mycoplasmas are phylogenetically too distantly related to produce visible precipitin reactions or that they are unrelated. The demonstration that acholeplasmas descended from streptococci and that several other mycoplasmas are rather distantly related or unrelated to streptococci, together with analysis of the fundamental lines of heterogeneity that cleave through the mycoplasmas, allowed us to show that the organisms comprising various other diverse mycoplasma subgroups similarly must have descended from other bacteria [32,74]. Consequently, the mycoplasmas are not a true phylogenetic class all of whose members have descended from a common ancestor. In fact, the fundamentally heterogeneous subgroups that can be discerned among the mycoplasmas [32,66] suggest that the genetic events that led to formation of the mycoplasmas occurred more than once. This does not negate the possibility that there can be clusters of phylogenetically related organisms among the mycoplasmas, and indeed the acholeplasmas themselves obviously are such a cluster. Previously, we suggested that acholeplasmas could be related to certain of the fermentative lactate-accumulating mycoplasmas in the same manner that streptococci are related to other lactic acid bacteria [32].

The immunological evidence indicates that acholeplasmas as a group diverged from the essentially sequential evolutionary path formed by the streptococci and are most closely related to the Group N and Group D streptococci [32,75]. Just when the acholeplasmas diverged from streptococci is uncertain. If the findings of Ibrahimi et al. [80] can be extended to other proteins, namely that a change of one immunological distance unit is equivalent to an amino acid sequence difference of 0.2%, then the streptococcal and acholeplasma aldolase subunits, which are composed of approximately 166 amino acids, may differ by as few as 30 amino acids. The close similarity between their shared enzymes suggests that this divergence occurred during the relatively recent evolutionary history of these enzyme proteins [75].

Our conclusion that mycoplasmas are not a true phylogenetic class is supported by others. Recently, Woese and co-workers [31] compared 16S ribosomal RNA oligonucleotide catalogs from four mycoplasmas and thermoplasmas to those of bacteria. They concluded that mycoplasmas evolved as a "branch of the subline of clostridial ancestry that led to bacillus and lactobacillus." They also concluded that mycoplasmas arose by degenerative evolution and that within the confines of the gram-positive spore-forming bacteria, the mycoplasma cluster is peripherally related to a subgroup defined by the genera *Bacillus, Lactobacillus,* and *Streptococcus.* They thus confirmed our conclusion that mycoplasmas arose from more complex walled bacteria by chromosomal losses and cited our work in support of theirs. The walled bacteria they identified as being most closely related to myocplasma, spiroplasma, and acholeplasma were two Group III clostridia [81], *Clostridium ramosum* and *Clostridium innocuum.* As Woese et al. noted, these two species had been shown by Johnson and Francis [81], using rRNA hybridization competition studies, to be unrelated to other clostridia. However, their analysis did not detect the close relationship between acholeplasmas and streptococci and their finding that *A. laidlawii* is more closely related to the Group III clostridia than to streptococci differs markedly from ours.

Subsequently, Fox et al. [82] in a summary paper published a phylogenetic tree for the gram-positive bacteria based on 16S RNA oligonucleotide sequence catalogs that confirmed previous immunological results that lactobacilli, pediococci, and streptococci evolved from a common ancestor [83]. However, the tree also indicated that acholeplasmas are closely related to the two Group III clostridia but are distant from the streptococci. We believe that analysis of 16S rRNA catalogs, pioneered by Woese, Fox, and co-workers, has considerable value and we were concerned when the procedure failed to detect the very close relationship that exists between acholeplasmas and streptococci. Clearly, it is imperative that the most specific bacterial antecedents of each mycoplasma group be identified in order to examine the evolutionary mechanism(s) that produced the mycoplasmas. We examined extracts from both clostridia and found that reactions with the *S. faecalis* anti-GA3P dehydrogenase antiserum were strong enough to carry out cross-match reactions against *C. innocuum* (GC content, 43%). The antiserum produced double-spur reactions of nonidentity between acholeplasma and *C. innocuum* extracts and also between streptococcal and *C. innocuum* extracts. These reactions support their observation that this Group III clostridium is related to the lactic acid bacteria, but the reactions of nonidentity between acholeplasmas and streptococci against the clostridium indicate that the clostridium is not as closely related to the acholeplasmas as the streptococci are. Further studies, ideally with specific antisera prepared against clostridial respiratory enzymes, will be required to determine the detailed relations among these bacteria.

With sufficient effort, it should be possible to identify the specific bacterial antecedents of each of the different subgroups that comprise the mycoplasmas. How widespread across the span of bacteria is the capacity to produce mycoplasmas? Thus far, the few close bacterial relatives of mycoplasmas that have been identified are all gram-positive. As noted already, the lipid composition of those mycoplasmas that have been examined is characteristic of gram-positive bacteria [77]. Also, tRNA sequences provide some information, and these, where determined for mycoplasmas [84-86], share a higher nucleotide sequence homology with *B. subtilis* than with *Escherichia coli*, and Walker concluded that these mycoplasmas could not be evolutionarily primitive bacteria [87]. Whether all mycoplasmas will prove to be descendants of gram-positive bacteria remains to be determined, since only fermentative mycoplasmas have been examined in detail. Even among the fermentative mycoplasmas there are physiological divergences; for example, certain of these mycoplasmas possess gliding motility [88]. The sequence of the 5S rRNA from the gliding organism *M. pneumoniae* has been determined by Walker (personal communication), and our analysis of this sequence utilizing the recently published generalized models for gram-positive and gram-negative 5S rRNA secondary structures [89] shows that this 5S rRNA is unusual in that it contains a combination of both gram-positive nucleotide signatures and signatures that are neither gram-positive nor gram-negative, indicating that its evolutionary history may differ from other mycoplasmas that are derived from gram-positive bacteria.

IV. EVOLUTION OF THE MYCOPLASMAS

A major question is, By what evolutionary mechanisms did mycoplasmas evolve from their progenitor bacteria? The detection of the specific progenitor-derivitive relationship between streptococci and acholeplasmas makes it possible to approach this question by identifying the existing cellular differences between these two groups and comparing them. Although acholeplasmas are closely related to streptococci, it is also clear that they are radically altered from streptococci. Aside from the absence of cell walls, one of the most striking and fundamental differences between the two groups is their genome size. Genome size values known for streptococci range from about 1200 to 1470 Mdal [90], and acholeplasma genome sizes, which cluster around 1000 Mdal, are 20-30% smaller than these streptococcal genomes. Evidently, some streptococci must have undergone massive reductions in genome size to produce acholeplasmas.

How did large reductions in genome size occur to produce the acholeplasmas and why do mycoplasma genome sizes not occur over a range, but rather all cluster to form two size classes of 500 or 1000 Mdal? Large reductions in genome size could have come about either through a series of individually small deletions or through losses of very large DNA segments. The occurrence of irregularities in chromosome replication, rearrangements of large chromosome segments [91], or the action of transposable elements [92] each could have contributed to large losses.

The absence of cell walls is the most conspicuous phenotypic character of mycoplasmas, and probably a significant portion of the lost genome segments was devoted to coding for wall structures or wall-associated processes. Losses of specific proteins that function in these processes have been identified. Acholeplasmas (and mycoplasmas), in contrast to streptococci, lack all penicillin-binding proteins [47], and losses of other proteins related to membrane function also appear to have occurred in acholeplasmas, since they lack a functional phosphoenolpyruvate-dependent phosphotransferase system [93] (however the latter may have been plasmid mediated [75]). The capacity to synthesize all wall-related components may not have been lost, however; the occurrence in certain acholeplasmas of free phospholipids that resemble the streptococcal lipid anchor for glycerol teichoic acid suggests the possible accumulation of a metabolic intermediate resulting from the inability to synthesize wall polymers [79].

In addition to genes coding for wall structure, it appears that rRNA genes were altered in the course of formation of mycoplasmas. Reff et al. [94] reported that the 16S rRNAs from all the mycoplasmas examined appeared to be smaller in size than the 16S rRNAs from bacteria (including an L-form) by about 12,000 daltons. (This would reflect the absence of about 37 nucleotides.) Also, Woese and co-workers [31] observed that a number of sequences normally highly conserved in bacterial 16S rRNA were absent from mycoplasma 16S rRNAs.

We compared the chromosomes of streptococci and acholeplasmas to determine what sorts of chromosomal alterations and losses occurred in acholeplasmas [95]. One of the most accessible measures of chromosome structure are ribosomal RNA genes. The number of ribosomal RNA gene sets in streptococci and acholeplasmas was estimated by hybridizing labeled 16S, 23S, and 5S rRNAs from *Streptococcus cremoris* to Southern blots bearing restriction fragments from streptococcal and acholeplasma chromosomes digested with various endonucleases. Five acholeplasma species have been examined, and we found that acholeplasma chromosomes each contain only two rRNA gene sets. In contrast, we estimated that there are at least five rRNA gene sets in *S. cremoris* and at least six rRNA gene sets in *Streptococcus lactis*. In certain restriction digests, these related streptococci shared at least two identically sized rDNA fragments bearing 16S, 23S, and 5S rRNA gene sequences. Some of the acholeplasmas shared equal-sized restriction fragments bearing both 16S and 23S rDNA sequences. Especially interesting was the fact that some of the acholeplasmas and streptococci shared single rDNA restriction fragments of apparent equal size; for example, one of the two *A. laidlawii* restriction fragments bearing 16S and 23S rDNA sequences was apparently the same size as one of the six *S. lactis* fragments [95].

These results indicate that acholeplasmas have two rRNA gene sets whereas their nearest bacterial relatives probably have at least five or six rRNA gene sets. It appears that the reduction in chromosome size of acholeplasmas relative to streptococci is accompanied by losses of entire rRNA gene sets, and perhaps as many as three or four rRNA gene sets were lost in the course of the transition to acholeplasmas [95]. (The number of rRNA gene copies in bacteria does not necessarily correlate with genome size, however; the archaebacterium *Halobacterium halobium*, for example, has only one rRNA gene set even though its genome size is 2600 Mdal [96]. *Thermoplasma* also contains only one copy of the 5S, 16S, and 23S RNA genes, but in contrast to eubacteria and eukaryotes, the genes appear to be unlinked [97].)

It seems likely that a parallel situation involving rRNA gene losses will be found to hold for other mycoplasmas. Information is available for the number of rRNA gene sets in only two mycoplasmas species, *Mycoplasma capricolum* [98] and *Mycoplasma mycoides* subspp. *capri* [99], and each has just two rRNA gene sets. In early work, Ryan and Morowitz [100] estimated by hybridization-saturation experiments that *M. capricolum* probably contained only one set of rRNA genes and one set of tRNA genes. It is now confirmed that there are two rRNA gene sets in *M. capricolum* (S. Razin, personal communication), and also that *A. laidlawii* has two gene sets.

A large number of studies provide detailed information on bacterial rRNA genes, but mainly for *E. coli* and *B. subtilis*. In *E. coli* it is now certain that there are exactly seven rRNA gene sets and each set is arranged as a transcription unit composed of a 16S, a 23S, and a 5S rRNA gene. The seven rRNA gene sets are arranged along a segment comprising 55% of the *E. coli* chromosome starting just to one side of and spanning across the origin of replication [101,102]. All seven of the rRNA gene operons contain tRNA genes encoded in spacer sequences located between the 16S and 23S rRNA genes; three of these rRNA gene sets each contain two tRNA genes, $tRNA_1^{Ile}$ and $tRNA_{1B}^{Ala}$, whereas the other four operons each contain a single $tRNA_2^{Glu}$ gene. Certain of the RNA transcription units also contain tRNA genes at the 3' end of the transcription unit. DNA sequencing studies have revealed that the *rrnD* gene set contains two 5S rRNA genes with a $tRNA^{Thr}$ gene located between them; possibly other ribosomal RNA transcription units (rrn) also have a similar 5S duplication, but it is certain that *rrnB*, *rrnC*, and *rrnH* have a single 5S rRNA gene. (For reviews, see Refs. 101, 103). In contrast, the gram-positive *B. subtilis* has 9 or, more probably, 10 rRNA gene sets [104,105]; however, only two gene sets contain spacer tRNAs and these are the same two tRNA genes (tRNA$_1^{Ile}$ and tRNA$_{1B}^{Ala}$) that are located together in *E. coli* and also in plant chloroplast rRNA genes [104].

Recently, a *B. subtilis* isolate was identified in which one of the 10 rRNA gene sets was deleted [106], and it was suggested that the loss may have resulted from recombination between tandemly repeated genes. An *E. coli* strain also has been isolated in which one rRNA gene set was deleted [107]. In *E. coli*, the scattering of the seven rRNA gene sets around the chromosome (rather than a tandem organization as appears to be the case in *B. subtilis* [P. Zuber, Ph.D. thesis, University of Virginia, 1982] may provide a mechanism to select against deletion or duplication of rRNA genes by unequal crossover [107].

Not only are several rRNA gene sets absent from mycoplasmas, but the remaining rRNA genes apparently are missing certain nucleotides or nucleotide sequences. In addition to the apparent absence of nucleotides from mycoplasma 16S rRNA already mentioned, nucleotide sequence analysis shows mycoplasma 5S rRNAs are shorter than any 5S rRNA from bacteria. 5S rRNA sequences from three mycoplasmas, *M. capricolum* [108], *M. mycoides* subsp. *capri*, and *Spiroplasma* sp. BC3 [109], have been determined and each is 107 nucleotides in length, indicating that mycoplasma 5S rRNAs also are missing several nucleotides. (5S rRNAs from gram-positive bacteria are usually 116 or 117 nucleotides long; those from gram-negative bacteria are generally 120 nucleotides long.) All three mycoplasma 5S rRNAs were recognized as being more closely related to gram-positive bacteria than to gram-negative bacteria and a few of the deletions responsible for the short chain lengths were identified. Comparison of the mycoplasma sequences to the generalized model for gram-positive bacterial 5S rRNA secondary structure confirms their gram-positive nature, and shows that each has sustained deletions at the base of helix V [89].

The apparent universality of missing rRNA sequences in mycoplasmas suggests that losses in rRNA genes, together with envelope gene losses, were important events in the formation of mycoplasmas [95].

Because the copies of the RNA operons are largely homologous, there is the potential for unequal recombination between these genes and such recombination could lead to extensive rearrangements of the chromosome. These rearrangements could take the form of tandem duplications of even deletions. The type of rearrangement would depend on the configuration of the interacting genes on the chromosome. The studies of Hill and co-workers [110-112] show that some of these alterations can be induced after ultraviolet mutagenesis in *E. coli*, although deletions have not yet been detected. Spontaneous tandem genetic duplications resulting from unequal recombination have also been observed in *Salmonella typhimurium* [113]. In *B. subtilis*, Anagnostopoulos and co-workers [114-116] have shown that very large chromosomal rearrangements (translocations and inversions) can occur. The rearrangements involve extensive regions of the bacterial chromosome (as much as one-third of the chromosome) and duplications, insertions, and deletions have been observed.

Based on the information presented previously, I believe a plausible working hypothesis to explain the genetic events leading to formation of mycoplasmas would include the following [95]: unequal crossing over between homologous rRNA genes could have resulted in losses of rRNA genes (of course, rRNA gene rearrangements could have occurred as well); this process may have been repeated several times. Genes located on the chromosome segments between rRNA genes undergoing unequal cross-over could have been lost in this process along with the rRNA genes. Ribosomal RNA genes are arranged tandemly on the chromosome of *Bacillus* and if RNA gene sets also occur tandemly in other gram-positive bacteria, then these bacteria could have a propensity for unequal crossing over. Similarly, if gram-negative bacteria have rRNA genes dispersed over approximately one-half their chromosomes, as is so in *E. coli*, then this dispersion could serve, as pointed out by Elwood and Nomura [107], as a mechanism to reduce, but not eliminate, the chance for unequal cross-over. Learning the location of envelope genes and tRNA genes on the chromosome relative to rRNA genes will be helpful in examining these possibilities.

V. CONCLUDING REMARKS

Unequal crossing over may not be the only process that has contributed to mycoplasma formation, but in light of the specific alterations evident in mycoplasma RNA genes, it seems plausible that it contributed in a large way to their formation. It is possible too, that recombination between other duplicated chromosome segments could have occurred. Further, events may have occurred in more than one sequence, and more than one pathway may have been followed to produce the mycoplasmas. Since these genetic events are not unique in time, does the possibility exist that events leading to formation of mycoplasmas could have occurred up to the present?

Added note: A review on wall-less prokaryotes [118] and two studies on 5S RNAs from clostridia and mycoplasmas appeared while this chapter was in press. Dams et al. [119] identified *C. bifermentans* as being related to lactobacilli and concluded that mycoplasmas evolved *from* lactic-acid bacteria. Rogers et al. [120] determined 5S RNA sequences from eight mycoplasmas and *C. innocuum*; they concluded that mycoplasmas are a coherent evolutionary group that evolved sequentially from clostridia and that *Mycoplasma* and *Ureaplasma* species arose from *Spiroplasma* through repeated independent events. Whether the altered mycoplasma 5S RNAs contain sufficient information to draw detailed branching is problematical, but immunological and 16S RNA sequence studies should resolve the paths of mycoplasma descent.

REFERENCES

1. Daneo-Moore, L. and Shockman, G. D. (1976). The bacterial cell surface in growth and division. *Cell Surf. Rev. 4*:1–205.
2. Ward, J. B. (1981). Teichoic and teichuronic acids: biosynthesis, assembly, and location. *Microbiol. Rev. 45*:211–243.
3. Koch, A. L., Higgens, M. L., and Doyle, R. J. (1982). The role of surface stress in the morphology of microbes. *J. Gen. Microbiol. 128*:927–945.
4. Mäkelä, P. H. and Stocker, B. A. D. (1981). Genetics of the bacterial cell surface in *Genetics as a Tool in Microbiology, Symposium of the Society for General Microbiology, 31.* (S. W. Glover and D. A. Hopwood, eds.), Cambridge University Press, Cambridge, pp. 219–264.
5. Easmon, C. S. F., Jeljaszewicz, J., Brown, M. R. W., and Lambert, P. A. (eds.). (1983). *Medical Microbiology*, vol. III, *Role of the Envelope in the Survival of Bacteria in Infection.* Academic, New York.
6. Sandler, N. and Keyman, A. (1981). Cell wall synthesis and inhibition of deoxyribonucleic acid replication in *Bacillus subtilis. J. Bacteriol. 148*: 443–449.
7. Mendelson, N. H. (1982). Bacterial growth and division. Genes, structures, forces, and clocks. *Microbiol. Rev. 46*:341–375.
8. Doyle, R. J., Koch, A. L., and Carstens, P. H. B. (1983). Cell wall-DNA association in *Bacillus subtilis. J. Bacteriol. 153*:1521–1527.
9. Smith, P. F. (1971). *The Biology of Mycoplasmas.* Academic, New York.
10. Smith, P. F. (1979). The composition of membrane lipids and lipopolysaccharides in *The Mycoplasmas*, vol. I. (M. F. Barile and S. Razin, eds.), Academic, New York, pp. 231–257.
11. Archer, D. B. (1981). The structure and functions of the mycoplasma membrane. *Int. Rev. Cytol. 69*:1–44.
12. Rottem, S. (1980). Membrane lipids of mycoplasmas. *Biochim. Biophys. Acta 604*:65–90.
13. Razin, S. (1982). Sterols in mycoplasma membranes in *Current Topics in Membranes and Transport*, vol. 17. Academic, New York, pp. 183–205.
14. Boatman, E. S. (1979). Morphology and ultrastructure of the mycoplasmatales in *The Mycoplasmas*, vol. I. (M. F. Barile and S. Razin, eds.), Academic, New York, pp. 63–102.
15. *The Mycoplasmas.* (1979). Vol. I–III. Academic, New York.
16. Zimmer, R. L. and Woollacott, R. M. (1983). Mycoplasma-like organisms: Occurrence with the larvae and adults of a marine bryozoan. *Science 220*: 208–210.
17. Razin, S. (1978). The mycoplasmas. *Microbiol. Rev. 42*:414–470.

18. Morowitz, H. J., Bode, H. R., and Kirk, R. G. (1967). The nucleic acids of mycoplasma. *Ann. N.Y. Acad. Sci. 143*:110-114.
19. Bak, A. L., Black, F. T., Christiansen, C., and Freundt, E. A. (1969). Genome size of mycoplasmal DNA. *Nature 224*:1209-1210.
20. Teplitz, M. (1977). Isolation of folded chromosomes from *Mycoplasma hominis. Nucleic Acids Res. 4*:1505-1512.
21. Darai, G., Zöller, L., Matz, B., Delius, H., Speck, P. T., and Flugel, R. M. (1982). Analysis of *Mycoplasma hyorhinis* genome by use of restriction endonucleases and by electron microscopy. *J. Bacteriol. 150*:788-794.
22. Sarov, I. and Becker, Y. (1969). Trachoma agent DNA. *J. Mol. Biol. 42*: 581-589.
23. Kingsbury, D. T. (1969). Estimation of the genome size of various microorganisms. *J. Bacteriol. 98*:1400-1401.
24. Weiss, E. (1982). The biology of Rickettsiae. *Ann. Rev. Microbiol. 36*: 345-370.
25. Myers, W. F. and Wisseman, C. L., Jr. (1980). Genetic relatedness among the Typhus group of Rickettsiae. *Int. J. Syst. Bacteriol. 30*:143-150.
26. Langworthy, T. A. (1979). Special features of Thermoplasma in *The Mycoplasmas*, vol. 1 (M. F. Barile and S. Razin, eds.), Academic, New York, pp. 495-513.
27. Mitchell, R. M., Loeblich, L. A., Klotz, L. C., and Loeblich, A. R. (1979). DNA organization of *Methanobacterium thermoautotrophicum. Science 204*:1082-1084.
28. Freundt, E. A. and Edward, D. G. (1979). Classification and taxonomy in *The Mycoplasmas*, vol. 1 (M. F. Barile and S. Razin, eds.), Academic, New York, pp. 1-41.
29. Black, F. T., Freundt, E. A., Vinther, O., and Christiansen, C. (1979). Flagellation and swimming motility of *Thermoplasma acidophilum. J. Bacteriol. 137*:456-460.
30. Tornabene, T. G. and Langworthy, T. A. (1979). Diphytanyl and dibiphytanyl glycerol ether lipids of methanogenic archaebacteria. *Science 203*:51-53.
31. Woese, C. R., Maniloff, J., and Zablen, L. B. (1980). Phylogenetic analysis of the mycoplasmas. *Proc. Natl. Acad. Sci. USA 77*:494-498.
32. Neimark, H. (1979). Phylogenetic relationships between mycoplasmas and other prokaryotes in *The Mycoplasmas*, vol. 1 (M. F. Barile and S. Razin, eds.), Academic, New York, pp. 43-61.
33. Hoyer, B. H. and King, J. R. (1969). Deoxyribonucleic acid sequence losses in a stable streptococcal L form. *J. Bacteriol. 97*:1516-1517.
34. Margulis, L. (1970). *Origins of Eukaryotic Cells.* Yale Univ. Press, New Haven.
35. Stanier, R. Y. (1974). The origins of photosynthesis in eukaryotes in *Evolution in the Microbial World. Symposium of the Society for General Microbiology, 24* (M. J. Carlile and J. J. Skehel, eds.), Cambridge University Press, Cambridge, pp. 219-240.
36. Margulis, L. (1981). *Symbiosis in Cell Evolution.* W. H. Freeman, San Francisco.

37. Lindmark, D. G. and Müller, M. (1973). Hydrogenosome, a cytoplasmic organelle of the anaerobic flagellate *Tritrichomonas foetus*, and its role in pyruvate metabolism. *J. Biol. Chem.* 248:7724–7728.
38. Whatley, F. R. (1981). The establishment of mitochondria: *Paracoccus* and *Rhodopseudomonas*. *Ann. N.Y. Acad. Sci. 361*:330–340.
39. Dillon, L. S. (1981). *Ultrastructure, Macromolecules and Evolution*, Plenum, New York and London, pp. 440–445; 504–510.
40. Cavalier-Smith, T. (1975). The origin of nuclei and of eukaryotic cells. *Nature 256*:463–468.
41. Schwartz, R. M. and Dayhoff, M. O. (1981). Chloroplast origins: inferences from protein and nucleic acid sequences. *Ann. N.Y. Acad. Sci. 361*:260–272.
42. Gray, M. W. and Doolittle, W. F. (1982). Has the endosymbiont hypothesis been proven? *Microbiol. Rev. 46*:1–42.
43. Delihas, N., Andresini, W., Andersen, J., and Berns, D. (1982). Structural features unique to the 5S ribosomal RNAs of the thermophilic cyanobacterium *Synechococcus lividus* III and the green plant chloroplasts. *J. Mol. Biol. 162*:721–727.
44. Herdman, M. and Stanier, R. Y. (1977). The cyanelle: Chloroplast or endosymbiotic prokaryote? *FEMS Lett. 1*:7–12.
45. Mucke, H., Löffelhardt, W., and Hohnert, H. J. (1980). Partial characterization of the genome of the "endosymbiotic" cyanelles from *Cyanophora paradoxica*. *FEBS Lett. 111*:347–352.
46. Jaynes, J. M. and Vernon, L. P. (1982). The cyanelle of *Cyanophora paradoxica*: Almost a cyanobacterial chloroplast. *Trends Biochem. Sci.* 7: 22–24.
47. Martin, H. H., Schilf, W., and Schiefer, H. (1980). Differentiation of mycoplasmatales from bacterial protoplast L-forms by assay for penicillin binding proteins. *Archiv. Microbiol. 127*:297–299.
48. Barbour, A. G., Ken-Ichi, A., Hackstadt, T., Perry, L., and Caldwell, H. D. (1982). *Chlamydia trachomatis* has penicillin binding proteins but not detectable muramic acid. *J. Bacteriol. 151*:420–428.
49. Preer, J. R. and Preer, L. B. (1984). Endosymbionts of protozoa in *Bergey's Manual of Determinative Bacteriology*, vol. 1, 9th ed. (J. G. Holt, ed.), Williams and Wilkins, Baltimore, pp. 795–811.
50. Soldo, A. T. and Godoy, G. A. (1974). The molecular complexity of *mu* and *pi* symbiont DNA of *Paramecium aurelia*. *Nucleic Acids Res. 1*:387–396.
51. Schmidt, H. J. (1982). Isolation of omicron-endosymbionts from mass cultures of *Euplotes aediculatus* and characterization of their DNA. *Exp. Cell Res. 140*:417–425.
52. Schwartz, R. M. and Dayhoff, M. O. (1978). Origins of prokaryotes, eukaryotes, mitochrondria, and chloroplasts. *Science 199*:395–403.
53. Dickerson, R. E. (1980). The cytochromes c: An exercise in scientific serendipity in *The Evolution of Protein Structure and Function* (D. S. Sigman and M. A. B. Brazier, eds.), Academic, New York, pp. 173–202.

54. Anderson, S., Benkier, A. T., Barrell, B. G., de Bruijn, M. H. L., Coulson, A. R., Drouin, J., Eperon, I. C., Nierlich, D. P., Roe, B. A., Sanger, F., Schreier, P. H., Smith, A. J. H., Staden, R., and Young, J. G. (1981). Sequence and organization of the human mitochondrial genome. *Nature* *290*:457-465.
55. Sanger, F. (1981). Determination of nucleotide sequences in DNA. *Bioscience Rep. 1*:3-18.
56. Farrelly, F. and Butow, R. A. (1983). Rearranged mitochondrial genes in the yeast nuclear genome. *Nature 301*:296-301.
57. Whatley, J. M., John, P., and Whatley, F. R. (1979). From extracellular to intracellular: The establishment of mitochondria and chloroplasts. *Proc. R. Soc. Lond. Ser. B 204*:165-187.
58. Finlay, B. J., Span, A. S. W., and Harman, J. M. P. (1983). Nitrate respiration in primitive eukaryotes. *Nature 303*:333-335.
59. MacKay, R. M., Salgado, D., Bonen, L., Stackebrandt, E., and Doolittle, W. F. (1982). The 5S ribosomal RNAs of *Paracoccus denitrificans* and *Prochloron*. *Nucleic Acids Res. 10*:2963-2970.
60. Delihas, N. and Anderson, J. (1982). Generalized structures of the 5S ribosomal RNAs. *Nucleic Acids Res. 10*:7323-7344.
61. Dienes, L., and Weinberger, H. J. (1951). The L-forms of bacteria. *Bacteriol. Rev. 15*:245-288.
62. Edward, D. G. (1960). Introduction. Biology of pleuropneumonialike organisms. *Ann. N.Y. Acad. Sci. 79*:308-311.
63. Klieneberger-Nobel, E. and Freundt, E. A. (1960). Discussion of the classification of PPLO. *Ann. N.Y. Acad. Sci. 79*:483-487.
64. Dienes, L. (1963). Comparative morphology of L forms and PPLO. *Rec. Prog. Microbiol. 8*:511-517.
65. Neimark, H. (1967). Heterogeneity among the mycoplasma and relationships to bacteria. *Ann. N.Y. Acad. Sci. 143*:31-37.
66. Neimark, H. (1970). Division of mycoplasmas into subgroups. *J. Gen. Microbiol. 63*:249-263.
67. Rodwell, A. W. (1960). Nutrition and metabolism of *Mycoplasma mycoides* var. *Mycoides*. *Ann. N.Y. Acad. Sci. 79*:499-507.
68. Neimark, H., and Pickett, M. J. (1960). Products of glucose metabolism by pleuropneumonia-like organisms. *Ann. N.Y. Acad. Sci. 79*:531-536.
69. Van Demark, P. J. (1967). Respiratory pathways in the mycoplasma. *Ann. N.Y. Acad. Sci. 143*:77-84.
70. Pollack, J. D., Merola, A. J., Platz, M., and Booth, Jr., R. L. (1981). Respiration-associated components of mollicutes. *J. Bacteriol. 146*:907-913.
71. Neimark, H., and Lemcke, R. M. Occurrence and properties of lactic dehydrogenases of fermentative mycoplasmas. *J. Bacteriol. 111*:633-640.
72. Neimark, H. (1973). Molecular evolutionary studies on mycoplasmas and acholeplasmas. *Ann. N.Y. Acad. Sci. 225*:14-21.
73. Neimark, H., and Tung, M. C. (1973). Properties of a fructose-1,6-diphosphate-activated lactate dehydrogenase from *Acholeplasma laidlawii* type A. *J. Bacteriol. 114*:1025-1033.

74. Neimark, H. (1974). Implications of the phylogenetic relationship between acholeplasmas and lactic acid bacteria. *Colloq. Inst. Natl. Sante Rech. Med.* *33*:71-78.
75. Neimark, H. and London, J. (1982). Origins of the mycoplasmas: Sterol-nonrequiring mycoplasmas evolved from streptococci. *J. Bacteriol. 150*: 1259-1265.
76. Shaw, N. and Baddiley, J. (1968). Structure and distribution of glycosyl diglycerides. *Nature 217*:142-144.
77. Shaw, N. (1974). Lipid composition as a guide to the classification of bacteria. *Adv. Appl. Microbiol. 17*:63-108.
78. Smith, P. F., Langworthy, T. A., and Mayberry, W. R. (1973). Lipids of mycoplasmas. *Ann. N.Y. Acad. Sci. 225*:22-27.
79. Smith, P. F., Patel, K. R., and Al-Shammari, A. J. N. (1980). An aldehydo-phosphoglycolipid from *Acholeplasma granularum. Biochem. Biophys. Acta 617*:419-429.
80. Ibrahimi, I. M., Prager, E. M., White, T. J., and Wilson, A. C. (1979). Amino acid sequence of California quail lysozyme. Effect of evolutionary substitution on the antigenic structure of lysozyme. *Biochemistry 18*:2736-2744.
81. Johnson, J. L. and Francis, B. S. (1975). Taxonomy of the clostridia: Ribosomal ribonucleic acid homologies among the species. *J. Gen. Microbiol. 88*:229-244.
82. Fox, G. E., Stackebrandt, E., Hespell, R. B., Gibson, J., Maniloff, J., Dyer, T. A., Wolfe, R. S., Balch, W. E., Tanner, R. S., Magrum, L. J., Zablen, L. B., Blakemore, R., Gupta, R., Bonen, L., Lewis, B. J., Stahl, D. A., Luerhsen, K. R., Chen, K. N., and Woese, C. F. (1980). The phylogeny of prokaryotes. *Science 209*:457-463.
83. London, J. and Kline, K. (1973). Aldolases of lactic acid bacteria. A case history in the use of an enzyme as an evolutionary marker. *Bacteriol. Rev. 37*:453-478.
84. Kimball, M. W., Szeto, K. S., and Söll, D. (1974). The nucleotide sequence of phenylalanine tRNA from Mycoplasma sp. (kid). *Nucleic Acids Res. 1*: 1721-1732.
85. Walker, R. T. and RajBhandary, U. L. (1978). The nucleotide sequence of formylmethionine tRNA from *Mycoplasma mycoides* sp. *capri. Nucleic Acids Res. 5*:57-70.
86. Kilpatrick, M. W. and Walker, R. T. (1980). The nucleotide sequence of glycine tRNA from *Mycoplasma mycoides* sp. *capri. Nucleic Acids Res. 8*: 2783-2786.
87. Walker, R. T. (1976). Mycoplasma tRNAs in *Proceedings of the International Conference on the Synthesis, Structure, and Chemistry of tRNAs and Their Components,* Poznan, Poland, pp. 291-305.
88. Bredt, W. (1979). Motility in *The Mycoplasmas,* vol. I (M. F. Barile and S. Razin, eds.), Academic, New York, pp. 141-155.
89. Neimark, H., Andersen, J. and Delihas, N. (1983). Unusual structural features of the 5S ribosomal RNA from *Streptococcus cremoris. Nucleic Acids Res. 11*:7569-7577.

90. Bak, A. L., Christiansen, C., and Stenderup, A. (1970). Bacterial genome sizes determined by DNA renaturation studies. *J. Gen. Microbiol.* 64:377-380.
91. Riley, M. and Anilionis, A. (1978). Evolution of the bacterial genome. *Annu. Rev. Microbiol.* 32:519-560.
92. Starlinger, P. (1980). IS elements and transposons. *Plasmid* 3:241-259.
93. Cirillo, V. P. (1979). Transport systems in *The Mycoplasmas*, vol. 1 (M. F. Barile and S. Razin, eds.), Academic, New York, pp. 323-349.
94. Reff, M. E., Stanbridge, E. J., and Schneider, E. L. (1977). Phylogenetic relationships between mycoplasmas and other prokaryotes based upon the electrophoretic behavior of their ribosomal ribonucleic acids. *Int. J. Syst. Bacteriol.* 27:185-193.
95. Neimark, H. (1983). Evolution of mycoplasmas and genome losses. Fourth International Congress, International Organization For Mycoplasmology, Tokyo, 1982. *Yale J. Biol. Med.* 56:377-383.
96. Hofman, J. D., Lau, R. H., and Doolittle, W. F. (1979). The number, physical organization and transcription of ribosomal RNA cistrons in an archaebacterium: *Halobacterium halobium*. *Nucleic Acids Res.* 7:1321-1333.
97. Tu, J. and Zillig, W. (1982). Organization of rRNA structural genes in the archaebacterium *Thermoplasma acidophilum*. *Nucleic Acids Res.* 10: 7231-7245.
98. Sawada, M., Osawa, S., Kobayashi, H., Hori, H., and Muto, A. (1981). The number of ribosomal RNA genes in *Mycoplasma capricolum*. *Mol. Gen. Genet.* 182:502-504.
99. Amikam, D., Razin, S., and Glaser, G. (1982). Ribosomal RNA genes in mycoplasma. *Nucleic Acids Res.* 10:4215-4222.
100. Ryan, J. L. and Morowitz, H. J. (1969). Partial purification of native rRNA and tRNA cistrons for mycoplasma sp. (KID). *Proc. Natl. Acad. Sci. USA* 63:1282-1289.
101. Morgan, E. A. (1982). Ribosomal RNA genes in *Escherichia coli*. *The Cell Nucleus* 10:1-29.
102. Ellwood, M. and Nomura, M. (1982). Chromosomal locations of the genes for rRNA in *Escherichia coli* K-12. *J. Bacteriol.* 149:458-468.
103. Lindahl, L. and Zengel, J. M. (1982). Expression of ribosomal genes in bacteria. *Adv. Genet.* 21:53-121.
104. Loughney, K., Lund, E., and Dahlberg, J. E. (1982). tRNA genes are found between the 16S and 23S rRNA genes in *Bacillus subtilis*. *Nucleic Acids Res.* 10:1607-1624.
105. Bott, K. F., Wilson, F. E., and Stewart, G. C. (1981). Characterization of *Bacillus subtilis* rRNA genes in *Sporulation and Germination* (H. S. Levinson, A. L. Sonenshein, and D. J. Tipper, eds.), American Society for Microbiology, Washington, D.C., pp. 119-122.
106. Loughney, K., Lund, E., and Dahlberg, J. E. (1983). Deletion of an rRNA gene set in *Bacillus subtilis*. *J. Bacteriol.* 154:529-532.
107. Ellwood, M. and Nomura, M. (1980). Deletion of a ribosomal ribonucleic acid operon in *Escherichia coli*. *J. Bacteriol.* 143:1077-1080.

108. Hori, H., Sawada, M., Osawa, S., Murao, K., and Ishikura, H. (1981). The nucleotide sequence of 5S rRNA from *Mycoplasma capricolum*. *Nucleic Acids Res.* 9:5407-5410.
109. Walker, R. T., Chelton, E. T. J., Kilpatrick, M. W., Rogers, M. J., and Simmons, J. (1982). The nucleotide sequence of the 5S rRNA from Spiroplasma species BC3 and *Mycoplasma mycoides* sp. *capri* PG 3. *Nucleic Acids Res.* 10:6363-6367.
110. Hill, C. W. and Harnish, B. W. (1982). Transposition of a chromosomal segment bounded by redundant rRNA genes into other rRNA genes in *Escherichia coli*. *J. Bacteriol.* 149:449-457.
111. Hill, C. W. and Harnish, B. W. (1981). Inversions between ribosomal RNA genes of *Escherichia coli*. *Proc. Natl. Acad. Sci. USA* 78:7069-7072.
112. Hill, C. W., Grafstrom, R. H., Harnish, B. W., and Hillman, B. S. (1977). Tandem duplications resulting from recombination between ribosomal RNA genes in *Escherichia coli*. *J. Mol. Biol.* 116:407-428.
113. Anderson, R. P. and Roth, J. (1981). Spontaneous tandem genetic duplications in *Salmonella typhimurium* arise by unequal recombination between rRNA (rrn) cistrons. *Proc. Natl. Acad. Sci. USA* 78:3113-3117.
114. Trowsdale, J. and Anagnostopoulos, C. (1975). Evidence for the translocation of a chromosome segment in *Bacillus subtilis* strains carrying the trpE26 mutation. *J. Bacteriol.* 122:886-898.
115. Anagnostopoulos, C. (1977). Genetic analysis of *Bacillus subtilis* strains carrying chromosomal rearrangements in *Modern Trends in Bacterial Transformation and Transfection* (A. Portoles, R. Lopez, and M. Espinosa, eds.), Elsevier/North-Holland, Amsterdam, pp. 211-230.
116. Schneider, A. and Anagnostopoulos, C. (1983). *Bacillus subtilis* strains carrying two non-tandem duplications of the *trpE-ilvA* and the *purB*-tre regions of the chromosome. *J. Gen. Microbiol.* 129:687-701.
117. Ogasawara, N., Seiki, M., and Yoshikawa, H. (1983). Replication origin region of *Bacillus subtilis* chromosome contains two rRNA operons. *J. Bacteriol.* 154:50-57.
118. Maniloff, J. (1983). Evolution of wall-less prokaryotes. *Ann. Rev. Microbiol.* 37:477-499.
119. Dams, E., Huysmans, E., Vanderberghe, A., and DeWachter, R. (1984). Primary structure of 5-S rRNA and phylogenetic position of *Clostridia* among the bacteria. *Arch. Int. Physiol. Biochem.* 92:B77.
120. Rogers, M. J., Simmons, J., Walker, R. T., Weisberg, W. G., Woese, C. R., Tanner, R. S., Robinson, I. M., Stahl, D. A., Olsen, G., Leach, R. H., and Maniloff, J. (1985). Construction of the mycoplasma evolutionary tree from 5S rRNA sequence data. *Proc. Natl. Acad. Sci. USA* 82:1160-1164.

3
L-Forms of Group D *Streptococcus*

JAMES R. KING
Division of Anti-Infective Drug Products, Center for Drugs and Biologics, Food and Drug Administration, Rockville, Maryland

I.	Introduction	43
II.	Morphology	44
III.	Recovery of L-type Growth	46
	A. Induction	46
	B. The Effect of Nutrition and Physical Environment on the Growth of L-Forms	47
	C. Reversion	49
IV.	Identification and Genetic Relatedness to the Parent Strain	50
V.	Biochemistry	51
	A. Production of Cell Wall Components	51
	B. Inhibition of Other Pathways	53
	C. Effects of Osmolality on Metabolism	53
	D. DNA Replication and Propagation of L-Forms	53
VI.	Growth of Group D L-Forms in Mammalian Cells	54
VII.	Concluding Remarks	55
	References	55

I. INTRODUCTION

This chapter is intended to give an insight into the nature of Group D streptococcal L-forms. To accomplish this end, key studies from many laboratories have been examined, and from those findings, the current status of research in selected topic areas has been synthesized. Other topics are not discussed in the same level of detail. In addition to discussing what is currently known, the reader will sometimes find brief guidelines for experimental approaches to fill in the breaks in our knowledge about Group D streptococcal L-forms.

Model systems using other L-forms were in existence before much of the research was done with Group D streptococcal L-forms. Findings were frequently derived from an application of an existing technique to the study of Group D L-forms. Thus, it is not surprising that many similar properties between Group D streptococcal L-forms and other L-forms have been described. Group A streptococcal L-forms are the most similar to Group D streptococcal L-forms. However, more detailed analysis of results revealed significant differences between Group A and Group D which made the separate study of Group D L-forms worthwhile. In this chapter, the author acknowledges the previous developmental work of others that led to many of the discoveries highlighted here, although specific references are sparse. Please consult the cited literature for the developmental flow of ideas leading to the work discussed below.

II. MORPHOLOGY

Among the earlier studies of Group D streptococcal L-form colonial morphology were those done by Hijmans and Kastelein [1] and Anderson [2]. Those studies showed that Group D streptococcal L-forms are not significantly different from other L-forms described by previous workers. Those two studies also show that the morphological observations were similar using two different fixation techniques. Hijmans and Kastelein used the formulation of the Dienes' stain [3] available at the time of studies. Anderson used a method of fixation based on organic acids with intensification from a series of rinses with concentrated hydrochloric acid [4]. Morphology of Group D L-forms in colonies is not profoundly dependent upon fixation and staining techniques. Therefore, the colonial morphology and developmental characteristics of Group D streptococcal L-forms can probably be duplicated from investigator to investigator as reflected in the works of Dienes [5], Young and Armstrong [6], Marro et al. [7], and Bibel and Lawson [8]. In other sections of this chapter, topics depending upon microscopic observation will be discussed in relationship to what is more properly the physiology of L-type growth.

Examination of Group D streptococcal L-forms by transmission electron microscopy did not require development of new procedures different from the techniques needed to preserve the cytoplasmic structures of other microorganisms. Ultra-thin sections of Group D L-forms produced knowledge about the similarity of organelles of the parent strains and their L-forms [7,9,10,11]. As with other L-forms, the most significant difference between Group D L-forms and their parent strains is the absence of a rigid cell wall in the L-form. Except during the lag phase, the genome of the L-form appears to have the same intracellular organization as a typical bacterial genome. Transmission electron microscopy was not required to demonstrate pleomorphism, which had already been demonstrated with light microscopy. Thus, Group D streptococcal L-forms are not morphologically unusual as L-forms.

On the other hand, there are some significant morphological differences between Group D L-forms and their parent strains. Aspects of this subject have been covered in electron microscopic studies by Wyrick and Gooder [11]. Briefly, they studied the growth of developing L colonies of *Streptococcus faecium* strain F24 on agar as well as L-type growth in broth. The broth-grown L-forms were studied throughout the full range of growth phases. The reversion process was studied in solid medium. They observed broth-grown L-forms undergoing internal genomic reorganizations during lag phase to produce discrete electron-opaque regions bounded by the electron-dense material. This is in contrast to the relatively loosely organized cytoplasm of the parent strain and other growth phases of broth-grown L-forms of *S. faecium* F24. "Core structures" were observed in the L-form during stationary phase. Corfield and Smith [12] also observed microtubular structures. To date, these "cores" have not been completely characterized. In addition, Wyrick and Gooder [11] observed reverting L-forms while loci of cell wall deposition were forming. These loci appeared to serve as a base for further polymerization of wall. Thus, several stages of cell wall defectiveness of *S. faecium* F24 were studied cytologically using the transmission electron microscope. Based on electron microscopic observations, Green et al. [13] proposed a life cycle for L-forms that has three branches, all of which have a common element as an electron-dense organism. The dense body can give rise to (1) simple budding which yields more dense bodies, (2) reversion, which leads to reverting L-forms and thus to revertant streptococci, and (3) vesiculation and growth into mother L-forms, from which elementary bodies escape and increase into more dense L-bodies.

Interactions of neighboring cells in a growing L-form colony had not been fully explored morphologically until the development of scanning electron microscopy (SEM). Bibel and Lawson [14] studied colonial growth of L-type colonies from protoplasts as well as from L-form inoculum. The textures of L-form bodies were observed to vary throughout growth of the colonies. In addition, the apparent pinching off or budding of new growth seemed to be evident, as had been suggested by earlier investigators looking at ultra-thin sections of L-type growth. In addition to growth on normal media, Bibel and Lawson studied growing L-colonies of strain F24 and *S. faecalis* var. *zymogenes* 30 (Z30L) on filter membranes by SEM [15]. The inoculum for these experiments was taken from the stationary phase as defined by the authors. Samples for examination by SEM were taken at intervals chosen to encompass the lag phase, log phase, and stationary phase. Group D L-forms growing on filter membranes had been studied by Wyrick and Gooder [16] and Dienes [5] using ultra-thin sections under transmission electron microscopy. Presumed filamentous growth forms were observed by transmission electron microscopy, but were initially obscured in SEM when the Millipore brand of filter membranes were used. However, colonies grown on the Nuclepore brand of filter membranes exhibited the apparent filamentous growth on top of the Nuclepore membrane instead of being imbedded, as in the Millipore membrane. In contrast to previous conclusions by Dienes [5], Bibel and Lawson [15] deduced that small granular elements could grow into larger L-phase bodies. As a result of the SEM studies briefly discussed above, it was feasible to obtain a direct three-dimensional visualization of L-type growth under conditions of high resolution instead of deduced visualization of three-dimensional L-type growth determined by transmission electron microscopy.

III. RECOVERY OF L-TYPE GROWTH

A. Induction

Group D streptococcal L-forms have been induced in vitro by only two well-defined mechanisms: i.e., by certain antibiotics affecting the cell wall and by muralytic enzymes. The antibiotics, such as penicillin, prevent synthesis of a complete cell wall. Under the proper osmotic conditions, the affected organism continues to survive without its rigid cell wall as the bacterial L-form. On the other hand, a muralytic enzyme, such as lysozyme, removes a portion of the cell wall or the entire detectable cell wall. With either a penicillin or muralytic enzyme induction system, complete removal of the wall is not necessary to induce L-type growth in the proper osmotically controlled environment. L-forms of Group D streptococci are similar to protoplasts with respect to the normal need for some protection of the membrane to prevent death of the wall-defective bacteria due to osmotic lysis. Typically, sucrose or salts such as sodium chloride or ammonium chloride were used in growth media for the Group D streptococcal L-forms obtained from penicillin induction, i.e., the agar trough method, as described by Sharp [17], Dienes and Sharp [18], and by a muralysin method [19,20] for Group A streptococci. In the penicillin induction studies by Young and Armstrong [6], 10 million units of penicillin in 1 liter of medium were used to induce L-colonies of *Streptococcus liquefaciens* in the presence of 15% sucrose. From a streptococcal suspension containing 10^8–10^9 colony-forming units (cfu) per milliliter, a maximum yield of 5×10^6 L-colonies per milliliter was obtained. This yield was not improved by changing the nutrient base in the agar or the osmotic stabilizer from sucrose to 3–5% sodium chloride. These variations in experimental conditions were designed to obtain a maximum yield of L-colonies from a streptococcal suspension. These studies demonstrated that penicillin induction is not an efficient induction method for Group D streptococci.

On the other hand, King and Gooder [21] were able to improve the efficiency of conversion to the L-state by plating protoplasts onto agar medium containing an added osmotic stabilizer rather than plating intact streptococci onto medium containing penicillin. In addition to an osmotic stabilizer, the medium was also fortified with 0.5% glucose and horse serum. The protoplasts of *S. faecium* strain F24 prepared essentially by the lysozyme method of Bibb and Straughn [22] were osmotically stabilized with 0.6 M sucrose. The growth medium contained either 2.0% (w/v) sodium chloride or 0.43 M ammonium chloride added to the medium. Either osmotic stabilizer worked well to produce 30-100% conversion of 2×10^9 streptococcal colony-forming units to L-colonies.

Normally, little interaction would be expected between the osmotic stabilizer in the medium and the osmotic stabilizer for the protoplast suspension. However, when 8% (w/v) polyethylene glycol 4000 (PEG 4000) was used instead of sucrose as the osmotic stabilizer for the protoplasts, only 0.43 M ammonium chloride could be used in the growth medium and still retain the efficient recovery of L-type growth from protoplast suspension. Another strain, *S. faecalis* E1, was tested and a similar conversion efficiency was observed. In subsequent experiments, PEG 4000 was used to stabilize protoplasts and ammonium chloride was used in the medium. Strain F24 was not the only strain for which the more efficient conversion could be seen. Spheroplasts rather than protoplasts of *S. faecalis* strain E1 were formed, but conversion efficiency was just as high. (This fact will be discussed further in a later discussion on reversion.) Further observations with other strains of enterococci showed that large yields of L-colonies could be obtained by treating the coccal form with lysozyme to form protoplasts or spheroplasts in the typical buffer-sucrose fluid.

One other variation on the theme of strain F24 protoplast conversion to L-colonies was done by Gooder [23]. Protoplasts of strain F24 were protected from lysis by spermine according to the method of Grossowicz and Ariel [24]. Those protoplasts were plated onto the typical induction medium and were efficiently converted to L-colonies. Those experiments were unusual because the protoplast suspension could be diluted in the absence of an osmotic stabilizer and still yield L-colonies in large numbers.

Gooder [25] also induced L-colonies of *S. faecalis* var. *liquefaciens* 31 using a Group D phage muralysin, although this system was not explored as fully as the F24 L form system.

B. The Effect of Nutrition and Physical Environment on the Growth of L-Forms

Glucose, the almost ubiquitous carbohydrate, is the most obvious sugar to use to fortify media, so the early studies on induction of L-colonies from protoplasts [21] were carried out with glucose in the media. During the course of those experiments, other carbohydrates and polyhydric alcohols were substituted for glucose as the prime carbon or energy source. None of the carbohydrates tested had a significant effect on the yield of L-colonies from a protoplast suspension, but the carbon source did have an impact on the size and texture of the L-colonies. Sodium acetate could be substituted for glucose on a weight basis, but not on a molar basis, i.e., 0.5% sodium acetate would produce the same robust colonies as observed with 0.5% glucose, but less acetate (i.e., the same molarity as glucose) only produced small highly granular colonies, instead of the typical large fried egg colonies obtained in the original induction system. Similar differences could be seen when the carbon source was varied in subculture medium. Complex media had been traditionally used to induce and propagate L-forms. Due to the undefined nature of these media, there was little opportunity to do quantifiable nutritional experiments. Even the less fastidious Group D L-forms required horse serum to produce typical robust colonies upon induction and propagation. The Group D L-forms could be induced with only 2% horse serum [21] instead of the 10% horse serum generally needed for efficient induction of Group A L-forms [19,20]. Therefore, robust colonies nearly always developed if the osmotically supplemented media had 2% horse serum and 0.5% glucose added. The precise roles of the added horse serum and added glucose have not been completely elucidated.

More quantifiable nutritional studies were possible with the advent of a completely synthetic broth medium for the growth of the F24 L-form and its parent strain. Gregory and Gooder [26] developed the medium and were able to show essentially identical growth parameters whether the parent strain or the L-form was grown in the medium. They observed doubling times of 64 and 65 min for the streptococcus and its L-form, respectively. The maximum turbidities, as measured in Klett units with a number 54 filter, were 268 and 249 for the streptococcus and the L-form, respectively. Therefore, the parent–L-form pair produced essentially equivalent amount of growth and doubled their numbers at the same rate.

On the other hand, Bibel and Lawson [27] reported that the physical environment has an effect on morphology of L-forms. Strain F24 L-forms growing imbedded in gelatin media produced exceedingly large bodies bounded by a single membrane. These bodies were visible to the unaided eye. By light microscopic techniques, the presence of various sizes of viable particles could be demonstrated inside the large individual L-bodies. The studies in gelatin provide a clue about the nature of the minimal reproductive unit of the Group D streptococcal L-form. Upon physical pricking of the membrane of the macroscopically visible large bodies, large numbers of quantifiable colony-forming units were released. These observations suggest that large body formation is followed by internal development of L-form elementary bodies. By scanning electron microscopy, Bibel and Lawson [8] had previously demonstrated an apparent pinching off of new growth from L-colonies. Wyrick and Gooder [11,28] have also demonstrated, by transmission electron microscopy of ultrathin sections, that apparent fission of the genome was occurring during growth of L-forms. These observations provide an argument in favor of the original conclusions of Dienes about L-form growth through large body subdivision rather than binary fission. Further studies of killing curves, such as a determination of the number of hits by radiation per individual element, in conjunction with specific staining studies of large bodies (as done by Kang and Casida [29]), would be an appropriate line of investigation to define the nature of the growth mechanism.

Early nutritional studies were aimed at developing the simplest broth medium available. Thus, a series of selective subcultures was begun with strain F24 L-form. Initially, the F24 L-forms were subcultured for approximately 100 times on agar medium containing added 0.43 M ammonium chloride, 0.5% (w/v) glucose, and 2% (v/v) horse serum. Medill and O'Kane [30] had shown what appeared to be a requirement for horse serum in L-form media. Furthermore, other typical L-form induction systems predating the Medill and O'Kane work seemed to require horse serum for vigorous growth of L-colonies, even when subcultured. The complex chemical nature of horse serum defied synthetic duplication, so the induced and repeatedly propagated L-forms of strain F24 were first adapted to growth in the absence of horse serum. Subsequently, the F24 L-form was adapted to growth without agar by decreasing the agar content of the medium at each successive passage until the L-form finally grew in the ammonium chloride and glucose-fortified broth. This history of the passage of strain of F24 L-forms is important for genetic reasons, to be discussed below, and for nutritional reasons. Nutritionally, the L-form colonies were significantly retarded in growth by each major change in medium composition, including some of the levels of agar concentrations. Gregory and Gooder [26] reported similar retardations in growth of L-forms when the L-forms were initially introduced into new media. Subsequent studies done by Cohen et al. [31] demonstrated that this L-form could be identified by comparison of biochemical test results from the L-form and its parent strain. Subsequently, Gregory and Gooder [26] demonstrated identical nutritional requirements for the F24 parent strain and its L-form.

C. Reversion

In general, reversion of penicillin-induced L-forms to the parent strain is not uncommon when penicillin is removed from the growth medium, even after many propagations as L-colonies. Usually, many subcultures are required before L-forms will stop reverting and become stable L-forms, i.e., before stable L-forms are selected out of the population. However, King and Gooder [32] demonstrated that only 4% of a population of lysozyme-induced *S. faecium* F24 L-colonies reverted when subcultured three times by a replica-plating technique.

The same type of experiment repeated with *S. faecalis* E1 showed that 18.5% reverted in three subcultures. The larger reversion percentage for strain E1 may be because spheroplasts instead of protoplasts were formed when this strain was treated with lysozyme. Continued propagation of strain E1 L-colonies could not be accomplished because the L-colonies were always overgrown by revertant streptococci and remaining L-forms could not be recloned. This is in contrast to strain F24, which had a low spontaneous reversion rate in three subcultures, and progeny selected for further propagation ceased to revert after about 30 subcultures.

The reversion rate of L-colonies is not quantitative when the L-colonies are freshly induced from protoplast suspensions plated onto agar medium. However, protoplasts immediately reverted to the coccal state with a higher frequency when the protoplasts were plated onto L-form medium solidified with gelatin instead of agar. King and Gooder [32] demonstrated that maximum reversion of protoplasts to the coccal state occurred at 25% and 35% (w/v) gelatin obtained from Difco and Eastman, respectively. Using either brand of gelatin, approximately 90% of protoplasts were recovered as the revertant cocci. Gooder [25] extended the studies of reversion of protoplasts on gelatin media to the use of media solidified with mixtures of 1% agar and gelatin in the concentrations discussed above. Reversion of protoplasts occurred even when agar was present. However, the protoplasts did not revert in the usual numbers when intact gelatin was removed from the mixtures by the action of gelatinase. Gooder concluded that the physical properties of the gelatin are the prime contributing factors to reversion of the protoplasts.

Reversion has also been studied with the electron microscope. Schönfeld and De Bruijn [33] studied the reversion of L-forms of *S. faecalis* 962 to the coccal state. These workers were able to observe the newly synthesized walls of the revertant streptococcus. However, later studies by Wyrick and Gooder [11] were able to show the synthesis of new wall from discreet loci in samples from reverting L-colonies of *S. faecium* F24. Eventually, the walls of the revertant strain F24 streptococci appeared similar to the walls of the revertant *S. faecalis* 962.

IV. IDENTIFICATION AND GENETIC RELATEDNESS TO THE PARENT STRAIN

If L-forms are isolated from sources other than a well-defined induction system, there is no morphological, single biochemical, or serological technique to provide positive identification. Three techniques have been proposed to differentiate an L-form isolate from other L-forms. Each is based on comparison with parent strains: (1) biochemical characterization, e.g., fermentation patterns, (2) polyacrylamide gel electrophoretic patterns of proteins, and (3) nucleic acid homology. Cohen et al. [31] developed a biochemical characterization of a large number of L-phase variants, including *S. faecalis (faecium)* F24. The major disadvantage of biochemical techniques for routine use is that a large number of characteristics should be examined to make an identification of Group D streptococci because the differentiating biochemical characteristics are not clear-cut for the parent strains, i.e., there are not always species-specific conclusive tests for the parent strains of Group D streptococci. Biochemical differentiation assumes that the biochemical genetic traits of a parent strain are conserved in the L-form progeny of the parent strain. Razin and Shafer [34], and King et al. [35] demonstrated that broth-grown L-forms could be identified to the level of genus by comparison of parent and L-form polyacrylamide gel electrophoretic patterns of proteins. The electrophoretic patterns of most of the parent–L-form pairs were not strictly superimposable. However, the patterns for the *S. faecium* F24 parent strain, protoplasts, and L-forms were almost indistinguishable, except for contaminating lysozyme bound to the membranes of protoplasts prepared with the enzyme. No further studies were done to catalogue the role of the individual protein bands in the scheme of the living cells. The precise identity of *S. faecium* F24 by biochemical and electrophoretic methods was particularly surprising in view of the differences in nucleic acid homology reported for this parent–L-form pair. Wittler and her associates [36] reported a loss of 20% of the F24 L-form genome, and Hoyer and King [37] reported a 4–6% loss. Even with the lesser reported degree of loss of genome by the stable L-form, it is remarkable that significant differences in biochemical characteristics or protein content were not observed. Therefore, the identification of an isolate of Group D streptococcal L-forms should not be assigned until all available tests have been done on a particular isolate. For management of a culture collection with well-defined biochemical characteristics and polyacrylamide gel patterns, either technique will probably work, although the polyacrylamide gel technique is only applicable to broth-grown L-forms. The nucleic acid homology technique is undesirable for routine use because the technique requires the use of radiolabeled DNA, which is expensive and time-consuming to prepare.

V. BIOCHEMISTRY

A. Production of Cell Wall Components

The presence of mucopeptide in Group D streptococcal L-forms has not been demonstrated. However, King et al. [38] were able to recover trace quantities of a formamide-insoluble residue from *S. faecium* strain F24 L-form. Such residues are composed of mucopeptide when obtained from normal bacteria or their isolated walls. The fraction was obtained by a modified method of James et al. [39]. Formamide-insoluble residues from whole cells of strain F24 L-form were analyzed chemically. Although amino sugar was found in the residue along with increased amounts of the mucopeptide amino acids, the molar ratios of the amino sugar and the amino acids usually associated with mucopeptide suggested that the residue was not mucopeptide. Additional amino acids not known to be wall-related were present in high proportions in the residue. Also, the fraction was soluble in phenol extracts as done by the method of Wheat et al. [40]. The residue may have been some type of aberrant mucopeptide, but no further characterization was attempted.

Mucopeptide is not the only well-characterized polymeric cell wall material synthesized by enterococci. Hijmans [41] demonstrated the absence of the cell wall polysaccharide-type hapten and group substance. These cell wall-associated antigens could not be demonstrated by the precipitin technique in culture supernatant fluids or by incorporating the antisera into culture media. The organisms were also extracted, but the extracts from L-forms of strains 27, 30, and D76 did not react with the antisera. However, both the group substance and the polysaccharide hapten were present in the revertant when strain D76 reverted to the parent strain. Group substance and cell wall polysaccharides could not be serologically demonstrated in *S. faecium* F24 L-forms (J. R. King and H. Gooder, unpublished results).

Clearly lacking a mucopeptide, the strain F24 L-form had an inheritable loss of synthetic capability. In unpublished results, King and Altenbern had shown the presence of UDP-muramylpeptides from broth cultures of *S. faecium*, strain F24 L-forms. However, Gregory and Gooder [42] studied the enzymes required for mucopeptide formation and demonstrated that the L-form was missing phospho-*N*-acetylmuramyl pentapeptide translocase. This is the enzyme needed to facilitate transfer of the *N*-acetylmuramyl peptides from the inside of the cell through the membrane to the point where the amino sugar backbone begins to be polymerized to form finished mucopeptide. Similarly, synthesis of rhamnose polymer appears to be blocked by the analogous mechanism. Therefore, the stable strain F24 L-form is biochemically inhibited between synthesis of the nucleotide precursors and the final cross-linking in the peptide portion of mucopeptide as well as the polymerization of rhamnose into cell wall polysaccharide.

There is no reason to believe that other stable strains of Group D streptococcal L-forms will be biosynthetically blocked at the same point as strain F24 L. In the future, there may be a simpler way to elucidate the specific enzyme deficiencies present in the L-forms. It may be possible to use certain antibiotics, particularly *beta*-lactam antibiotics, when their abilities to bind to specific so-called "penicillin-binding proteins" and the precise functions of those specific penicillin binding proteins have been unequivocally defined. Other antibiotics also may be useful as probes, such as bacitracin, cycloserine, and vancomycin.

B. Inhibition of Other Pathways

Montgomerie et al. [43] demonstrated the apparent increased in vitro susceptibility of *S. faecalis* L-forms to various antibiotics. Almost universally, the antibiotics tested (except penicillin) were more active against the derived L-form than the parent strain. Although L-forms are generally more susceptible to antimicrobial agents than their bacterial counterparts, some interpretive caution is in order, because the precise standardization of L-form inoculum in relation to bacterial inoculum is essential before accurate susceptibility data can be generated.

In addition to inhibition by the usual anti-infective drugs, other growth inhibitors have an effect on L-forms. King [44] showed that *S. faecium* F24 parent strain could be released from the action of the DNA inhibitors [45,46] phenylethyl alcohol (PEA), and *para*-fluorophenylalanine (FPA), whereas the F24 L-form could be released from the inhibition of FPA only. The F24 L-forms were lysed by the PEA [47]. Thus, L-forms could retain viability after treatment with FPA; however, subsequent studies revealed that protoplasts could be plated on L-form induction medium containing FPA, and no L-form colonies developed. If agar blocks were cut from the plates no later than 1-2 hr after plating, and immersed in broth L-form growth medium to dilute the FPA, then L-colonies would develop on the agar blocks in the biphasic growth medium. The recovery of L-colonies could not be quantitated with respect to the number of protoplasts plated, but the phenomenon was observed frequently. These observations suggest that it would be technologically possible to develop a series of tests based on selective media to determine if true L-forms (L-phase variants by the nomenclature of McGee et al., ref. 48) were present in clinical specimens from certain chronic infections. Further laboratory work may be fruitful in this direction.

C. Effects of Osmolality on Metabolism

Montgomerie et al. [49] demonstrated that in the absence of sucrose the unsaturated fatty acid C18.1 increased while C18 and C19 fatty acids decreased in membranes of L-forms. Sucrose normally functions as an osmotic stabilizer for *S. faecalis* protoplasts or spheroplasts, because *S. faecalis* does not metabolize sucrose. Montgomerie et al. [50] demonstrated that internal sodium and potassium content is lower in L-forms adapted to growth without sucrose than in L-forms not adapted.

D. DNA Replication and Propagation of L-Forms

A series of unpublished reports by Lentsch and Lawson appear to define the relationship of DNA replication to cell growth of the L-form of *S. faecium* F24 in an environment leading to growth of extraordinarily large bodies. These investigators have shown that most of the DNA synthesis occurs within approximately 28 hr after inoculation into media, but cell compartmentalization and formation of large bodies continues. Large body growth can continue, even when mitomycin C, an inhibitor of DNA synthesis, is added at 36 hr. In addition, these workers showed that normal growth of the L-form occurs until critical levels of adenosine 3',5'-cyclic monophosphate (cAMP) are reached, when normal compartmentalization of L-forms ceases. Large bodies continue to increase in size under those conditions. Lentsch and Lawson also showed that a factor in gelatin controls the growth and development of the large bodies.

VI. GROWTH OF GROUP D L-FORMS IN MAMMALIAN CELLS

Clasener [51] thoroughly explored all available data on the pathogenicity of bacterial L-forms, including tissue culture systems. In addition to reporting the results of the studies reviewed, Clasener also critically evaluated the original authors' interpretations of their data, and came to the final conclusion that the precise role of L-forms in pathogenicity has not been elucidated. Group D streptococcal L-forms fitting the definition of McGee et al. [48] are no exception. Clasener recognizes the probable role of some type of pleiomorphic state in infections. From later studies, a good example may be normal isolates of *Haemophilus influenzae* [52]. However, further work needs to be done. To prove the presence of L-phase variants may not necessarily require the isolation of L-forms or some other cell wall-defective variant. With proper media containing specific metabolic inhibitors as probes, it may be possible to design a regimen of treatment of clinical specimens followed by selective plating that would yield a colony recovery pattern from which the type of cell wall-defective variant could be deduced. As discussed by Clasener [51], the effect of simple osmotic adjustments alone on a differential recovery of bacteria are insufficient to establish the presence of the type of a cell wall-defective variant.

Seemingly mundane studies may be important. King and McGee [53] showed that L-forms of *S. faecium* F24 could usually be quantitatively recovered on a viable count basis after centrifugation. Similarly, Clasener et al. [54] working with several L-forms including *S. faecalis* B9, showed that tissue spiked with L-forms could be homogenized without losing viability in the inoculum. Wyrick and Gooder [16] determined that strain F24 L-form could pass through a filter with a pore size of 0.22 μm, whereas protoplasts of the parent strain could pass only through a pore diameter of 0.45 μm. However, the filtration experiments showed a loss in viability as opposed to the homogenization and centrifugation experiments of Clasener et al. [54] and King and McGee [53], respectively.

Studies of such laboratory procedures may reveal the deleterious effect of some manipulations not otherwise expected to be deleterious.

Tissue culture work with *S. faecium* F24 is now feasible, since R. S. Foster and H. Gooder (unpublished results) have shown that intracellular infection of tissue culture cells can be monitored. Nevertheless, any exposition on the survival of Group D streptococcal L-forms in animals should take into consideration the observation by McGee and his associates [55] of an antibody-complement system that killed L-phase variants in serum. J. R. King (unpublished data) extended these observations to *S. faecium* F24 (see Chap. 13).

VII. CONCLUDING REMARKS

This chapter has been devoted to L-forms of Group D streptococci. The corollary work with other organisms has not been included because that work will be covered thoroughly in other portions of this volume. More recent publications should be available for any subsequent editions of this book.

The aim of this chapter is to stimulate the study of streptoccal L-forms. In drafting the chapter, the minutiae of details was avoided. The flow of ideas in the development of the field of Group D streptococcal L-forms should be apparent, while enough details were provided in the chapter to be informative. Occasionally, review articles terminate with a recitation of unresolved questions. These have been sprinkled liberally throughout the text of this chapter. With good fortune those deficiencies in knowledge will be filled and other questions will continue to draw the interest of scientists toward L-forms and to Group D streptococcal L-forms in particular.

ACKNOWLEDGMENTS

I gratefully thank Dr. Priscilla B. Wyrick for many hours of thoughtful discussion about the chapter.

REFERENCES

1. Hijmans, W. and Kastelein, M. J. (1960). The production of L forms of enterococci. *Ann. N.Y. Acad. Sci.* 79:371-373.
2. Anderson, R. J. (1968). Microscopic morphology of an enterococcal L form. *Can. J. Microbiol.* 14:746-747.
3. Dienes, L. (1967). Permanent stained agar preparation of mycoplasma and of L forms of bacteria. *J. Bacteriol.* 93:689-692.
4. Anderson, R. J. (1967). Acid treatment modification for the preparation of permanent slides of L forms and mycoplasmas. *J. Bacteriol.* 93:493-494.
5. Dienes, L. (1967). Morphology and reproductive processes of the L forms of bacteria. I. Streptococci and staphylococci. *J. Bacteriol.* 95:672-687.

6. Young, L. S. and Armstrong, D. (1969). Induction, colony morphology, and growth characteristics of the L form of *Streptococcus liquefaciens*. *J. Infect. Dis.* *120*:281-291.
7. Marro, R. V., Pfister, R. M., Rheins, M. S., and Kapetonavic, I. (1971). The morphology of induced wall-defective variants of *Streptococcus faecalis* as studied by light and electron microscopy. *Can. J. Microbiol.* *17*:365-371.
8. Bibel, D. J. and Lawson, J. W. (1972). Development of streptococcal L-form colonies. *J. Bacteriol.* *112*:602-610.
9. Thorsson, K. G. and Weibull, C. (1958). Studies on the structure of bacterial L forms, protoplasts and protoplast-like bodies. *J. Ultrastruct. Res.* *1*:412-427.
10. Corfield, P. S. and Smith, D. G. (1970). Ultrastructural changes during propagation of a group D streptococcal L-form. *Arch. Mikrobiol.* *75*:1-9.
11. Wyrick, P. B. and Gooder, H. (1977). Reversion of *Streptococcus faecium* cell wall-defective variants to the intact bacterial state. In *Spheroplasts, Protoplasts and L-forms of Bacteria* (J. Roux, ed.), Ed. INSERM, vol. 64. Paris, pp. 59-88.
12. Corfield, P. S. and Smith, D. G. (1968). Microtubular structures in group D streptococcal L-forms. *Arch. Mikrobiol.* *63*:356-361.
13. Green, M. T., Heidger, Jr., P. M., and Domingue, G. (1974). Proposed reproductive cycle for a relatively stable L-phase variant of *Streptococcus faecalis*. *Infect. Immun.* *10*:915-927.
14. Bibel, D. J. and Lawson, J. W. (1971). A simple method for scanning electron microscopy of L-form colonies grown on agar. *Can. J. Microbiol.* *17*: 822-823.
15. Bibel, D. J. and Lawson, J. W. (1972). Scanning electron microscopy of L-phase streptococci. II. Growth in broth and upon Millipore filters. *Can. J. Microbiol.* *118*:1179-1184.
16. Wyrick, P. B. and Gooder, H. (1971). Filterability of streptococcal L-forms. *J. Bacteriol.* *105*:284-290.
17. Sharp, J. T. (1954). L-colonies from *beta*-haemolytic streptococci. New technique in the study of L-forms of bacteria. *Proc. Soc. Exp. Biol. Med.* *87*:94-97.
18. Dienes, L. and Sharp, J. T. (1956). The role of high electrolyte concentration in the production and growth of L-forms of bacteria. *J. Bacteriol.* *71*: 208-213.
19. Gooder, H. and Maxted, W. R. (1961). External factors influencing structure and activities of *Streptococcus pyogenes* in *Microbial Reaction to the Environment* (G. C. Meynell and H. Gooder, eds.), University Press, Cambridge, pp. 151-173.
20. Freimer, E. H., Krause, R. M., and McCarty, M. (1959). Studies of L-forms and protoplasts of group A streptococci. I. Isolation, growth and bacteriologic characteristics. *J. Exp. Med.* *110*:853-874.
21. King, J. R. and Gooder, H. (1970). Induction of enterococcal L-forms by the action of lysozyme. *J. Bacteriol.* *103*:686-691.
22. Bibb, W. R. and Straughn, W. R. (1964). Inducible transport system for citrulline in *Streptococcus faecalis*. *J. Bacteriol.* *87*:815-822.

23. Gooder, H. (1964). L-type growth of Streptococcal protoplasts. *Bacteriol. Proc.*, p. 60.
24. Grossowicz, N. and Ariel, M. (1963). Mechanism of protection of cells by spermine against lysozyme-induced lysis. *J. Bacteriol. 85*:293-300.
25. Bibel, D. J. and Lawson, J. W. (1975). Morphology and viability of large bodies of streptococcal L-forms. *Infect. Immun. 12*:919-930.
26. Gregory, W. W. and Gooder, H. (1977). Identical nutritional requirements of *Streptococcus faecium* F24 and a derived stable L-phase variant. *J. Bacteriol. 129*:1151-1153.
27. Gooder, H. (1968). Streptococcal protoplasts and L-form growth induced by muralytic enzymes in *Microbial Protoplasts, Spheroplasts, and L-forms* (L. B. Guze, ed.), Williams & Wilkins, Baltimore, pp. 40-51.
28. Wyrick, P. B. and Gooder, H. (1971). Growth of streptococcal protoplasts and L-colonies on membrane filters. *J. Bacteriol. 105*:646-656.
29. Kang, K. S. and Casida, L. E. (1967). Large bodies of *Mycoplasma* and L-form organisms. *J. Bacteriol. 93*:1137-1142.
30. Medill, M. A. and O'Kane, D. J. (1954). A synthetic medium for the L type colonies of Proteus. *J. Bacteriol. 68*:530-533.
31. Cohen, R. L., Wittler, R. G., and Faber, J. E. (1968). Modified biochemical tests for the characterization of L-phase variants of bacteria. *Appl. Microbiol. 16*:1655-1662.
32. King, J. R. and Gooder, H. (1970). Reversion to the streptococcal state of enterococcal protoplasts, spheroplasts, and L-forms. *J. Bacteriol. 103*: 693-696.
33. Schönfeld, J. K. and De Bruijn, W. C. (1973). Ultrastructure of the intermediate stages in the reverting L-phase organisms of *Staphylococcus aureus* and *Streptococcus faecalis. J. Gen. Microbiol. 77*:261-271.
34. Razin, S. and Shafer, Z. (1969). On the determination of the L-phase parentage by the electrophoretic patterns of cell proteins. *J. Gen. Microbiol. 58*:338-339.
35. King, J. R., Theodore, T. S., and Cole, R. M. (1969). Generic identification of L forms by polyacrylamide gel electrophoretic comparison of extracts from parent strains and their derived L forms. *J. Bacteriol. 100*: 71-77.
36. Wittler, R. G., McGee, Z. A., Williams, C. O. Burris, C., Cohen, R. L., and Roberts, R. B. (1968). Identification of L-forms: Problems and approaches in *Microbial Protoplasts, Spheroplasts, and L forms* (L. B. Guze, ed.), Williams & Wilkins, Baltimore, pp. 333-339.
37. Hoyer, B. H. and King, J. R. (1969). Deoxyribonucleic acid sequence losses in a stable streptococcal L form. *J. Bacteriol. 97*:1516-1517.
38. King, J. R., Prescott, B., and Caldes, G. (1970). Lack of murein in a formamide-insoluble fraction from the stable L-form of *Streptococcus faecium. J. Bacteriol. 102*:296-297.
39. James, A. M., Hill, M. J., and Maxted, W. R. (1965). A comparative study of the bacterial cell wall, protoplast membrane, and L form envelope of *Streptococcus pyogenes. Antonie van Leeuwenhoek J. Microbiol. Serol. 31*: 423-432.

40. Wheat, R. W., Rollins, E. L., Leatherwood, J. M., and Barnes, R. L. (1963). Studies on the cell wall of *Chromobacterium violaceum*: the separation of lipopolysaccharide and mucopeptide by phenol extraction of whole cells. *J. Biol. Chem. 238*:26-29.
41. Hijmans, W. (1962). Absence of the group-specific and the cell-wall polysaccharide antigen in L-phase variants of group D streptococci. *J. Gen. Microbiol. 28*:177-179.
42. Gregory, W. W. and Gooder, H. (1978). Inhibition of peptidoglycan biosynthesis at a postcytoplasmic reaction in a stable L-phase variant of *Streptococcus faecium*. *J. Bacteriol. 135*:900-910.
43. Montgomerie, J. Z., Kalmanson, G. M., and Guze, L. B. (1966). The effects of antibiotics on the protoplast and bacterial forms of *Streptococcus faecalis*. *J. Lab. Clin. Med. 68*:543-551.
44. King, J. R. (1970). Survival of *Streptococcus faecium* F24 and its stable L-form after treatment with inhibitors of DNA synthesis. *Bacteriol. Proc.*, p. 37.
45. Silver, S. and Wendt, L. (1967). Mechanism of action of phenylethyl alcohol: Breakdown of the cellular permeability barrier. *J. Bacteriol. 93*:560-566.
46. Carpenter, C. and Binkley, S. B. (1968). Effect of p-fluorophenylalanine on chromosome replication in *Escherichia coli*. *J. Bacteriol. 96*:939-949.
47. King, J. R. (1974). Lysis of enterococcal L-forms by phenylethyl alcohol. *Antimicrob. Agents Chemother. 5*:98-100.
48. McGee, Z., Wittler, R., Gooder, H., and Charache, P. (1971). Wall-defective microbial variants: terminology and experimental design. *J. Infect. Dis. 123*: 433-438.
49. Montgomerie, J. Z., Kalmanson, G. M., and Guze, L. B. (1973). Fatty acid composition of L-forms of *Streptococcus faecalis* cultured at different osmolalities. *J. Bacteriol. 115*:73-75.
50. Montgomerie, J. Z., Kalmanson, G. M., Hubert, E. G., and Guze, L. B. (1972). Osmotic stability and sodium and potassium content of L-forms of *Streptococcus faecalis*. *J. Bacteriol. 110*:624-627.
51. Clasener, H. (1972). Pathogenicity of the L-phase of bacteria. *Ann. Rev. Microbiol. 26*:55-84.
52. Klein, R. D. and Luginbuhl, G. H. (1977). Ampicillin-induced morphological alterations of *Haemophilus influenzae* type b. *Antimicrob. Agents Chemother. 11*:559-562.
53. King, J. R. and McGee, Z. A. (1974). Viability of L-phase variants after centrifugation. *Infect. Immun. 9*:964-965.
54. Clasener, H. A., Ensering, H. L., and Hijmans, W. (1970). Persistence in mice of the L-phase of three streptococcal strains adapted to physiological osmotic conditions. *J. Gen. Microbiol. 62*:195-202.
55. McGee, Z. A., Ratner, H. B., Bryant, R. E., Rosenthal, A. S., and Koenig, M. G. (1972). An antibody-complement system in human serum lethal to L-phase variants of bacteria. *J. Infect. Dis. 125*:231-242.

4
Macromolecular Synthesis, Survival, and Cytotoxicity of an L-Form of *Streptococcus pyogenes*

CHARLES PANOS
Department of Microbiology, Jefferson Medical College, Thomas Jefferson University, Philadelphia, Pennsylvania

I. Introduction	59
II. Inhibition of Macromolecular Synthesis	60
A. Peptidoglycan	60
B. Teichoic and Lipoteichoic Acids	65
III. Altered Osmotic Fragility and Survival	74
IV. Effect on Host Cells and Immunosuppressed Mice	81
A. Latent Infection vs. Cytotoxicity	81
B. Cytotoxicity	85
C. Adherence to Host Cells	88
D. Defective Collagen Biosynthesis	89
V. Summary	91
References	92

I. INTRODUCTION

L-forms of bacteria have been studied sporadically since the initial isolation of an L-form by Klieneberger in 1935 [1]. Although most of the early studies dealt with morphology, growth conditions, or serology, relatively little, if any, concern was given to changes in the biochemistry or cellular physiology of these resulting aberrant forms [2]. But it was not long before it was realized that many bacteria could be converted to an L-form by a variety of agents, including certain antibiotics, and most notably penicillin [3]. Further, when it was observed that the resulting L-form was now resistant to penicillin, speculation quickly arose as to the possible role of such aberrant forms from microbial pathogens in recurring human infection. However, when experiments failed to elicit a disease state in animals, interest in the L-form as an infectious agent waned [4,5].

This laboratory began comparative biochemical studies of an osmotically fragile L-form and its parental *Streptococcus pyogenes*, type 12, in 1957. More recently our efforts have concentrated on two broad, fundamental, and, at times, interrelated areas of study. They are: resulting physiologic changes after conversion to the L-form and the survival and/or pathogenic potential of such an L-form in vivo. In so doing, our direction has centered on answers to particular questions at the molecular level. They are: (1) To what extent does the macromolecular mechanism(s) for cell wall synthesis still function in an L-form? (2) Does an osmotically fragile L-form have the capability of altering its membrane so as to grow or survive in a physiologically isotonic environment? and (3) Is an L-form of a pathogen capable of adhering to, and eventually destroying, monolayers of human host cells in tissue culture?

This overview is based upon our attempts to answer these questions. As a result it stresses only certain of our studies done within each of these broad areas of interest. In so doing, the topics indicated above have been selected and our biochemical findings emphasized.

At the outset, it should be made clear that this L-form, which in the "early" literature was referred to as the AED L-forms (examples in Refs. 6,7). lacks completely the bacterial cell wall as determined by physical, chemical, and serological means. Initially, it was derived from *S. pyogenes* type 12 using a solid hypertonic (3% w/v NaCl) medium with horse serum (10% v/v) and penicillin as the inducer. Since then it has remained stabilized, that is, nonreverting to the parental streptococcus from which it was derived. Finally, our investigations have always included the parental coccus for comparative purposes. In so doing, much new information has accumulated relative to this human pathogen. However, and because of topic concern and space limitation, selected findings pertinent to only this L-form are emphasized.

II. INHIBITION OF MACROMOLECULAR SYNTHESIS

A. Peptidoglycan

Earlier biochemical studies had established the lack of a rigid cell wall and the absence of amino sugars and C-polysaccharide as structural components of this osmotically fragile L-form [6,7]. Still earlier, Park and Johnson and Park had reported on the accumulation of amino sugar-containing uridine nucleotides in *Staphylococcus aureus* treated with penicillin and of their precursor relationship to bacterial peptidoglycan formation [8-11]. Therefore, to obtain some insight into the extent of cell wall inhibition in a stabilized streptococcal L-form induced by this antibiotic, a study of its acid-soluble nucleotide content and composition was undertaken [12]. In retrospect, the use of this organism for these studies was fortuitous because like *S. aureus*, but unlike *Escherichia coli*, for example, cell wall nucleotide precursors continued to accumulate in these organisms after cessation of cell wall formation by penicillin. Of interest was the initial finding that, on an equivalent weight basis, no significant difference in the total extractable, acid-soluble, ultraviolet-absorbing material was observed from *S. pyogenes* and its L-form during logarithmic growth [12]. Nevertheless, two cell wall nucleotide precursors were found accumulating within the L-form and one of these, UDP-muramyl-peptide, predominated. Chemical analyses of this accumulating nucleotide showed it to contain glutamic acid, lysine, and excess alanine. However, the isomeric configuration of this excess alanine component was not determined at the time [12]. Prior to these studies, it had been established that UDP-muramyl-peptide from other organisms was unusual in that it contained the natural as well as the unnatural isomers of this amino acid and that its terminus was D-alanyl dipeptide. Also, that this was the ultimate nucleotide for cell wall synthesis at the cytoplasmic level. Therefore, it was thought that an inability of this L-form to resynthesize its rigid cell wall might very well be due to an enzyme defect or deficiency affecting the racemization of alanine or in an inability to synthesize the D-alanyl-D-alanine dipeptide portion of this terminal nucleotide. This postulated defect in alanine metabolism was heightened at the time when it was discovered that the teichoic acid from the L-form also lacked D-alanine while that from the parental coccus contained this amino acid [13]. Therefore, comparative studies were undertaken to examine the isomerization of L-alanine as well as the formation of the dipeptide, D-alanyl-D-alanine, in this L-form and its parental *S. pyogenes* type 12 [14].

Extensive enzymatic and chromatographic studies established that the two crucial enzymes, alanine racemase and D-alanyl-D-alanine synthetase, were present and that this dipeptide was being formed from L-alanine in this stabilized L-form. Likewise, it was observed that the combined rate of the racemase and synthetase enzymes by cell-free preparations from these organisms was similar: specific activities of 1.2 nmol/min/mg protein for the coccus and 1.0 nmol/min/mg protein for the L-form. The importance of the isomers of alanine and of D-alanyl-D-alanine in bacterial cell wall formation is well known and will not be pursued here. But the detection of these two reactions still functioning unabated in this stabilized L-form was highly significant. It demonstrated that the lack of cell wall synthesis in this wall-less bacterial derivative was not due to an inability to (1) isomerize the natural isomer of alanine or (2) to form the required alanyl dipeptide portion of the ultimate nucleotide precursor necessary for continued cell wall synthesis. Also, these results established that the initial phase for cell wall synthesis, nucleotide precursor formation within the cytoplasm, was intact and still functioning in this stabilized coccal L-form.

Earlier, it had been shown that alanine racemase persisted after conversion of *Proteus mirabilis* to either a stable or an unstable L-form [15]. Thus, while this enzyme continues to persist in L-forms of gram-negative and gram-positive organisms, a possible need for it, at least in this streptococcal L-form, may be for the anticipated return of cell wall formation by this organism. The finding of a functional alanine racemase within this stabilized L-form also proved that this enzyme was not responsible for the lack of D-alanine in the teichoic acid of only the L-form. More about this later.

It is not possible to generalize with respect to inhibition of cell wall synthesis in bacterial L-forms. Earlier, for example, Foder had examined 20 penicillin-induced L-forms from *S. aureus* strain 100 [16]. He observed that these L-forms (1) synthesized very little mucopeptide and that (2) the quantity of N-acetyl amino sugar containing acid-soluble nucleotides produced by these L-forms varied considerably. He suggested that mucopeptide biosynthesis in these L-forms "... are inhibited at different stages of cell wall mucopeptide synthesis. The block could be before, beyond, or at the site of penicillin action." Conversely, others had been unable to even demonstrate mucopeptide precursors in a penicillin-induced L-form of another *S. aureus* [17]. Therefore, these collective streptococcal and staphylococcal L-form studies serve to illustrate that inhibition of cell wall formation in bacterial L-forms from different as well as from the same parental organism is by no means biochemically uniform.

In the membrane, the pathway by which peptidoglycan is synthesized from uridine-5'-diphospho-N-acetyl-D-muamyl-L-Ala-D-iso-Glu-L-Lys-D-Ala-D-Ala (UMPPMp) and uridine-5'-diphospho-N-acetyl-D-glucosamine (UDP-GlcNAc) is well established. Of prime importance for this sequence of events to occur is the presence of an acceptor lipid, undecaprenyl phosphate ($C_{55}OP$). During cell wall formation, this lipid undergoes a cyclic series of metabolic events, culminating in the degradation of undecaprenol pyrophosphate (C_{55}-OPP) by a specific phosphatase, thereby insuring the reintroduction of carrier lipid into the pathway for peptidoglycan formation, i.e., at the translocase level. Also, when the pool of carrier lipid becomes rate limiting, peptidoglycan formation may be accelerated by endogenous undecaprenyl ($C_{55}OH$) being phosphorylated by isoprenoid alcohol phosphokinase. These reactions are catalyzed by membrane-bound enzymes. The metabolism of undecaprenol in bacteria is summarized in Figure 1.

Prior to these studies, evidence had been obtained suggesting the existence of a specific lesion at the membrane level for the formation of group-specific polysaccharide that is covalently linked to peptidoglycan in this streptococcal L-form. This evidence centered about the almost complete inability of L-form membrane fragments, but not those from the parent coccus, to accept rhamnose from TDP-rhamnose [18]. Thus, a comparative investigation of peptidoglycan formation by membrane fragments from *S. pyogenes* and its L-form was initiated to document possible L-form defects in the pathway leading to the

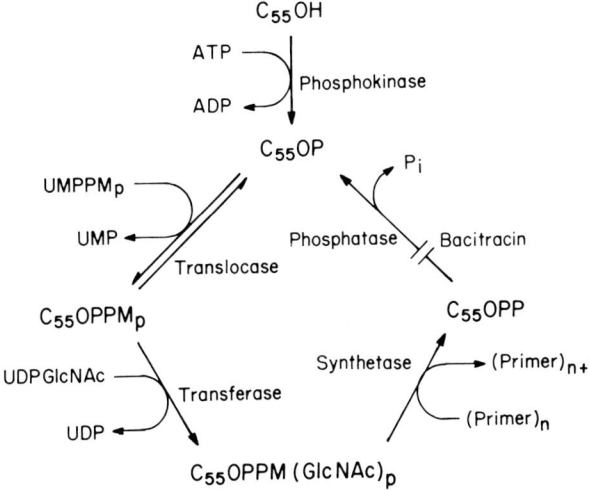

Figure 1 The metabolism of C_{55}-isoprenoid alcohol in bacteria. The enzymes involved in this pathway are: isoprenoid alcohol phosphokinase; phospho-N-acetyl-D-muramyl-pentapeptide translocase; UDPGLcNAc:undecaprenyl-pyrophosphoryl-N-acetyl-D-muramyl-peptapeptide N-acetylglucosaminyl transferase; peptidoglycan synthetase; isoprenoid alcohol pyrophosphate phosphatase.

synthesis of this polymer. These enzymatic studies were aimed primarily at elucidating whether defective synthesis of membrane lipid intermediates might account for the inhibition of peptidoglycan formation in this particular stabilized L-form [19].

Using reaction mixtures with appropriate radiolabeled nucleotide substrates and streptococcal membrane fragments, synthesis of undecaprenyl pyrophosphoryl-N-acetly-D-muramyl-L-Ala-D-iso-Glu-L-Lys-D-Ala-D-Ala (C_{55}-OPPMp) and peptidoglycan was demonstrated (Fig. 1). In striking contrast to this, when membrane fragments prepared from the L-form were assayed peptidoglycan formation was not observed and only a small amount of radioactivity was detected that corresponded to C_{55}-OPPMp, indicating the presence of suboptimal amounts of translocase activity in the L-form membrane and confirming the earlier results of UDP-muramyl-pentapeptide formation. Also, when streptococcal transferase enzyme was assayed using UMPPMp, UDP-[^{14}C]GlcNAc and ATP as substrates, the synthesis of radioactive lipid containing [^{14}C]GlcNAc was observed. The synthesis of this lipid was consistent with the presence of transferase activity (Fig. 1). Conversely, when L-form membranes were assayed for UMPPMp-dependent incorporation of [^{14}C]GlcNAc with ATP, no enzymatic activity was found, suggesting that the isolated L-form membranes lacked the transferase activity. Next, studies with the coccal membrane fragments were undertaken to examine the role of ATP in the stimulation of lipid and/or peptidoglycan polymer formation. Although radioactivity could be transferred from $[\gamma\text{-}^{32}P]$ATP into lipid when UMPPMp was present, this did not occur when L-form membranes were assayed. Therefore, the L-form membrane lacked observable phosphokinase activity under conditions where this enzyme could be demonstrated for streptococcal membranes [19].

These studies with ATP were designed to establish the synthesis of C_{55}-OP from endogenous C_{55}-OH (see Fig. 1) directly through use of $[\gamma\text{-}^{32}P]$ATP. This proved initially difficult because of the large amounts of ATPase activity (>139 nmol/min/mg) associated with the parental coccal membrane, a property also exhibited by L-form membrane preparations. But, unlike the L-form, this kinase reaction could be demonstrated for the streptococcal membrane if UMPPMp was also present in the reaction mixture. Preincubation of these coccal membranes with large amounts of ATP did not eliminate this need for ATP. This result is consistent with conditions under which C_{55}-OP synthesis can be observed only if UMPPMp is available to "trap" the C_{55}-OP as it is being formed. These data implied that rapid degradation of C_{55}-OP occurs in the coccal membrane and that the level of C_{55}-OP is regulated by the availability of UMPPMp which can serve to remove the C_{55}-OP from degradative influences through the translocase reaction. Again, these results could not be obtained with reaction mixtures containing L-form membrane fragments.

The lack of phosphokinase and transferase activities in the L-form persisted despite the fact that high concentrations of unlabelled ATP appeared to stimulate suboptimal incorporation of PM[^{14}C]p into some L-form preparations. Also, considerable effort was spent in these studies trying to optimize the conditions for synthesis of lipids and peptidoglycan by these L-form membrane preparations. However, all efforts met with little success in raising the levels of incorporation above that initially observed for C_{55}-OPPMp formation (<50 pmol/mg protein) (Fig. 1).

From these results it was concluded that the in vitro properties of the peptidoglycan synthesizing system for this coccus were similar to those already described for other bacteria. However, it was not possible to conclude whether the specific lesions in this coccal L-form existed at the level of the enzyme molecules or the endogenous lipid substrates, even though 50-fold higher levels of lipid intermediates which serve as membrane-bound substrates for peptidoglycan synthesis were synthesized in reaction mixtures containing coccal membranes than with similar preparations from the L-form. But the results did suggest that the L-form membrane is incapable of synthesizing significant quantities of the lipid substrates for peptidoglycan synthesis from exogenous nucleotide substrates.

Other specific defects might also explain this L-forms inability to form lipid intermediates. For example: (1) an inability to form $C_{55}OH$, (2) excessive degradation of $C_{55}OP$ by a specific phosphatase, or (3) the synthesis of a structurally altered lipid acceptor that would remain nonfunctional. In any event, the continued accumulation of UDP-muramyl-peptide in this L-form supports the fact that the membrane of this organism is unable to use nucleotide sugars efficiently for the peptidoglycan pathway [19].

The streptococcal in vitro system utilized in these enzymological studies for peptidoglycan synthesis was sensitive to sodium chloride, the osmotic stabilizer necessary for growth of this osmotically fragile streptococcal L-form. However, while the concentration of salt markedly inhibiting this synthesis was similar to that added to the L-form growth medium, it is not true that use of this osmotic stabilizer is responsible for the inability of this L-form to synthesize peptidoglycan. The parent streptococcus continued to synthesize a cell wall even when grown in the L-form medium. Also, this L-form was unable to reinitiate cell wall formation after being adapted to grow in physiologically isotonic media or when other stabilizers (both ionic and nonionic) served in lieu of NaCl [19].

It must be pointed out that the results obtained with this streptococcal L-form are not universally applicable to all L-forms. For example, others had shown that the cell wall defect in a stable L-form of *S. aureus* appeared to reside at a point in the pathway *after* formation of the peptidoglycan chain [17]. Here, membranes prepared from this staphylococcal L-form were able to form peptidoglycan in vitro but could not synthesize the interpeptide bridges necessary for cross-linking to occur. This, in turn, prevented the anchoring of these newly formed chains and the formation of a stable cell wall. By comparison, in this streptococcal L-form the lesion is clearly earlier in the pathway for cell wall formation and, indeed, may involve more than one lesion [19]. Therefore, in addition to the nucleotide variations, cell wall defects may also occur at the membrane level. Relatively recently, abnormalities in the "soluble-branch" and in the "membrane-bound branch" for cell wall synthesis have been documented in several L-forms of *B. licheniformis* and *B. subtilis* [20]. These results support the findings with the stabilized streptococcal L-form and demonstrate that a given L-form may possess discrete, multiple lesions. In conclusion, results thus far have demonstrated multiple, specific enzymatic defects in the lipid metabolism of the membrane-bound branch of an osmotically stabilized streptococcal L-form of *S. pyogenes* type 12, namely, a lack of phosphokinase, translocase, and transferase activities [19].

B. Teichoic and Lipoteichoic Acids

Prior to the initiation of these biochemical studies some work had been done on the teichoic acid (TA) of the Group A streptococci. Also, varied information was available concerning this polymer in bacterial L-forms. For example, in 1959 McCarty reported on the occurrence of polyglycerol phosphate (glycerol TA) as an antigenic component *in some but not all* of the gram-positive bacteria examined [21]. Polyglycerol phosphate was found in the Groups A–G streptococci. Later, Matsuno and Slade detailed the composition and serological properties of a glycerol TA from a Group A streptococcus (strain Richards, type 3) [22]. Further studies also led these investigators to conclude that it was likely ". . . that this TA is associated with the protoplast membrane." Conversely, Hijmans was unable serologically to detect the Group D antigen, which is an intracellular glycerol TA, in L-forms of the Group D streptococci [23]. However, others did find this antigen in these same L-forms but only when grown without penicillin and after the glucose content of the medium had been increased, with most of the antigen being found in solution [24]. In retrospect, this is an interesting observation since it has now been documented that the amount of intracellular and extracellular LTA produced by several bacteria may be profoundly affected by changes in the growth conditions [25]. However, in another study Pratt was unable to find either a glycerol or ribitol-type TA by chemical means in L-forms of *S. aureus* or in their spent medium [26].

Although inhibition of peptidoglycan formation had been substantiated in an osmotically fragile streptococcal L-form [12,19], nothing was known concerning its continued ability to synthesize TA or whether structural changes had occurred in this anionic polymer after loss of the rigid cell wall. Shortly after a report of a possible relationship between TA synthesis and peptidoglycan formation had appeared in the literature [27], the TA of an L-form and its parental *S. pyogenes* was quantitated and characterized for the first time [13]. It was hoped that, as a result of this comparison, any major differences between these two organisms would be a result of inhibition of cell wall formation in the L-form. This, indeed, proved to be the case.

These initial studies employed extraction of intact cells with trichloroacetic acid to reveal the continued presence of TA in this streptococcal L-form [13]. Based upon column chromatographic analyses, the molecular weight of TA from both organisms was determined to be between 5,000 to 10,000. However, much less of this anionic polymer was found in the L-form than in the parental coccus; specifically, yields of 8.7 and 1.1 mg/g dry weight cells for the coccus and L-form, respectively. No changes in these results were observed when the L-form was grown with or without penicillin. Also, molar ratio determinations of highly purified TA from each organism showed the first major difference; namely, that alanine was missing in the TA from the L-form. This signified that a structural alteration had occurred. Characterization of alanine from the TA extracted and purified from the parental coccus by identical procedures had shown it to be of the unnatural or D configuration. Also, this amino acid was esterified to the glycerol moiety of the polyol backbone from this organism. Necessary precautions had been taken to assure that the known alkaline lability of this bond was not compromised during the isolation and preparation of this polymer from the L-form. Therefore, the lack of this amino acid in the TA from the L-form was not the result of a laboratory manipulation.

The separation of organic phosphates, after NaOH hydrolysis of TA from both of these organisms, was achieved on DEAE-cellulose columns. Of the three compounds resolved and later characterized, the one of major importance was diglycerol triphosphate [13]. The finding of this hydrolytic product established the glycerol TA in these organisms as a 1,3-phosphate-linked glycerophosphate polymer. Also, characterization of a diphosphorylated product from such hydrolysates with a molar ratio of glucose-phosphorus-glycerol of 1:1.98:2.98 proved that the small amount of D-glucose originally detected in the glycerol TA from this coccus and its L-form was not a contaminant. This particular finding was to have other implications and I shall return to this point later. Finally, the chain length of the TA from each of these organisms was determined and, surprisingly, they were also different: streptococcus, averaging 25 glycerolphosphate units in length; L-form, averaging 11 such units long. Because of this difference it should, perhaps, be mentioned that the chain length of bacterial TA may be dependent upon the method of isolation used. However, in this study identical procedures for the extraction of this polymer from the coccus and L-form were rigidly adhered to. Therefore, this difference in the TA from these two organisms is meaningful and is not thought to be a procedural artifact. Therefore, two major structural differences had now become apparent as a result of these studies; that the TA of the L-form lacked D-alanine and that this polymer was appreciably shorter in length than that of its parental *S. pyogenes*. Also, the finding of glycerol TA in this stabilized L-form from *S. pyogenes*, which is completely devoid of a cell wall, illustrated that the formation of this anionic polymer was independent of peptidoglycan synthesis in this Group A streptococcus. The proposed structure for TA from *S. pyogenes* and its L-form is summarized in Figure 2.

A possibility existed that the absence of alanine in the TA of the L-form was due to the high "salt" content of its growth medium. To attempt to resolve this point, *S. pyogenes* was grown in L-form medium and its TA isolated and characterized as before. Briefly, the TA yield obtained was in close agreement with that from this coccus when grown in the usual manner. Also, appropriate analyses showed the continued presence of alanine. Therefore, just as the presence of an increased amount of NaCl in itself did not inhibit peptidoglycan formation, nor was it sufficient to inhibit the insertion of alanine into the glucosylpolyglycerol phosphate of the L-form [13].

As already indicated, it had been established that extracts of this L-form continued to isomerize L-alanine [14]. Therefore, the lack of D-alanine in only the TA from this organism was not due to the absence of alanine racemase. At

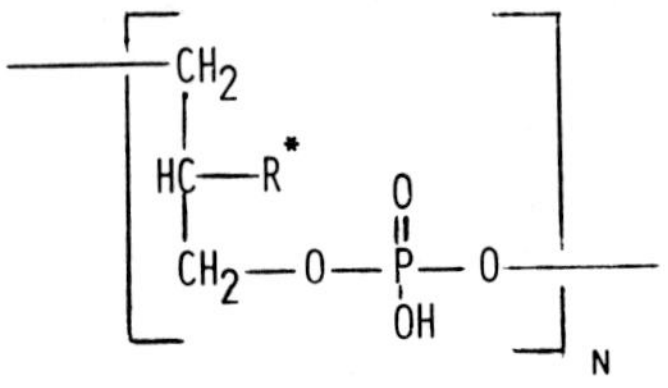

$$\left[\begin{array}{c} -CH_2 \\ | \\ HC-R^* \\ | \\ CH_2-O-\overset{O}{\underset{OH}{P}}-O- \end{array} \right]_N$$

	CHAIN LENGTH (AVERAGE)	R^*
STREPTOCOCCUS PYOGENES	N=25	GLUCOSE EVERY 14 UNITS, D-ALANINE EVERY 1.4 UNITS
L-FORM	N=11	GLUCOSE EVERY 14 UNITS, NO ALANINE

Figure 2 Proposed structure of teichoic acid from *Streptococcus pyogenes* and its stabilized L-form.

about this time, others had shown the presence of a new enzyme, membrane acceptor ligase, in a lactobacillus that was capable of inserting D-alanine into its membrane glycerol TA [28,29]. In addition, it was observed that this enzyme required a proper membrane protein to TA conformation for this insertion to occur. However, what was missing in our repertoire of knowledge then was whether a membrane acceptor ligase was also present in the Group A streptococci and, if so, whether its absence or inhibition might be responsible for this lack of D-alanine in the TA of the L-form. Or conversely, and because of this need for a proper membrane conformation for enzymic activity, the possibility existed that membrane structural or conformational changes might have also occurred after conversion of this coccus to its L-form to account for this defect. Actually, credence that this latter thought was more than mere speculation came from previous studies which had shown marked quantitative differences in the membrane protein patterns of this coccus and its L-form by disc gel electrophoresis and amino acid analyses [30]. Additional support was subsequently obtained when electron spin resonance spectroscopy studies also detailed differences in the membrane fluidity of these two organisms [31].

Earlier studies by McCarty [32] and Matsuno and Slade [22] had shown that D-alanine was an antigenic determinant of Group A streptococcal TA. As mentioned above, Hijmans had failed to detect serologically the Group D antigen, an intracellular glycerol TA, in L-forms of the Group D streptococci [23]. Therefore, and in light of these findings with an L-form of *S. pyogenes*, a possible lack of D-alanine may have been responsible for this initial lack of detection in these Group D coccal L-forms.

Concomitant with these initial studies were those performed with protoplasts of *S. pyogenes* obtained by a phage-associated lysin technique [13]. The results showed that (1) at least some of the enzymes concerned with TA formation resided in the membrane, (2) that most, if not all, of the glycerol TA in this Group A coccus was probably associated with the membrane, but (3) this TA was loosely associated between the cell wall and membrane, like that reported earlier for the Group D (glycerol TA) antigen from protoplasts of *S. faecalis* [33]. This latter point was in contrast to the L-form that continued to form a small amount of glycerol TA which was firmly attached to its membrane, suggesting an essential role for this entity.

By this time the in vitro incorporation of D-alanine into the membrane TA of *Lactobacillus casei* had been demonstrated [28,29,34]. In these studies, it was observed that this incorporation by membrane fragments was dependent upon two enzymes for the linkage of D-alanine to membrane TA: stimulator or D-alanine activating enzyme, and D-alanine:membrane acceptor ligase. The reaction of labeled product formed by this in vitro system with antiserum containing globulin specific for polyglycerolphosphate confirmed that the labeled alanine incorporated was covalently linked to membrane TA.

To determine whether these two enzymes were associated with the lack of D-alanine in the L-form, it was necessary first to define the system in *S. pyogenes* responsible for the incorporation of D-alanine into membrane TA [35]. Chromatographic and enzymological approaches quickly showed that the in vitro incorporation of D-alanine into membrane fragments of *S. pyogenes* required ATP, Mg^{2+}, and supernatant fraction. Boiled membranes were inactive. However, a similar system composed of preparations from the L-form failed to incorporate D-alanine. In an attempt to determine the reason for the L-form systems failure to incorporate D-alanine, supernatant fraction from the coccus was used with membrane fragments from the L-form, without positive results being noted. However, when coccal membrane fragments were combined with supernatant fraction from the L-form, appreciable incorporation of D-alanine into coccal membranes was observed. The rate of incorporation of alanine into coccal membrane fragments as a function of coccal or L-form supernatant fraction was nearly linear when varying amounts of supernatant fractions were used. Also, a linear relationship was obtained when coccal supernatant fraction was used with varying amounts of membrane preparations. Finally, the same relationship was noted when L-form supernatant fraction combined with differing amounts of coccal membrane fragments.

The pH optimum for the incorporation of D-alanine into coccal membrane fragments by supernatant fraction from the coccus and L-form was similar (between pH 6.3–6.9). Likewise, the effect of D-alanine concentration on the rates of incorporation for these supernatant fractions from these two organisms was nearly identical, K_m values of 26 and 28 μM with supernatant fractions from the coccus and L-form, respectively. Supernatant fraction from the coccus and L-form were also assayed for their D-alanine activation activity. The specific activity for this enzyme in these two fractions was the same; 1141 and 1110 nmol/h/mg. Also, the amount of D-alanine capable of being incorporated into coccal membrane fragments by each supernatant fraction was close—0.34 and 0.21 nmol D-alanine/h/mg supernatant fraction of the coccus and L-form, respectively. Finally, the separation, by column chromatography, of D-alanine activating enzyme and D-alanine:membrane acceptor ligase from the supernatant fractions of the coccus and L-form and the replacement of supernatant fraction by the addition of these two enzymes for D-alanine incorporation into coccal membrane fragments established the requirement of two soluble components for the incorporation of this amino acid in *S. pyogenes* [35].

The above results implied that the system previously established by others for the incorporation of D-alanine into the membrane of a lactobacillus was also functioning in *S. pyogenes*, it being:

Enzyme + D-alanine + ATP $\longleftrightarrow$ Enzyme AMP-D-alanine + PPi

Enzyme AMP-D-alanine + membrane acceptor $\xrightarrow{\text{ligase}}$ D-alanyl-membrane-acceptor + Enzyme + AMP

As already explained, only the system utilizing either supernatant fraction from the L-form or coccus together with coccal membrane fraction incorporated D-alanine, and none other. Therefore, this established that although the L-form did, indeed, possess the required soluble components for D-alanine incorporation, its membrane did not function as acceptor even though it contained D-alanine-deficient membrane TA. Incidentally, these in vitro studies were done under physiologically isotonic conditions. Thus, the presence of excessive salt was not a factor in the inability of these L-form membrane fragments to incorporate D-alanine. These results had shown that the defect in the L-form system for incorporation of D-alanine resided in the inability of its membrane to function as an acceptor. Earlier, it had been established that the glucose containing TA from this L-form is shorter in length than that from the parental coccus (11 vs. 25 glycerophosphate units) [13]. Therefore, this shorter chain length in the L-form may have resulted in a conformational change in its membrane TA. Conversely, it was also possible that the formation of a specific

TA complex, like lipoteichoic acid (LTA), may be necessary for alanine incorporation and that this was defective in the L-form. But since D-alanine incorporation was completely inhibited when the membrane was denatured by heat, the role of an as yet unknown membrane enzyme(s) could not be discarded either. Therefore, this inability of L-form membrane fragments to incorporate D-alanine may be due to: (1) an alteration in the acceptor TA, (2) a change in its conformation, or (3) the lack of an essential enzyme(s) associated with the membrane.

Differences in the membrane complex lipids and fatty acids between *S. pyogenes* and its L-form had been demonstrated in the past [36,37]. However, while electron microscope studies failed to reveal significant differences in thickness between these two membranes, electron spin resonance spectroscopy, using spin-labeled fatty acids as probes, did show a pronounced difference in the mobility of the lipids within the membranes of this coccus and L-form [31]. These findings added credence to a possible membrane structural alteration in the L-form to account for its nonfunctional D-alanine incorporation system. These electron spin resonance spectroscopy studies will be enlarged upon later.

These studies were not the first to suggest that the membrane of this L-form might be biochemically defective. A component of the Group A coccal cell wall is the group C-polysaccharide which is largely composed of two carbohydrates: L-rhamnose and N-acetyl-D-glucosamine, with L-rhamnose predominating. In 1966, extracts of this coccus and its L-form were shown to synthesize a proposed precursor, TDP-rhamnose, for C-polysaccharide formation [38]. However, membrane fragments of the L-form were capable of only 10% uptake of labeled rhamnose from this nucleotide as compared with coccal membrane fragments. Surprising, however, once bound both membrane fragments polymerized rhamnose to the same extent [18]. It was concluded that the L-form's inability to accept rhamnose was due to either a lack of membrane rhamnose acceptor sites, to membrane enzymes necessary for the effective transfer of ribonucleotide rhamnosyl units to acceptor sites, or to both. These findings remained unaltered when 11 years later more detailed enzymic studies of "group polysaccharide" synthesis in these same two organisms led to a working hypothesis that in *S. pyogenes* "... a group A-specific polysaccharide proceeds at the cellular membrane with the nonordered addition of rhmanosyl and N-acetylglucosaminyl residues to a membrane acceptor that contains a neutral lipid anchor." Under identical conditions, L-form membrane fragments again were still not able to accept these carbohydrates from appropriate nucleotide substrates [39]. Once more, decreased acceptor activity implied that an active acceptor was unavailable in the L-form, appropriate enzymes were lacking, or both. Therefore, profound membrane changes had indeed occurred after conversion of *S. pyogenes* to an L-form.

Since other studies had established the presence of glycerol TA in the membrane of a stabilized L-form of *S. pyogenes*, attention now turned to determining just how this polymer was attached to the membrane. Earlier, it had been shown that the membranes of most gram-positive bacteria contained glycerol TA in association with lipid as a lipid complex, lipoteichoic acid (LTA) [40–47]. Also, a rather novel complex lipid, a phosphoglycolipid, identified as phosphatidyl kojibiosyl diglyceride, had been established as the lipid portion of LTA from *S. faecalis* by Ganfield and Pieringer [43]. This lipid seemingly possessed the necessary physicochemical properties for anchoring the long hydrophilic glycerol phosphate polymer of LTA to the hydrophobic environment of the bacterial membrane [44]. Earlier, a probable TA-lipid complex had been found capable of sensitizing erythrocytes [45,46], and the suggestion had been made of the possible involvement of this streptococcal component in the pathogenesis of rheumatic fever and glomerulonephritis [46,47]. Therefore, the finding of LTA in the L-form would add to its potential armament and tend to increase the speculation of a role for all such aberrant forms in pathogenesis. Therefore, proof was sought for the continued presence of LTA in this stabilized L-form of *S. pyogenes*.

Earlier TA studies had employed a trichloroacetic acid extraction procedure that hydrolyzed the linkage between lipid and TA to obtain the TA from *S. pyogenes* and its L-form [13]. Now, a cold phenol extraction method was used to extract intact LTA from these two organisms [48]. The data obtained, in conjunction with an earlier study [13], clearly showed that all of the TA present in these two organisms was in the form of LTA; the yield of LTA from intact cells of the coccus and L-form was 0.97 and 0.19%, respectively. In addition, duplicate analyses of this L-form recently adapted to grow in physiological isotonic media (see Sect. III), and the coccus from hypertonic L-form medium, showed no change in the amount of TA or LTA obtained (depending upon the extraction method used), indicating that the hypertonic environment of the osmotically fragile L-form was not responsible for its low LTA (or TA) content. The coccal-to-L-form LTA ratio was 5.7:1. These studies with *S. pyogenes* and its L-form also showed for the first time the continued formation of LTA in an L-form that lacks a rigid cell wall, confirming earlier TA results by showing that synthesis of LTA is independent of cell wall formation in this Group A coccus [48]. Previously, others had shown that mucopeptide and TA formation within the cell wall of bacteria may be interrelated; the turnover rates of these two are identical in certain bacilli [27,49]. However the absolute concentration of this membrane component did decrease drastically (by 80%) when synthesis of the rigid cell wall was inhibited (i.e., in the stabilized L-form) [48].

At this point, I should like to dwell on a facet of the purification of LTA that pertains to the continued presence of ester linked D-alanine and utilizes deoxyribonuclease and ribonuclease to remove contaminating nucleic acids [48]. The reaction mixture employing these enzymes was routinely adjusted to pH 8.0 *before* the addition of crude extracts of LTA. Upon addition of these L-forms or coccal extracts, the pH dropped to between pH 7.0-7.2. A comparison of the molar ratios of TA (obtained by acidic procedures) and LTA (by the cold phenol procedure) after purification showed no change in the alanine content, suggesting that no (or insignificant) loss of this amino acid had occurred in the LTA after enzymic treatment (unpublished results). I make this point here because of a misprint in one of our papers which indicates that the pH of the reaction mixture *during* treatment of LTA with these nucleases remained at pH 8.0, which, if true, would have resulted in considerable loss of alanine during this purification step [48]. Subsequent comparative studies of the purified TA and LTA of a Group B coccus treated in identical fashion confirmed the results obtained with LTA from *S. pyogenes* (i.e., no loss of alanine); Group B streptococcal molar ratio of phosphorus-glycerol-D-alanine-glucose of $1.00:1.02 \pm 0:0.58 \pm 0.13:0.02 \pm 0.01$ for TA and $1.00:1.05 \pm 0.07:0.48 \pm 0.09:0.11 \pm 0$ for LTA [84].

Chemical and chromatographic analyses of lipid of LTA indicated that glycerophosphoryldiglucosyl diglyceride, a phosphoglycolipid similar but not identical to that from the LTA of *S. faecalis* already mentioned above, was the lipid component of LTA from this *S. pyogenes* and its L-form [48]. A major difference between these novel complex lipids is the number of long-chain fatty acyl groups present—that from *S. faecalis* and *S. pyogenes* possessing four and two long-chain fatty acyl groups, respectively.

Glycerophosphoryldiglucosyl diglyceride had been found in *S. pyogenes* prior to these studies [50]. Also, it should perhaps be emphasized that on the basis of calculated values, the maximum amount of this phosphoglycolipid in 1 g (dry wt) of the coccus and its L-form was low—0.16 and 0.07%, respectively [48]. This low yield from either organism probably accounted for an earlier inability to detect this novel lipid when the complex membrane lipids of these two organisms was detailed [37]. However, in this early study it was shown that the glycolipid content (diglycosyl diglyceride) in the membrane of the L-form was twice as high as that of the parental coccus. Subsequently, Pieringer and co-workers did establish that this glyceride glycolipid was involved in the synthesis of the phosphoglycolipid (phosphatidylkojibiosyl diglyceride) moiety of the LTA in *S. faecalis* [51,52]. Therefore, it is most probable that the accumulation of diglycosyl diglyceride in the L-form membrane is also indicative of a precursor role for lipid of LTA in *S. pyogenes*.

The L-form's continued ability to synthesize a small amount of LTA, which remains firmly attached to its membrane, was now established. But a reason for this seemingly important need, even in the complete absence of peptidoglycan formation, was obscure. Much had appeared concerning the involvement of this anionic polymer as a scavenger of divalent cations and that the D-alanine component of this polymer regulated this activity [53]. Therefore, it was thought that a possible need for this continued synthesis of LTA by this L-form might be for the control of its magnesium ion concentration at the membrane. In addition, lack of alanine in only the LTA from the L-form would, according to theory, maximize the amount of divalent cations capable of being bound by this polymer. Surprisingly, however, atomic absorption spectroscopy studies of *S. pyogenes* and its physiologic isotonic L-form (i.e., L-form adapted to grow in physiologically isotonic growth media, see Section III) revealed that both organisms accumulated magnesium ions to the same extent (approximately 1.50 μg/mg cell protein), in spite of the L-form containing only one-sixth of the LTA of the coccus. Therefore, the binding of magnesium ion by the L-form was not affected by its greatly reduced LTA content and loss of the cell wall. Further, calculations from these and earlier findings indicated that the magnesium ion concentration capable of being bound by all of the TA (and LTA) present in the coccus and L-form only accounted for 34 and 0.07%, respectively, of the total actually found in these organisms. This suggested that the importance or involvement of LTA for magnesium ion accumulation in this coccus was low and for its L-form practically nonexistent, and, obviously, that other components of the cell wall or membrane were also binding this cation (F. Varga and C. Panos, unpublished results). Therefore, a need for the continued presence of the small amount of LTA in the L-form had to await the eventual completion of tissue culture studies.

III. ALTERED OSMOTIC FRAGILITY AND SURVIVAL

Earlier, a few reports had appeared on the adaptation to low salt media of osmotically fragile L-forms of *S. pyogenes*. But only one, to my knowledge, had detailed the frequency of successive transfers needed to achieve this goal. This was done with an osmotically fragile L-form of *S. pyogenes*, strain 8 [54]. This adaptation required a time period of over 6 months, some 200 transfers, and involved periodic stepwise reductions in the salt content of the medium to achieve growth of this L-form near physiological isotonicity. A different approach was attempted utilizing as its basis observations with two different types of organisms. Gallin et al. had shown the occurrence of significant increases in the concentration of serum lipids (triglycerides, free fatty acids, or both) in patients with infection by gram-negative bacteria [55]. Also, the osmotic fragility of various mycoplasmas (*Acholeplasmas*) could be markedly decreased by incorporation into their membranes of preformed monoenoic acids from the growth medium [56]. Therefore, we endeavored to see if the use of oleic acid, an unsaturated fatty acid ubiquitous in human tissues, together with a regulated decrease in the NaCl content of the medium would result in the rapid adaptation of our L-form to grow in media capable of supporting the parental coccus. However, before initiating this approach the inability of the L-form to oxidize long-chain fatty acids (i.e., lacking β-oxidation), in order to negate the degradation of long-chain fatty acids absorbed from the growth medium, had to be determined. After this was established, a final concentration of oleic acid that would not inhibit L-form growth in the albumin-containing medium being used had to be found. The experimentally determined value eventually chosen was 2 μg/ml medium (Fig. 3).

Briefly, growth of the L-form at a final NaCl concentration of 0.85% w/v with the use of oleic acid was achieved [57]. The transition from 3.5 to 0.85% NaCl in the presence of this monoenoic acid required approximately 20 transfers (in time, about 2.5 weeks) and was a far cry from the 200 transfers required by others for the same result without the use of a fatty acid. This newly adapted L-form, now capable of growth in media with a final concentration of 0.85% NaCl, was termed the physiological isotonic L-form. The eventual omission of this temporary oleic acid requirement was easy. After subculturing the L-form in the presence of oleic acid for 10 times, it was simply omitted from the medium without any apparent ill effect being noted. It had been reported by

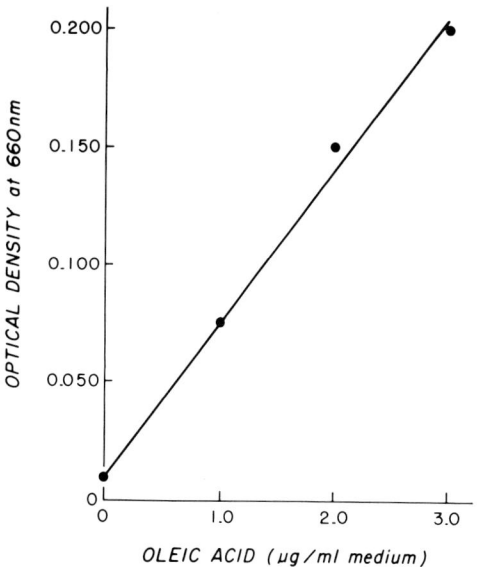

Figure 3 Temporary requirement for oleic acid by a newly adapted L-form of *Streptococcus pyogenes* growing in a lipid-extracted medium with 1.2% (w/v) sodium chloride.

others that once adapted to grow at a particular concentration of NaCl, growth of an L-form could not be maintained in broth containing higher or lower concentrations of this electrolyte. This was not the case here. The physiological isotonic L-form grew readily when returned to the original hypertonic medium. However, its inability to continue to grow in isotonic media once transferred several times in the hypertonic medium indicated that adaptation to growth in an isotonic environment was not analogous to that of an L-form made to grow in liquid medium. Once achieved, the ability to grow in broth from agar is never lost.

The temporary need for oleic acid by the L-form growing with 1.2% NaCl and with the new isolates of the physiological isotonic L-form was quantitated using the same medium after being lipid-extracted. A typical concentration dependent growth response curve was obtained over the concentrations of oleic acid indicated in Figure 3. However, oleic acid remained a permanent requirement when the L-form was adapted to grow in lipid extracted or nonextracted medium with a NaCl content of 0.5%.

This need for oleic acid by the physiological isotonic L-form could not be replaced by various concentrations of saturated fatty acids (palmitic or myristic acids) or by cholesterol. Also, no synergistic effect was observed when various mixtures of oleic and palmitic acids replaced this temporary octadecenoic acid requirement [57].

As already indicated, during these studies several L-forms capable of growing at various concentrations of NaCl (3.5, 1.2, 0.85, and 0.5% with oleic acid) were obtained and their comparative growth characteristics compared. Figure 4 shows: (1) the changes in cell yields and generation times of established midlogarithmically growing cells and (2) their maximal optical densities when entering the stationary phase of growth as the NaCl content of the growth medium was lowered. As is apparent, protein content and optical densities decreased while the generation times increased as adaptation to growth at lesser concentrations of NaCl was realized. It should be mentioned here that while growth of the physiological isotonic L-form in terms of colony-forming units was comparable to that of the osmotically fragile L-form from which it was derived (10^7 to 10^9 CFU/ml), its cellular yields and final optical density attained were approximately 20% lower [57].

Detailed fatty acid analyses were an integral part of these adaptation studies to correlate changes in osmotic fragility with membrane fatty acid alterations. During the adaptation to physiological isotonicity the amount of oleic acid incorporated from the growth medium accounted for 30-35% of the total fatty acid content of the L-form. But once established (i.e., after omission of exogenous oleic acid supplied to the medium), the octadecenoic acid content of the physiological isotonic L-form dropped to approximately 15%. The predominant saturated fatty acid in the L-form during these investigations was always palmitic acid.

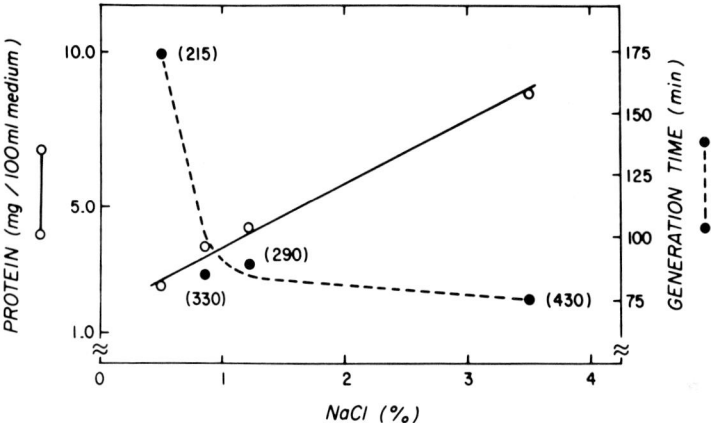

Figure 4 Changes in yields (protein) and generation times during midlogarithmic growth of established L-forms in lipid-extracted growth medium with different concentrations of sodium chloride. Numbers in brackets indicate maximum optical density (660 nm) of each culture entering the stationary phase of growth.

Of interest was the finding that although the fatty acid composition remained similar, established L-forms growing with NaCl concentrations of 3.5, 1.2, and 0.85% showed differing saturated/unsaturated fatty acid ratios (Fig. 5). Therefore, as the NaCl content of the growth medium was reduced, more saturated but less unsaturated long-chain fatty acids were being formed. Since the fatty acid content of these organisms remained constant, 4.0-4.5% of the dry weight of each intact organism, we were observing preferential and not excessive synthesis of long-chain fatty acids [57].

The isolation of a streptococcal L-form able to grow in media with only 0.5% NaCl *but* only if oleic acid was supplied exogenously was interesting. The saturated/unsaturated fatty acid ratio of this "lowest salt-oleic acid requiring" L-form was 0.89 (Fig. 5). Therefore, the spread in the saturated/unsaturated fatty acid ratio noted between the osmotically fragile L-form and those capable of growing at various decreasing concentrations of NaCl seemingly reflected a versatility in membrane stability to different environments, from maximal flexibility at the lowest NaCl concentration with the required -enoic acid to maximum rigidity in isotonic media without the need for an exogenously supplied unsaturated acid [57].

Salt-requiring or osmotically fragile L-forms have less phospholipids than salt-nonrequiring L-forms, and it has been hypothesized that this need for salt may be for the condensation and solidification of their phospholipids by metal ions

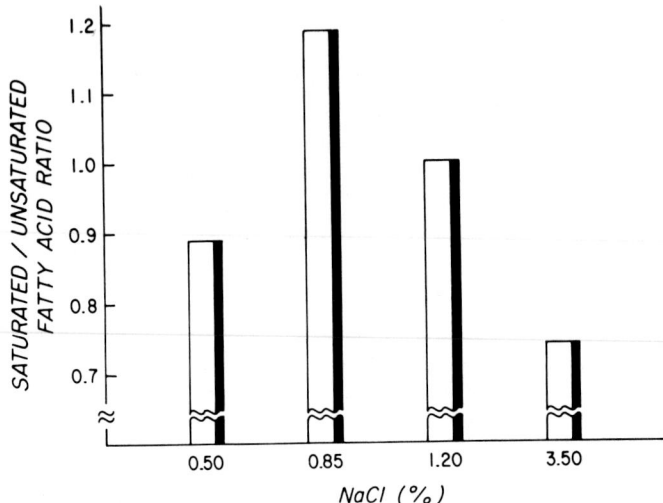

Figure 5 Saturated to unsaturated fatty acid ratio of the established streptococcal L-form growing with different concentrations of sodium chloride. The L-form growing with a sodium chloride concentration of 0.5% (w/v) requires the presence of oleic acid (2 µg/ml).

[58]. During the adaptation procedure to lower salt concentrations with the temporary use of oleic acid, the data obtained seemingly suggested a biphasic response to this end. First, the membrane became highly elastic, as evident by its massive (over 30%) increase in oleic acid, and this was confirmed by electron spin resonance spectroscopy data. Then, once established (i.e., after withdrawal of added oleic acid) the saturated/unsaturated fatty acid ratio changed, as stated above, to now show a decreasing unsaturated fatty acid content in cells, from hypertonicity to physiological isotonicity. A possible explanation for this decreased fragility was that the L-form was slowly strengthening its membrane by increasing the packing mode of its fatty acid content through the production of more saturated fatty acids so as to minimize the solidification and condensation effect by NaCl. This would explain why it was not possible for the physiological isotonic L-form to grow in the isotonic medium after being returned to the hypertonic medium for several transfers as mentioned earlier [57]. In addition, earlier electron spin resonance spectroscopy findings had corroborated these results by showing that the lipid chain rigidity of the membrane had also changed markedly (see below and Ref. 31). In this regard, and as stated earlier, parallel electron microscopic measurements of thin sections of the osmotically fragile and physiological isotonic L-forms and of the parental coccus failed to show a correlation between membrane thickness and increased osmotic stability.

Since the total fatty acid content did not change, a reason for the effective use of this exogenous oleic acid seemed to be to allow a gradual altering of the L-forms saturated/unsaturated fatty acid ratio and possibly for rearranging or redistributing its membrane lipids and proteins for maximum osmotic stability [57]. It had been shown with the *Acholeplasmas* that preformed long-chain unsaturated fatty acids, when added to the growth medium, increased membrane elasticity and decreased osmotic fragility [56,60]. These organisms do not synthesize long-chain unsaturated fatty acids. However, since the L-form is capable of both saturated and unsaturated fatty acid formation, but not degradation, the addition of an exogenous unsaturated fatty acid into the growth medium probably alters preferentially the de novo synthesis of its long-chain fatty acids and, in turn, the physical state of the L-form membrane.

As is known, membrane fluidity is not solely dependent upon the lipids and some information has appeared on quantitative membrane protein differences after conversion of their microorganism to an L-form [30,59]. In these fatty acid adaptation studies, changes in the protein profile of the cytoplasm with decreasing concentrations of NaCl were also noted with this coccal L-form [57]. These findings may be analogous to those observed with several mycoplasmas and possibly with the conclusions that protein changes may influence the physical state of the membrane lipids [56].

Physical studies played a part in corroborating the conclusions drawn from biochemical findings; i.e., the emergence of a "tougher" membrane in the physiological isotonic L-form. Since electron spin resonance spectroscopy had been used for the study of membrane structure and function, this technique was employed to compare the lipid organization and changes in the physical state of the membrane of *S. pyogenes* and its osmotically fragile L-form with this same L-form now adapted to grow under physiologically isotonic conditions [31]. As is common practice, this technique is used in conjunction with paramagnetic reporter molecules ("spin labels"), which are analogous to the optically absorbing or fluorescent groups so useful in other spectroscopic procedures. The reporter group is either covalently linked to specific functional groups in the system being investigated or, as in these studies, allowed to diffuse into the regions of interest. Two types of fatty acid spin label probes were used in these studies: type I (m,n) were N-oxyl-4′,4′-dimethyloxazolidine derivatives of 5-ketostearic where (m,n) is $(1,14)$, $(5,10)$, and $(12,3)$ and type II which is the 2,2,6,6-tetramethylpiperidine-1-oxyl derivative of stearamide.

Briefly, these comparative studies showed that the lipid chain rigidity of these membranes was of the order: physiological L-form > osmotically fragile L-form > streptococcus. Also, signal intensity vs. temperature analyses showed two transitions for these membranes, the first with melting points of 45, 26, and 36°C and the second at 70, 63, and 60°C for the physiological L-form, osmotically fragile L-form, and streptococcal membranes, respectively. This same order of membrane lipid chain rigidity was seen from the cooperativities obtained for each of these systems from analyses based on the expression of an n-order reaction. Also, the use of the type I (12,3) and other probes with the paramagnetic group close to the methyl end of the molecule suggested that this difference resided in the area closer to the lipid head group region rather than in the hydrophobic lipid core of the membrane [31].

As already indicated, no qualitative differences were evident in the fatty acid analyses of the membranes of these three organisms. However, quantitative changes in the ratio of saturated/unsaturated fatty acids were documented between these two L-forms [57]. As is known, the distribution of fatty acid probes used in any membrane is unknown and one cannot draw conclusions on the extent or arrangement of the assumed lipid bilayers of a membrane. Therefore, it is possible that the differences observed here might be related to quantitative changes in lipid composition or changes in the structure of the membrane associated protein. Similar findings with *Mycoplasma hominis* and *Acholeplasma laidlawii*, labeled with the same fatty acid probe used in these studies, I (12,3), had indicated that membrane proteins do influence the physical state of membrane lipids [61]. Nevertheless, this change in lipid chain rigidity provided an explanation to account for the survival of the L-form at physiological isotonicity and focused on changes in the physical nature of the membrane of this organism.

Even though the physiological isotonic L-form was capable of growth in ordinary media and a change in its lipid chain rigidity had been documented, information was still needed as to its increased longevity or survival in environments that would not permit cellular division. During these studies, it had been established that while the parental coccus divided in tissue culture medium containing serum its physiological isotonic L-form did not [57]. Therefore, changes in survival time (i.e., increased longevity) with increased membrane osmotic stability were assessed by suspending the physiological isotonic L-form and the L-form capable of growing at 0.5% NaCl with oleic acid in this tissue culture milieu (which was felt to be a more simulated in vivo environment), and comparing their survival time with that of the osmotically fragile L-form. As expected, viability decreased fastest, in minutes, when the osmotically fragile L-form (3.5% NaCl, control) was tested. In contrast, the same survival time was noted with the physiological isotonic L-form and the L-form capable of growth with 0.5% NaCl plus oleic acid, viability being demonstrable up to 4.5–5.0 days (see Fig. 3, Ref. 57). Therefore, these viability studies corroborated the increase in survival time of these "low-salt" L-forms that was expected from the biochemical and physical data obtained earlier.

Finally, in an earlier conversion of an osmotically fragile L-form of *S. pyogenes* to growth in physiologically isotonic media, Clasener et al. had reported that hemolysis production by the L-form disappeared with successive transfers ". . . of the low-salt GL-8 L-strain" [62]. In contrast to these results, this physiological isotonic L-form continues to be β-hemolytic [57].

IV. EFFECT ON HOST CELLS AND IMMUNOSUPPRESSED MICE

A. Latent Infection vs. Cytotoxicity

It has been established that osmotically fragile L-forms are inducible in vivo. Also, it is likely that once formed they may be sequestered in particular areas of the host and protected from an array of host mechanisms capable of destroying them. Therefore, the continued ability to make toxins and antigens clearly establishes the L-form as a potential pathogen *IF* its survival or multiplication is feasible within a host.

Schmitt-Slomska et al. were successful in inducing L-forms in human diploid cells infected by Group A streptococci and of establishing a chronically infected cell system for several months [63,64]. Later, Green et al. demonstrated the survival of stable L-forms of *S. faecalis* and of their subsequent reversion in human embryonic kidney cells [65]. Thus, latent infections of tissue monolayers by streptococcal L-forms had been documented. Therefore, the almost complete destruction of human heart cell monolayers in tissue culture after infection by our physiological isotonic L-form for 3-4 days was totally unexpected [57]. At the end of this time, it was noted that the few adhering heart cells still remaining were conspicuous by their atypical morphology; namely, large and deeply stained nuclei relative to their cytoplasmic volume as compared with uninfected heart cell controls. Finally, although the infectivity ratio of L-form to heart cells used in these studies was from 50 to 100:1, the results obtained from viable cell counts and confirmed by the use of the L-form labeled with oleic acid, established that infectivity resulted in (1) uptake and subsequent release of the L-form after cell destruction and (2) that the number of organisms remaining was less than the initial inoculum size used, indicating that destruction of heart cell monolayers was due to L-form survival and not cell division. Earlier, it was indicated that this L-form was unable to multiply in tissue culture medium with serum. Obviously, the presence of growing heart cells failed to alter this condition. In contrast, the parental coccus very quickly overgrew the tissue culture when used as the inoculum [57].

During these studies it was found by electron microscopy that the L-form was capable of binding to the surface as well as being found within these infected heart cells. This penetration was established by the use of viable L-forms now labeled with potassium tellurite, which caused heavy black deposits of metallic tellurium or tellurium oxide to appear on and near the inside of the L-form cytoplasmic membrane. This approach was necessary to distinguish quickly and easily the intracellular L-form from the internal structures of the heart cells when thin sections of infected monolayers were examined by electron microscopy after infection. The results obtained established beyond doubt the presence of the physiological isotonic L-form within heart cell monolayers. Therefore, it would seem that the L-form is capable of intracellular parasitism [57].

Earlier studies with lyophilized preparations of this same osmotically fragile L-form had shown that, when injected into the hearts of rabbits, they caused granulomas at the site of injection that differed from those induced by streptococcal cell walls or by sonic extracts [5]. In tissue culture studies, however, infection by the L-form with time always resulted in the almost complete loss of intracellular detail within the host cell and was reminiscent, microscopically, of the cytopathic effect of tissue culture cells infected with certain viruses [57]. A similar cytopathic effect was observed when a heat-killed L-form inoculum was employed. Therefore, although based on only a relatively few completed studies, it would seem that the L-forms of the Group A streptococci are not predictable in their actions toward human cell monolayers in tissue culture, the effects noted thus far ranging from latent infection to rapid cytotoxicity.

As a perusal of the literature will indicate, the adaptation of an osmotically fragile L-form to grow in physiological conditions does not necessarily imply that its survival in vivo will be comparable to that of the parental organism. As indicated earlier, Clasener et al. found that L-forms of Group A streptococci so adapted were unable to persist in mice beyond approximately 60 min following intraperitoneal or intravenous injection [62]. But Schmitt-Slomska et al., after injecting mice intraperitoneally with osmotically fragile coccal L-forms, were able to isolate these organisms for the duration of their study, 25 days [66]. By comparison, Group A streptococci can persist in the tissues of rabbits in the absence of bacteremia for up to 104 days after intravenous injection [67].

There is evidence that the defense mechanisms of a host are instrumental in helping to eliminate rapidly bacterial L-forms in vivo. This is exemplified by both human and animal sera which are lethal for L-forms, protoplasts, and spheroplasts [68-70]. However, no information had been available on the overt pathogenic or persistent capability of an L-form in a host whose immune response has been suppressed. Therefore, and because of the cytopathic effect of the physiological isotonic L-form on human heart cells in tissue culture, the pathogenicity, persistence, and change in morphology of this L-form when injected into immunosuppressed mice was investigated [71].

The earlier results of others were confirmed. Namely, that isolation of the L-form from nonimmunosuppressed mice (controls) was possible for up to 2 hr with only an occasional isolate up to 24 hr. However, maximum time of detection of the L-form in the peritoneal cavity by fluorescent antibody, after intraperitoneal injection, was greater, 3 days. Finally, newborn mice, believed to be more susceptible to infection, were still able to clear the viable L-form from the peritoneal cavity 8 hr after intraperitoneal injection. Also, no viable organisms were recovered from the liver, spleen, or kidneys and each of these was devoid of antigen by indirect fluorescent antibody when examined for from 2 hr to 1 month after intraperitoneal injection. When injected intravenously into newborn mice, however, these same organs were positive for L-form infectivity by indirect fluorescent antibody up to 72 hr. Some viable L-forms were obtained, on occasion, from these and from blood after 24 hr but not thereafter. Thus, these results indicated that this lack of L-form persistence in vivo was not due to osmotic lysis and that the immune response of the host was probably instrumental in removing the L-form [71].

Viability and detection of the L-form by fluorescent antibody was greatly prolonged in 3-week-old mice when the immune response was compromised with methylprednosolone sodium succinate. Since the L-form was detected for a longer period of time and isolated in far greater numbers from various organs after intraperitoneal injection, this route of injection was used throughout these studies [71]. By comparison with nonimmunosuppressed mice, viable L-forms persisted in the peritoneal cavity of the immunosuppressed mice for up to 14 days and showed a close correlation between decreasing viability and loss of host immunosuppression. Incidentally, this substantiated an initial belief that the rapid decrease in viability in nonimmunosuppressed mice was due, in part, to the defenses of the host [71]. However, while no organisms could be isolated from any of the organs indicated above after 14 days, L-form antigen was still detectable up to 17 days after injection by indirect fluorescent antibody. Finally, heat-killed L-forms were only detectable for 3 days in these immunosuppressed mice. Therefore, the persistence of viable cells for at least 2 weeks was not due to just the lack of clearance by this compromised host. Also, the ability of these mice to remove rapidly the heat-killed L-form indicated that cellular factors were not significantly depressed and that humoral factors were necessary for viable L-form removal. As mentioned earlier, humoral factors such as antibody and complement are cidal to L-forms. However, these are probably not necessary for the elimination of heat-killed L-form cells since they were rapidly removed even in the immunosuppressed mice.

It should be emphasized here that at no time was there any indication of illness in these nonimmunosuppressed or immunosuppressed mice after L-form injection and all of their organs at autopsy appeared to be normal by visual inspection. Therefore, overt pathogenesis was not a characteristic of this particular L-form when injected into a suitable host, even after its immune response had been compromised [71]. However, as with adaptation to grow in liquid media, it may be that the physiological isotonic L-form needs prolonged or continued passage in these immunosuppressed mice for reversion to the parental coccus or for overt pathogenesis to be demonstrable.

The microscopic morphology of the L-form after isolation from immunosuppressed mice changed drastically. They were predominately and rather uniformly coccal in appearance and remained so up to 3 days after isolation (see Fig. 2A, in Ref. 71). However, after this time the typical microscopic L-form morphology reappeared. Most L-forms of gram-positive bacteria require an osmotic stabilizer for growth, and this need for their survival in vivo may be supplied by mucin or spermine, ingredients normally found in many tissues and purported to be necessary for membrane stability. Also, as had been seen with this particular L-form, the presence of a free unsaturated fatty acid can profoundly alter the osmotic fragility of an L-form [57]. However, the need for osmotic stabilization may not be as important in vivo as in vitro since there are sites in vivo where the osmotic pressure is greater than that of serum.

The data obtained from these studies and the wide use of immunosuppressive drugs in medicine strongly supports the possibility that bacterial L-forms are quite capable of surviving in immunologically suppressed individuals. If so, this would enhance considerably the role of the L-form in pathogenesis by, perhaps, increasing the probability of reversion to the bacterial form or by sensitizing appropriate tissues. Of interest in this regard is a report of stabilized L-forms of certain gram-negative bacteria reverting to the bacterial form only after passage in rat kidney [72]. The tissue-damaging properties of streptolysin S and its possible involvement in renal damage are well known. Thus, it was of considerable interest to find that the reisolated L-form, after 6 days in the immunosuppressed mouse, had increased its production of streptolysin S significantly, culminating in at least a 16-fold rise in hemolytic units per milliliter when the L-form had reached the stationary phase of growth [71]. However, this increase decreased to that before mouse passage after the L-form was cultured in broth for 3 days. Based on cellular protein, the rise in hemolytic units per milligram of L-form protein was equally as impressive, increasing from 59 to 160 after from 2-10 hr of growth in liquid medium. In contrast, hemolytic activity in the L-form before mouse passage was low and only noted at the stationary phase of growth (see Fig. 7, in Ref. 71). Such an increase in vivo could be of great consequence to a host, especially when it is realized that streptolysin S may become complexed to carrier molecules (serum, albumin, RNA, etc.) and transferred from one carrier to another. By comparison, no M protein as a cellular component was detected serologically in extracts prepared from 80 mg dry weight of L-form cells before or after being in immunosuppressed mice for 6 days [71].

B. Cytotoxicity

A streptococcal L-form adapted to grow in physiological isotonic media had been shown capable of destroying human heart cells in vitro [57]. Therefore, a series of studies were initiated to examine the destructive effect of this L-form on growing tissues with a predilection for the Group A streptococci [73]. Because of the relationship between streptococcal infection and acute glomerulonephritis primary human embryonic kidney cells were used. Also, the same established Girardi human heart and human liver cells as before were included for comparative purposes. Again, L-form infectivity (L-form infectivity ratio of 100:1) resulted in primary kidney monolayer destruction after 4 days' incubation. Other effects noted were the appearance of enlarged, heavily staining nuclei, spindle-shaped cytoplasm, presence of giant cells, and the appearance of dinucleated cells. Similar results were also observed after infection of the established cell line of human liver cells. Likewise, some cell damage characterized by vacuolated cytoplasm, enlarged nuclei, and granulation within the cytoplasm were observed with these two cell lines after 7 days' incubation when an equivalent amount of heat-killed L-form cells served in lieu of viable cells. Therefore, the death of human kidney and liver cells in vitro seemed to show that the L-form was equally as effective against established and primary cell lines with a predilection for the Group A streptococci [73].

A comparison of these morphological findings with previous results using human heart cells showed that only kidney and liver cells became enlarged and/or dinucleated after L-form infection. Likewise, with an L-form infectivity ratio of 40:1 (to decrease or minimize the rapid destruction of host cells observed with the higher, 100:1, infectivity ratio), live L-form cells could be recovered at 10-12 days after infection from infected liver and kidney monolayers. Earlier, the L-form had been detected by fluorescent antibody for a maximum of 17 days in various organs from immunosuppressed mice. In contrast, use of L-form-infected kidney and liver monolayers extended this time period of detection beyond 1 month [73].

In addition to morphological changes, biochemical alterations also occurred when human heart cells were infected with the L-form. For example, the altered protein profile (determined by polyacrylamide disc gel electrophoresis) of these infected heart cells was reminiscent of the results of others showing protein alterations in liver cell membranes during infection with *Coxiella burnetii*. Also, on a dry weight basis, although the fatty acid content of these infected cells increased (by 62%), their fatty acid composition remained unaltered. Thus, these results, together with earlier electron microscope findings illustrating marked intracellular deterioration of the heart cells after infection, clearly reveal a capability by supposedly innocuous wall-less organisms of pathogens to induce profound morphological and biochemical changes in an infected host [73].

Earlier, heat-killed L-form preparations had been shown to be cytotoxic for human heart, liver, and kidney monolayers in tissue culture, suggesting a toxic cellular component [57,73]. Also, the compositional and structural differences existing between the LTA isolated and purified from *S. pyogenes* and its osmotically fragile L-form had been detailed [13,48]. Now, these LTAs were tested to determine if they would mimic the morphological changes and death of human kidney cell monolayers caused by the intact L-form [73]. These early studies were performed in tissue culture medium containing 10% serum, an ingredient now known to minimize or significantly lessen the toxic effect(s) of LTA (I. Ginsburg, personal communication). This is an important point because, in our hands, subsequent data were to show that whereas 50 μg/ml of streptococcal LTA, for example, was not deleterious for a variety of cell monolayers in tissue culture medium with 10% serum after 24-48 hr, cytotoxic effects were easily apparent with from 8 to 12 μg/ml of streptococcal LTA under identical conditions when the serum content was decreased to 0.5 to 1.0%. Conversely, lesser amounts of LTA (1-5 μg/ml) in the presence of low levels of serum (0.1%) instead stimulated proliferation of HeLa and mouse fibroblast cells in tissue culture (O. Leon and C. Panos, unpublished results). Others had also shown that LTA stimulates cell division [74]. Nevertheless, in these early studies 250 μg/ml of LTA was sufficient to destroy human kidney cell monolayers after 3 days' incubation in medium with 10% serum; with lesser amounts causing proportionally less destruction (e.g., 142 μg/ml causing 50% destruction) [73]. The results obtained with the LTA from the coccus and L-form were identical, with complete destruction being characterized by less than 10% of the initial cell population still being attached and their atypical appearance being as described earlier for kidney cells infected with the viable L-form after 4 days' incubation.

Structural alterations of LTA affected cytotoxicity. Streptococcal LTA with its fatty acids and alanine removed and deacylated L-form LTA failed to elicit a cytotoxic response or alter the growth rate of the human heart, liver, and kidney monolayers. A maximum concentration of 285 μg/ml of deacylated LTA from the coccus or L-form was inactive. These findings were the first to show the marked destruction capable by LTA for human cells in tissue culture and to indicate that L-form cytotoxicity was, at least in part, due to its LTA content. In addition, it was clear that although loss of D-alanine and a significantly shorter glycerol phosphate chain length did not affect the toxicity of LTA, deacylation by chemical means did. Therefore, although changes in the teichoic acid moiety of LTA did not seemingly affect its toxicity, changes in its lipid component did [73]. At the conclusion of these experiments, one could not help but note the similarity in this lipid-toxicity relationship of LTA with that of another amphiphile, lipopolysaccharide, from the gram-negative bacteria.

In a previous section (Sect. II.B), it had been emphasized that a hydrolytic product of TA from both *S. pyogenes* and its L-form had been isolated that had a molar ratio of glucose-phosphorus-glycerol of 1:1.98:2.98, proving that the small amount of D-glucose present was not a contaminant [13]. However, this aspect has been overlooked by others who, in reference to this work had erroneously stated that the polyglycerophosphate backbone of *S. pyogenes* LTA was devoid of all glycosyl units and that, "The only sugar in *S. pyogenes* LTA resides in the glycerophosphoryldiglucosyl diglyceride moiety at one end of this amphipathic molecule" [74,75]. This is an important point that bears on the cytotoxicity of L-form and coccal LTA. Recently, Simpson et al. concluded ". . . that the glucose moieties of *S. pyogenes* (their strain 1RP41) LTA must be intact for the toxic activity against human heart cells to be expressed." Also, that deacylated LTA ". . . killed heart cells" [74]. Earlier, their studies had also shown the LTA from this strain of *S. pyogenes* to be 56 glycerol phosphate units long and its polyglycerophosphate backbone to be devoid of glycosyl residues [76]. These results indicated obvious structural and compositional and cytotoxic differences between the LTA from this organism and that from *S. pyogenes*, type 12, and its L-form. However, although the glucose moieties and not the acyl groups were judged responsible for the cytotoxicity of LTA by these investigators, several aspects make this assumption difficult to comprehend, namely, the extremely low glucose content of this long polymer, the failure of periodate oxidation to nullify completely the cytotoxicity of deacylated LTA and LTA, and the massive amount of each needed to cause maximum cytotoxicity (to wit, "At a concentration of 1 mg/ml LTA (or dLTA) was found to be toxic as manifested by reduced incorporation of radiolabeled nucleotides and leucine."). Clearly, this was not the case with LTA isolated from this L-form or its parental *S. pyogenes*. Instead, these LTAs when deacylated, still contained the diglucosyl component of the complex lipid *plus* the glucose units of the TA portion of the molecule, but they were noncytotoxic. Also, a very much smaller amount of LTA, even in the presence of 10% serum, was used to affect maximum cytotoxicity (almost 100%) as determined by cell monolayer destruction and cell detachment and confirmed by the dye exclusion method with Erythrosin B [73]. Although the moiety responsible for the toxicity of LTA may seem unclear, recent studies in this laboratory have indicated that intact L-form or coccal LTA may possess a dual cytotoxic mechanism for cells in tissue culture with from 0.5 to 1.0% serum, small amounts (10–50 $\mu g/ml$) causing metabolic disturbances in host cells with death occurring after several days, and larger amounts (75–250 $\mu g/ml$) causing perturbations of the cell membrane, probably as a result of its acyl groups, with death of attached cells resulting after only 0.5–4 hr (O. Leon and C. Panos, unpublished results). Nevertheless, L-form and streptococcal LTA does mimic the cytotoxicity resulting from host cell infection by the intact and viable L-form.

C. Adherence to Host Cells

A prerequisite for pathogenesis is the attachment of the infectious agent to a suitable host. Also, one study has detailed the ability of a streptococcal L-form to adhere to host cells [73]. By comparison much work had appeared on the binding of the Group A streptococci to exfoliated cells from appropriate donors [77,78]. However, in very early comparative studies between *S. pyogenes* and its L-form, it had been decided to avoid the use of such cells because of the following reasons: (1) normal bacterial flora could not be easily removed, (2) viability of such cells was variable and, most critically, (3) receptors on these cells for bacterial attachment could vary from donor to donor. To overcome these difficulties human cells grown in tissue culture were used instead.

As may be recalled, the attachment of the L-form to the surface of infected heart cells had been demonstrated earlier by electron microscopy [57]. Therefore, studies were begun to assess the ability of LTA to inhibit coccal binding to a host cell with a predilection for *S. pyogenes* [73]. It was observed that human kidney cells first treated with coccal or L-form LTA inhibited attachment of *S. pyogenes*; an average of not more than one organism per tissue culture cell was counted. Without such treatment, kidney cells bound suspensions of *S. pyogenes* and its physiological isotonic L-form equally; 42 ± 6 streptococci bound per human kidney cell as compared with 50 ± 19 for the L-form. However, pretreatment of kidney cells with deacylated LTA (1 mg/ml) prepared from L-form LTA did not prevent or lessen coccal binding to these kidney cells, indicating the need of the long-chain fatty acids of the complex lipid component of this amphiphile for binding activity. By demonstrating the binding of the L-form to a host cell, the new tensile strength of a membrane once responsible for the osmotic fragility of this intact organism was obvious. Also, this corroborated the membrane changes obtained earlier by electron spin resonance spectroscopy. The demonstration of L-form adherence to a human cell in tissue culture had now been confirmed by light microscopy (Fig. 6) [73].

These binding studies also showed that a rigid cell wall was not necessary for host cell adherence. Therefore, the binding of this L-form, which lacks M protein as a structural component, to these kidney cells and the inhibition of coccal binding by exogenously supplied LTA showed that LTA, and not M protein, was involved in the binding of *S. pyogenes*, type 12 (and most likely its L-form), to a susceptible host cell. Others had shown that the fimbriae of gram-positive bacteria are involved in bacterial adherence to the mammalian membrane [79]. While the binding substance on the fimbriae of the Group A cocci is LTA, no such fimbriae have been found thus far on the surface of an L-form of a gram-positive bacterium.

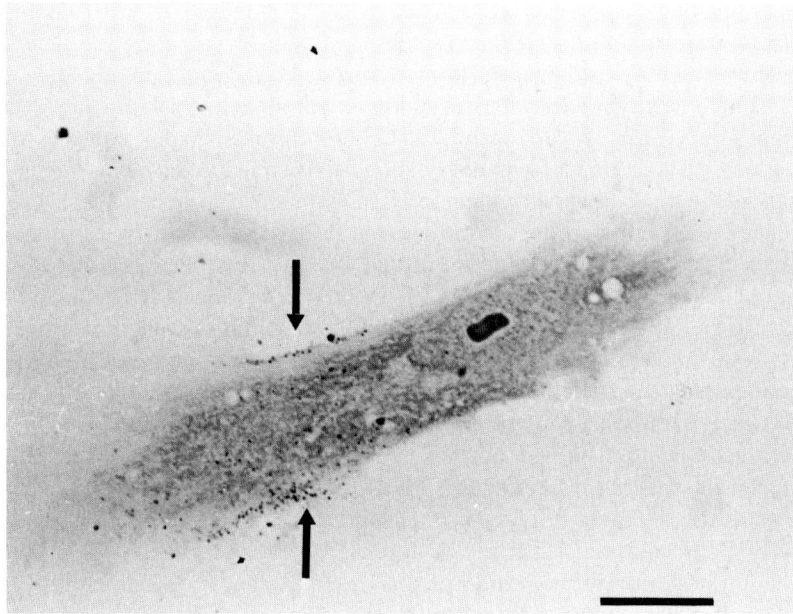

Figure 6 An individual human kidney cell with the much smaller isotonic L-form attached (Giemsa stain). Arrows indicate areas of maximum attachment. Bar, 25 μm.

D. Defective Collagen Biosynthesis

In addition to the binding and cytotoxic properties of LTA from *S. pyogenes* and its L-form already mentioned, most recent work has also shown that this amphiphile causes the formation of defective collagen by mouse fibroblasts in tissue culture in the absence of serum [80]. Although this work was performed with LTA from the parental coccus, at this writing there is no reason to believe that duplicate results would not be obtained with LTA from the L-form. Because of the known secretion of LTA by *S. pyogenes* during growth and after penicillin treatment and the possible secretion and/or exposure of LTA as a surface component of L-forms or cell wall-defective organisms in vivo, a synopsis of these results has been incorporated into this treatise.

Using isotopic, chromatographic, and enzymic methods, mouse fibroblasts in tissue culture treated with LTA (17.5 μg/ml) in the absence of serum for 24 hr were found to increase their production and accumulation of collagenous protein by an astounding 450%. However, this protein was practically hydroxyproline-free, as compared with that from control cells. It is known that under-hydroxylated collagen is secreted at a markedly reduced rate. The amount of collagen secreted into the medium by fibroblast monolayers before and after treatment with LTA was the same. However, secreted collagenous protein also showed a significantly reduced content of hydroxyproline (by 24%) as compared with that from cells not treated with LTA. Column chromatographic comparisons of secreted collagen whose hydroxylation had been reduced by exposure to a,a'-dipyridyl with collagenous protein secreted by monolayers exposed to LTA confirmed our chemical analyses indicating that the latter was defective (under-hydroxylated). These studies led to the conclusion that LTA does not affect the amount of collagenous protein secreted. However, it does increase the amount of collagen formed and retained by this cell line in tissue culture as well as causing a reduction in the hydroxylation of proline in both intracellular and secreted collagenous material. These findings are detailed elsewhere [80].

Collagen is a major macromolecule of most connective tissue and a component of the basement membrane of the kidney. As is known, this membrane has a profound role in glomerular filtration. Poststreptococcal glomerulonephritis is often a sequelae of Group A, type 12, infections, a disease thought to be related to immunologic disorder. However, to our knowledge, no information is available on possible defects in the collagenous component of the glomerular basement membrane in this streptococcal disease. The probable reason for this is amply expressed in the following quotation: "Only fragmentary and incomplete data on the biochemistry of glomerular basement membrane is available concerning specific glomerulopathies. This area of investigation has been compromised by lack of availability of tissue for study in the early stages of disease and the formidable problems encountered in obtaining purified material for study in patients with advanced disease. Not surprisingly then, the results of chemical analysis of such tissue has often been confusing and contradictory. In addition, many of the studies have been conducted in extremely heterogenous populations of patients with 'chronic glomerulonephritis'" [81].

Acute glomerulonephritis in children may be accompanied by swelling of the glomerular basement membrane and an impairment of the glomerular process, possibly as a result of immune complex depositions [82]. In the results just briefly discussed, the synthesis and accumulation of large amounts of abnormal intracellular collagenous material, by a small amount of LTA, for mouse fibroblast monolayers in tissue culture was established [80]. In a concurrent study, it was also shown that intact, growing mouse glomeruli in tissue culture are destroyed by LTA from *S. pyogenes*, type 12, and its L-form. However, preceding this destruction, electron microscopic and enzymological techniques revealed that a two- to four-fold thickening of the glomerular basement membrane had occurred and that no region was normal in thickness [83]. These collective results in the absence of complement or specific antibody suggest a nonimmune-LTA-mediated mechanism for kidney damage that may be related to abnormal or defective collagen formation. In addition, they entice the speculation of coccal L-forms, once sequestered in vivo, eventually adhering to, and helping to destroy host cells with the aid of this anionic membrane component.

V. SUMMARY

This compendium focuses on the effects of inhibition of cell wall synthesis on the continued formation of selected macromolecules by an L-form of *S. pyogenes*, type 12. Also, it documents this L-form's ability to destroy a variety of human cells in tissue culture. The information presented indicates that the changes that have occurred within this L-form are many, varied, and complex and that they cannot be generalized for all L-forms. It emphasizes that in spite of change portions of the cell wall "machinery" continue to be perpetuated and are, or can be, made active in an L-form already stabilized for many years, perhaps attesting to the tenacity with which the L-form hopes to revert eventually to the parental bacterium. Also, changes in the composition and structure of lipoteichoic acid illustrates that the membrane is affected after *S. pyogenes* is converted to an L-form. Likewise, the ability of the L-form to increase the rigidity of its membrane permanently points to an adaptive capability that is noteworthy. Because of this change, the adaptation of an osmotically fragile L-form to grow in physiologically isotonic media was realized, suggesting the possible presence of an innate and perhaps rudimentary mechanism for survival (and eventual multiplication?) in vivo. The possibility of such an adaptation occurring in other "wall-less or defective" organisms is, therefore, inferred. In addition, the ability to bind to a variety of human cell monolayers and to destroy them, to survive in immunosuppressed mice, and to destroy glomeruli in tissue culture points to a cytotoxic capability and illustrates a potential for pathogenesis previously unrealized for an L-form. The continued synthesis of a greatly reduced but structurally altered lipoteichoic acid by the L-form suggests a vital role or need for this amphiphile which, at the moment, seems to be primarily associated with the adherence and destructive capabilities of this organism. From the data available, the function of the lipoteichoic acid within this L-form does not appear to be essential for the accumulation of necessary ions for metabolic purposes.

ACKNOWLEDGMENTS

Over the years these investigations have been supported by Public Health Grants (AI-11161 and AI-1117) from the National Institute of Allergy and Infectious Diseases and a contract (NR 136-756) from the Office of Naval Research.

REFERENCES

1. Klieneberger, E. (1935). The natural occurrence of pleuropneumoniae-like organisms in apparent symbiosis with *Streptobacillus moniliformis* and other bacteria. *J. Path. Bact. 40*:93–105.
2. Dienes, L. and Weinberger, H. J. (1951). The L-forms of bacteria. *Bacteriol. Rev. 15*:245–288.
3. Smith, P. F. (1971). Relationship of mycoplasmas to bacterial L-phase in *The Biology of Mycoplasmas* (P. F. Smith, ed.), Academic Press, New York, p. 16.
4. Hijmans, W. (1968). Present methods for the study of L-forms in *Current Research on Group A Streptococcus* (R. Caravano, ed.), Excerpta Medica Foundation, New York, pp. 305–312.
5. Ginsburg, I. (1972). Mechanisms of cell and tissue injury induced by group A streptococci: Relation to poststreptococcal sequelae. *J. Infect. Dis. 126*: 294–456.
6. Sharp, J. T., Hijmans, W., and Dienes, L. (1957). Examination of the L-forms of group A streptococci for the group-specific polysaccharide and M protein. *J. Exp. Med. 105*:153–159.
7. Panos, C., Barkulis, S. S., and Hayashi, J. A. (1959). Streptococcal L-forms II. Chemical composition. *J. Bacteriol. 78*:863–867.
8. Park, J. T. and Johnson, M. J. (1949). Accumulation of labile phosphate in *Staphylococcus aureus* grown in the presence of penicillin. *J. Biol. Chem. 179*:585–592.
9. Park, J. T. (1952). Uridine-5′-pyrophosphate derivatives. I. Isolation from *Staphylococcus aureus*. *J. Biol. Chem. 194*:877–884.
10. Park, J. T. (1952). Uridine-5′-pyrophosphate derivatives. II. A structure common to three derivatives. *J. Biol. Chem. 194*:885–895.
11. Park, J. T. (1952). Uridine-5′-pyrophosphate derivatives. III. Amino acid-containing derivatives. *J. Biol. Chem. 194*:897–904.
12. Edwards, J. and Panos, C. (1962). Streptococcal L-forms. V. Acid-soluble nucleotides of a group A streptococcus and derived L-form. *J. Bacteriol. 84*:1202–1208.
13. Slabyj, B. M. and Panos, C. (1973). Teichoic acid of a stabilized L-form of *Streptococcus pyogenes*. *J. Bacteriol. 114*:934–942.
14. Pandhi, P. N. and Panos, C. (1972). Biosynthesis of D-alanyl-D-alanine from L-alanine by extracts of a stabilized L-form from *Streptococcus pyogenes*. *J. Gen. Microbiol. 71*:487–494.
15. Platt, R. von. and Kandler, O. (1964). Vorkommen und Bedeutung der alanin-racemase bei *Proteus mirabilis*, dessen L-phasen und bei Mycoplasma. *Z. Naturforsch. 19b*:1135–1142.
16. Fodor, M. (1965). Studies on the cell wall mucopeptide synthesis of staphylococcal L-forms. *Naturwissenschaften 52*:522.
17. Chatterjee, A. N., Ward, J. B., and Perkins, H. R. (1967). Synthesis of mucopeptide by L-form membranes. *Nature 214*:1311–1314.

18. Cohen, M. and Panos, C. (1971). Cell wall polysaccharide biosynthesis by membrane fragments from *Streptococcus pyogenes* and stabilized L-form. *J. Bacteriol.* 106:347–355.
19. Reusch, V. M., Jr. and Panos, C. (1976). Defective synthesis of lipid intermediates for peptidoglycan formation in a stabilized L-form of *Streptococcus pyogenes*. *J. Bacteriol.* 126:300–311.
20. Ward, J. B. (1975). Peptidoglycan synthesis in L-phase variants of *Bacillus licheniformis* and *Bacillus subtilis*. *J. Bacteriol.* 124:668–678.
21. McCarty, M. (1959). The occurrence of polyglycerophosphate as an antigenic component of various gram-positive bacterial species. *J. Exp. Med.* 109:361–378.
22. Matsuno, T. and Slade, H. D. (1970). Composition and properties of a group A streptococcal teichoic acid. *J. Bacteriol.* 102:747–752.
23. Hijmans, W. (1962). Absence of the group-specific and the cell wall polysaccharide antigen in L-phase variants of group D streptococci. *J. Gen. Microbiol.* 28:177–179.
24. Smith, D. G. and Shattock, P. M. F. (1964). The cellular location of antigens in streptococci of groups D, N and Q. *J. Gen. Microbiol.* 34:165–175.
25. Jacques, N. A., Hardy, L., Campbell, L. K., Knox, K. W., Evans, J. D., and Wicken, A. J. (1979). Effect of carbohydrate source and growth conditions on the production of lipoteichoic acid by *Streptococcus mutans* Ingbritt. *J. Bacteriol.* 26:1079–1087.
26. Pratt, B. C. (1966). Cell-wall deficiencies in L-forms of *Staphylococcus aureus*. *J. Gen. Microbiol.* 42:115–122.
27. Maucks, J., Chan, L., and Glaser, L. (1971). Turnover of the cell wall of gram-positive bacteria. *J. Biol. Chem.* 246:1820–1827.
28. Reusch, V. M., Jr., and Neuhaus, F. C. (1971). D-alanine: membrane acceptor ligase from *Lactobacillus casei*. *J. Biol. Chem.* 246:6136–6143.
29. Linzer, R. and Neuhaus, F. C. (1973). Biosynthesis of membrane teichoic acid: a role for the D-alanine-activating enzyme. *J. Biol. Chem.* 248:3196–3201.
30. Panos, C., Fagan, G., and Zarkadas, C. G. (1972). Comparative electrophoretic and amino acid analyses of isolated membranes from *Streptococcus pyogenes* and stabilized L-forms. *J. Bacteriol.* 112:285–290.
31. Chevion, M., Panos, C., and Paxton, J. (1976). Membrane studies of *Streptococcus pyogenes* and its L-form growing in hypertonic and physiologically isotonic media: An electron spin resonance spectroscopy approach. *Biochim. Biophys. Acta* 426:288–301.
32. McCarty, M. (1964). The role of D-alanine in the serological specificity of group A streptococcal glycerol teichoic acid. *Proc. Natl. Acad. Sci. USA* 52:259–265.
33. Slade, H. D. and Shockman, G. D. (1963). The protoplast membrane and the Group D antigen of *Streptococcus faecalis*. *Iowa State J. Sci.* 38:83–96.

34. Neuhaus, F. C., Linzer, R., and Reusch, V. M., Jr. (1974). Biosynthesis of membrane teichoic acid: role of the D-alanine-activating enzyme and D-alanine:membrane acceptor ligase. *Ann. N.Y. Acad. Sci. 235*:502–518.
35. Chevion, M., Panos, C., Linzer, R., and Neuhaus, F. C. (1974). Incorporation of D-alanine into the membrane of *Streptococcus pyogenes* and its stabilized L-form. *J. Bacteriol. 120*:1026–1032.
36. Panos, C., Cohen, M., and Fagan, G. (1966). Lipid alterations after cell wall inhibition. Fatty acid content of *Streptococcus pyogenes* and derived L-form. *Biochemistry 5*:1461–1468.
37. Cohen, M. and Panos, C. (1966). Membrane lipid composition of *Streptococcus pyogenes* and derived L-forms. *Biochemistry 5*:2385–2392.
38. Panos, C. and Cohen, M. (1966). Cell wall inhibition in a stable streptococcal L-form. *Biochem. Biophys. Acta 117*:98–106.
39. Reusch, V. M., Jr. and Panos, C. (1977). Synthesis of "Group Polysaccharide" by membranes from *Streptococcus pyogenes* and its stabilized L-form. *J. Bacteriol. 129*:1407–1414.
40. Wicken, A. J. and Knox, K. W. (1975). Lipoteichoic acids: A new class of bacterial antigen. *Science 187*:1161–1167.
41. Wicken, A. J. and Knox, K. W. (1980). Bacterial cell surface amphiphiles. *Biochem. Biophys. Acta 604*:1–26.
42. Shockman, G. D. (1981). Cellular localization, excretion and physiological roles of lipoteichic acid in gram-positive bacteria in *Chemistry and Biological Activities of Bacterial Surface Amphiphiles* (G. D. Schockman and A. J. Wicken, eds.), Academic Press, New York, p. 21–40.
43. Ganfield, M-C.W. and Pieringer, R. A. (1975). Phosphatidylkojibiosyl diglyceride—the covalently linked lipid constituent of the membrane lipoteichoic acid from *Streptococcus faecalis (faecium)* ATCC 9790. *J. Biol. Chem. 250*:702–709.
44. Pieringer, R. A. and Ganfield, M-C.W. (1975). Phosphatidylkojibiosyl diglyceride: Metabolism and function as an anchor in bacterial cell membranes. *Lipid 10*:421–426.
45. Jackson, R. W. and Moskowitz, M. (1966). Nature of a red cell sensitizing substance from streptococci. *J. Bacteriol. 91*:2205–2209.
46. Moskowitz, M. (1966). Separation and properties of a red cell sensitizing substance from streptococci. *J. Bacteriol. 91*:2200–2204.
47. Knox, K. W. and Wicken, A. J. (1973). Immunological properties of teichoic acids. *Bacteriol. Rev. 37*:215–257.
48. Slabyj, B. M. and Panos, C. (1976). Membrane lipoteichoic acid of *Streptococcus pyogenes* and its stabilized L-form and the effect of two antibiotics upon its cellular content. *J. Bacteriol. 127*:855–862.
49. Rogers, H. J. and Perkins, H. R. (1968). *Cell Walls and Membranes*, E. and F. M. Spon Ltd., London.
50. Fischer, W., Ishizuka, I., Landgraf, H. R., and Herrmann, J. (1973). Glycerophosphoryl diglycosyl diglyceride, a new phosphoglycolipid from streptococci. *Biochem. Biophys. Acta 296*:527–545.

51. Ambron, R. T. and Pieringer, R. A. (1971). The metabolism of glyceride glycolipids. V. The identification of the membrane lipid formed from diglucosyl diglyceride in *Streptococcus faecalis* ATCC 9700 as an acylated derivative of glyceryl phosphoryl diglucosyl glycerol. *J. Biol. Chem. 246*: 4216-4225.
52. Pieringer, R. A. (1972). Biosynthesis of the phosphatidyl diglycosyl diglyceride of *Streptococcus faecalis* (ATCC 9790) from diglucosyl diglyceride and phosphatidyl glycerol or diphosphatidyl glycerol. *Biochem. Biophys. Res. Commun. 49*:502-507.
53. Lambert, P. A., Hancock, I. C., and Baddiley, J. (1977). Occurrence and function of membrane teichoic acids. *Biochim. Biophys. Acta 472*:1-12.
54. Maekawa, S. and Hayashi, T. A. (1973). L-phase variants of group A hemolytic streptococci not requiring high osmolarity. *Jpn. J. Microbiol. 17*: 228-229.
55. Gallin, J. L., Kaye, D., and O'Leary, W. M. (1969). Serum lipids in infection. *N. Engl. J. Med. 281*:1081-1086.
56. Rottem, S. (1979). Molecular organization of membrane lipids in *The Mycoplasmas I. Cell Biology* (M. F. Barile and S. Razin, eds.), Academic Press, New York, pp. 260-285.
57. Leon, O. and Panos, C. (1976). Adaptation of an osmotically fragile L-form of *Streptococcus pyogenes* to physiological osmotic conditions and its ability to destroy human heart cells in tissue culture. *Infect. Immun. 13*: 252-262.
58. Smith, P. F. and Rothblat, G. H. (1962). Comparison of lipid composition of pleuropneumonia-like and L-type organisms. *J. Bacteriol. 83*:500-506.
59. Gilpin, R. W., Young, F. E., and Chatterjee, A. N. (1973). Characterization of a stable L-form of *Bacillus subtilis* 168. *J. Bacteriol. 113*:486-499.
60. Rottem, S. and Panos, C. (1969). The effect of long chain fatty acid isomers on growth, fatty acid composition and osmotic fragility of *Mycoplasma laidlawii* A. *J. Gen. Microbiol. 59*:317-328.
61. Rottem, S. and Samuni, A. (1973). Effect of proteins on the motion of spin-labeled fatty acids in mycoplasma membranes. *Biochim. Biophys. Acta 298*:32-38.
62. Clasener, H. A., Ensering, H. L., and Hijmans, W. (1970). Persistence in mice of the L-phase of three streptococcal strains adapted to physiological osmotic conditions. *J. Gen. Microbiol. 62*:195-202.
63. Schmitt-Slomska, J., Bové, A., and Caravano, R. (1966). A carrier state in human diploid cell cultures infected with L-forms of group A streptococcus in *Current Research on Group A Streptococcus* (R. Caravano, ed.), Excerpta Medica Monograph, New York, pp. 352-359.
64. Schmitt-Slomska, J., Bové, A., and Caravano, R. (1972). Induction of L-variants in human diploid cells infected by group A streptococci. *Infect. Immun. 5*:389-399.
65. Green, M. T., Heidger, P. M., Jr., and Domingue, G. (1974). Demonstration of the phenomena of microbial persistence and reversion with bacterial L-forms in human embryonic kidney cells. *Infect. Immun. 10*:889-914.

66. Schmitt-Slomska, J., Sacquet, E., and Caravano, R. (1967). Group A streptococcal L-forms. I. Persistence among inoculated mice. *J. Bacteriol.* 93:451–455.
67. Denny, F. W., Jr. and Thomas, L. (1955). Persistence of group A streptococci in tissues of rabbits after infections. *Proc. Soc. Exp. Biol. Med. 88*: 260–263.
68. McGee, Z. A., Ratner, H. B., Bryant, R. E., Rosenthal, A. S., and Koenig, M. G. (1972). An antibody-complement system in human serum lethal to L-phase variants of bacteria. *J. Infect. Dis. 125*:231–242.
69. Muschel, L. H. and Jackson, J. E. (1966). The reactivity of serum against protoplasts and spheroplasts. *J. Immunol. 97*:46–51.
70. Montgomerie, J. Z., Kaplan, D., Schotz, M., and Guze, L. B. (1976). Effect of serum on phospholipids of L-forms of *Streptococcus faecalis*. *Infect. Immun. 14*:951–954.
71. Fernandes, P. B. and Panos, C. (1976). Persistence, pathogenesis and morphology of an L-form of *Streptococcus pyogenes* adapted to physiological isotonic conditions when in immunosuppressed mice. *Infect. Immun.* 14:1228–1240.
72. Winterbauer, R. H., Gutman, L. T., Turck, M., Wedgwood, R. J., and Petersdorf, R. G. (1967). The role of penicillin-induced bacterial variants in experimental pyelonephritis. *J. Exp. Med. 125*:607–618.
73. DeVuono, J. and Panos, C. (1978). Effect of L-form *Streptococcus pyogenes* and of lipoteichoic acid on human cells in tissue culture. *Infect. Immun. 22*:255–265.
74. Simpson, W. A., Dale, J. B., and Beachey, E. H. (1982). Cytotoxicity of the glycolipid region of streptococcal lipoteichoic acid for cultures of human heart cells. *J. Lab. Clin. Med. 99*:118–126.
75. Courtney, H. S., Simpson, W. A., and Beachey, E. H. (1983). Binding of streptococcal lipoteichoic acid to fatty acid-binding sites on human plasmic fibronectin. *J. Bacteriol. 153*:763–770.
76. Simpson, W. A., Ofek, I., and Beachey, E. H. (1980). Binding of streptococcal lipoteichoic acid to the fatty acid binding sites on serum albumin. *J. Biol. Chem. 255*:6092–6097.
77. Ofek, I., Beachey, E. H., Jefferson, W., and Campbell, G. L. (1975). Cell membrane-binding properties of group A streptococcal lipoteichoic acid. *J. Exp. Med. 141*:990–1003.
78. Beachey, E. H. (ed.) (1980). *Bacterial Adherence*, Chapman and Hall, New York.
79. Alkan, M., Ofek, I., and Beachey, E. H. (1977). Adherence of pharyngeal and skin strains of group A streptococci to human skin and oral epithelial cells. *Infect. Immun. 18*:555–557.
80. Leon, O. and Panos, C. (1983). Cytotoxicity and inhibition of normal collagen synthesis in mouse fibroblasts by lipoteichoic acid from *Streptococcus pyogenes*, type 12. *Infect. Immun. 40*:785–794.
81. Glassock, R. J. (1978). Pathology of basement membranes, alterations in diabetes and other disease states in *Biology and Chemistry of Basement Membranes* (N. A. Kefalides, ed.), Academic Press, New York, pp. 421–444.

82. Mims, C. A. (ed.) (1982). *The Pathogenesis of Infectious Disease*, Academic Press, New York, p. 185.
83. Tomlinson, K., Leon, O., and Panos, C. (1983). Morphological changes and pathology of mouse glomeruli infected with a streptococcal L-form or exposed to lipoteichoic acid. *Infect. Immun. 42*:1144–1151.
84. Goldschmidt, J. C., Jr. and Panos, C. (1984). Teichoic acids of *Streptococcus agalactiae*: Chemistry, cytotoxicity, and effect on bacterial adherence to human cells in tissue culture. *Infect. Immun. 43*:670–677.

5
L-Forms of *Bacillus*

RICHARD W. GILPIN*
Department of Microbiology and Immunology, The Medical College of Pennsylvania, Philadelphia, Pennsylvania

FRANK E. YOUNG†
Department of Microbiology, University of Rochester School of Medicine and Dentistry, Rochester, New York

I. Introduction	99
II. L-Form Induction and Reversion	100
III. *Bacillus* L-Form Replication	104
IV. L-Form Membrane Chemistry	108
V. *Bacillus* L-Form Genetics	117
VI. Concluding Remarks	120
References	121

I. INTRODUCTION

Research with L-forms of the *Bacillus subtilis* genospecies (*Bacillus subtilis, Bacillus licheniformis, Bacillus amyloliquifaciens,* and *Bacillus pumilus*) increased dramatically in recent years because *Bacillus* spp. have a cell wall that is less complex than the cell wall of gram-negative bacteria; chromosomal markers can be mapped by generalized and specialized transduction as well as by DNA-mediated transformation [1], and their cell wall can be removed by growth in the presence of penicillin [2] or by treatment with lysozyme, N-acetylmuramyl hydrolase [3]. Therefore this model system can be studied readily. Protoplasts resulting from these treatments can be induced to grow as L-form colonies that may or may not form a cell wall and revert to classical, cell

---

*Present affiliation: Department of Biochemistry, Jefferson Medical College, Thomas Jefferson University, Philadelphia, Pennsylvania
†Present affiliation: Office of the Commissioner, U.S. Food and Drug Administration, Washington, District of Columbia

wall-containing bacilli. L-form colonies that do not revert to bacilli are termed "stable L-forms," whereas those that do revert are termed "unstable L-forms."

II. L-FORM INDUCTION AND REVERSION

Landman and Halle [4] used penicillin or lysozyme to induce L-forms of *B. subtilis* by plating protoplasts on minimal salts agar medium containing an osmotic stabilizer (0.5 M sodium succinate). L-form colonies developed after 3 days of incubation at 30°C. The authors found that reversion was promoted on medium containing 2% agar or 30% gelatin, but medium containing lower concentrations of agar or gelatin promoted L-form growth instead. Reversion was also inhibited by several D-amino acids, D-methionine being the most effective. Ryter and Landman [5] observed irregularly shaped L-forms that reverted to bacilli by invagination of the membrane followed by synthesis of cell wall material and septa. Fodor and Rogers [6] found that L-forms induced from *B. licheniformis* with penicillin, cycloserine, or methicillin and transferred 15 times on agar medium with antibiotic would then grow without reversion after the antibiotic was omitted. If the concentration of agar was increased from 0.9 to 2.5%, however, some reversion did occur. They also observed that the parent bacillus and L-form would not form colonies where streak lines of the two organisms crossed. The inhibitory factor was associated with freeze-thaw extracts, but not with mechanically disrupted cell extracts of the parent bacillus. The factor was heat-labile and nondialyzable. Miller et al. [7] followed the stages of L-form induction in lysozyme-treated *B. subtilis* cultures. They found that bacilli first became osmotically sensitive, then they became spherical spheroplasts, and finally became protoplasts with no cell wall material on their surface. Bacilli in the spheroplast stage formed L-form colonies when cultured on agar medium containing D-methionine, but they reverted to bacilli on medium without D-methionine.

Burmeister and Hesseltine [8] found that *B. subtilis* NRRLB-3275 (*B. pumilus*, Ref. 9) could be induced to produce L-forms by growing the bacillus at room temperature in tryptone minimal salts broth medium containing 1.2 M NaCl. L-forms grew without reverting in medium containing 0.3 M NaCl. This was the first report of bacillus L-form induction in liquid medium without using cell wall antibiotics or enzymes. Dienes [10] reported the induction of *Bacillus* L-forms on agar medium containing 0.4 M NaCl and penicillin that subsequently became stable without reverting when penicillin was removed. He also reported that bacilli grown on high salt medium had a coiled, pleomorphic morphology even though they did not become L-forms. A similar morphology was found when *B. subtilis* BR151 was grown in tryptone liquid medium containing 1.2 M NaCl (Fig. 1). Young et al. [11] reported the induction of a stable L-form (*sal-1*) of *B. subtilis* 168 strain BR151 with or without treatment

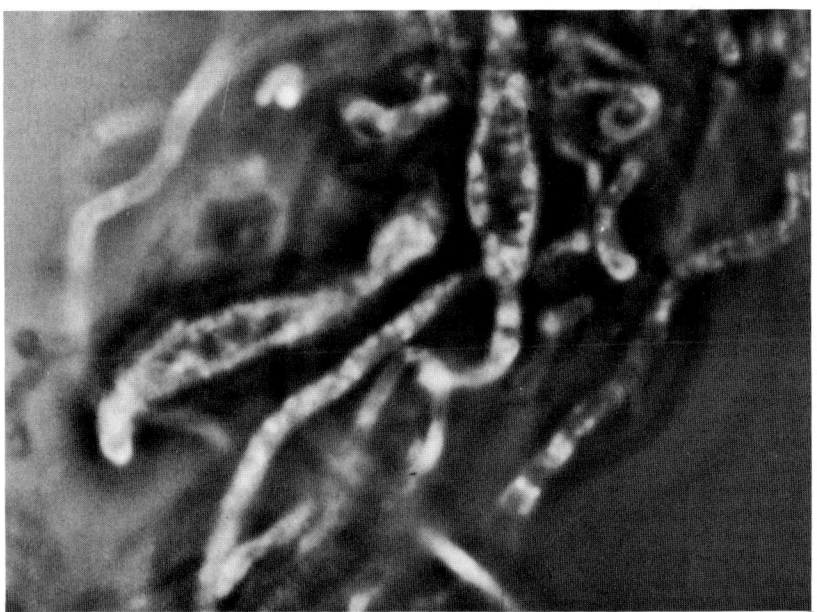

Figure 1 Morphology of *B. subtilis* strain BR151 grown in minimal salts medium containing 1.2 *M* NaCl. Magnification approximately × 3000.

with 100 µg of *N*-methyl-*N'*-nitro-*N*-nitrosoguanidine per milliliter followed by incubation with 200 µg of lysozyme per milliliter and plating on agar medium containing 2000 U of penicillin per ml. Clones were adapted to liquid minimal salts tryptone medium containing 1.2 *M* NaCl. After many subcultures, *sal-1* did not revert when penicillin was omitted from the medium. Lovett [12] also reported the induction of L-forms from *B. pumilus* using a high concentration of NaCl in liquid medium. These L-forms reverted when the NaCl concentration was decreased to 0.5 *M*. This *B. pumilus* BpBl strain had a high rate of spontaneous mutation at certain areas of the chromosome, which might have contributed to the relative ease of L-form induction. Forsberg and Ward [13], working with penicillin-induced L-forms of *B. licheniformis* maintained in osmotically stabilized liquid medium containing methicillin, found that *N*-acyl muramyl-L-alanine amidase was associated with the cytoplasmic membrane fraction of lysed L-forms. They found no detectable muramic acid or diaminopimelic acid associated with these membranes. The authors also reported that *N*-acyl muramyl-L-alanine amidase activity [13] was associated with protoplast and mesosome membrane fractions isolated on sucrose density gradients. L-form colonies produced zones of clearing, an indication of autolytic activity, on osmotically stabilized agar containing procion red-conjugated cell walls. Therefore, it was highly probable that the membrane-associated amidase activity was also present on the membranes of intact L-forms. Forsberg and Ward also found that membranes from lysed L-forms had a low level of autolytic activity unless the membranes were first treated with 0.05% Triton X-100. When L-form membranes were washed with buffer alone, protein was slowly removed, but amidase activity remained. If $MgSO_4$ was added to the buffer, protein loss decreased and so did autolysin activity. The addition of 1 M NaCl to the buffer during the membrane washing step resulted in a greatly increased level of autolytic activity when the membranes were assayed in the presence of Triton X-100. Washing L-form membranes in 1.5 M NaCl or 3.0 M LiCl did not remove autolytic activity from the membranes. Washing with sodium lauryl sulfate or Sarkosyl produced a loss of amidase activity. The authors also found that L-forms grown in the presence of *B. licheniformis* cell walls did not revert to bacilli. But there was a substantial transfer of autolytic activity from the L-forms to the cell walls. The authors concluded that the amidase was bound to L-form membranes by nonionic bonds, which permitted its transfer to cell walls where it formed ionic bonds. Wyrick and Rogers [14] found that lysozyme-protoplasts of *B. subtilis* and *B. licheniformis* became stable L-forms when plated and transferred for several months on minimal salts agar medium with methicillin and 0.5 M sodium succinate for osmotic stabilization. These stable L-forms would also grow in liquid medium without reverting. Soft agar overlays, containing 3 mg/ml of procion-conjugated cell walls from *B. licheniformis*, placed over stable L-form colonies resulted in zones of clearing around the colonies. The authors suggested that the L-forms produced autolytic enzyme even though they did not produce any biochemically detectable cell wall polymer.

Wyrick and Rogers [14] followed the reversion of unstable *B. licheniformis* L-forms by electron microscopy. The first visible sign of reversion was the presence of electron-dense material, external to the membrane, that became thicker and ultimately resulted in the formation of rod-shaped bacilli with the usual cell wall morphology. Elliott et al. [15] studied teichoic acid and peptidoglycan synthesis during reversion of lysozyme-induced protoplasts of *B. licheniformis* plated on agar medium supplemented with radioactively labeled N-acetylglucosamine. Peptidoglycan with a short chain length was produced during the early stages of reversion. Peptidoglycan later increased in length and in the extent of peptide cross-linking between adjacent chains. Soluble peptidoglycan isolated from the reversion medium seemed to be a product of autolysis and not excreted cell wall precursor. Elliott et al. [16] used ferritin-conjugated anti-peptidoglycan antibody and freeze-etch techniques to study reverting protoplasts. They discovered that protoplasts synthesized lysozyme-sensitive cell wall polymer at an earlier stage of reversion than was previously detected by electron microscopic observation of thin sections.

Landman and Forman [17] found that casein hydrolysate enhanced reversion if protoplasts were incubated on 2.5% gelatin-containing minimal medium. Chloramphenicol, puromycin, and actinomycin D blocked the reversion-stimulatory effect of casein hydrolysate, but penicillin or lysozyme did not. The authors concluded that protein and RNA synthesis was required to produce the casein hydrolysate-stimulated reversion. Once casein hydrolysate-treated protoplasts were placed on gelatin medium, however, reversion was not inhibited by chloramphenicol. Reversion was delayed, however, by puromycin, actinomycin, penicillin, or cycloserine. Chloramphenicol and puromycin inhibit protein synthesis, but their specific modes of action are quite different. Treatment of cell wall-containing bacteria with 100 μg/ml of chloramphenicol often resulted in the formation of thick, lysozyme-resistant cell walls. The inability of chloramphenicol to inhibit the later stages of reversion may be related to its ability to promote the overproduction of peptidoglycan.

Clive and Landman [18] found that reversion of *B. subtilis* L-forms could be stimulated by autoclaved bacteria or boiled cell wall preparations. Landman et al. [19] summarized their research by concluding that induction of unstable L-forms of *B. subtilis* did not have a genetic origin because the L-forms reverted after penicillin or lysozyme was removed from the culture. They proposed that cell wall residues may act as a primer for reversion and that incubation of L-forms with casein hydrolysate would stimulate reversion at a faster rate. At high protoplast concentrations, however, reversion to bacilli was inhibited. The inhibitory factor was heat-sensitive, nondialyzable, sensitive to 0.4% sodium laural sulfate, Pronase, and trypsin, but not to 0.1% Triton X-100. Because 600 μg of trypsin per milliliter stimulated reversion, they suggested that the reversion inhibitor was a protein related to cell wall autolytic enzyme. DeCastro-Costa and Landman [20] found that *B. subtilis* protoplasts would revert more rapidly when trypsin or Pronase was added to the casein hydrolysate-containing reversion medium. They found that reversion was inhibited by β-mercapto-ethanol, which they suggested was a result of a stimulation of the rate of autolysis of newly synthesized cell wall polymer. The authors proposed that protoplasts secrete autolysin (amidase), which may delay or prevent the accumulation of a threshold level of peptidoglycan required for reversion. Therefore, manipulations that would decrease or block autolytic activity during the early stages of reversion would accelerate the reversion process.

L-forms may be placed into two groups, those that become stable and those that are unstable (revert back to bacillary morphology). The former seem to have a phenotypic or genetic block because they do not revert under conditions that promote reversion of unstable L-forms (2.5% agar, 25% gelatin, trypsin, Pronase, reduction of salt concentration, addition of autoclaved bacteria, or boiled cell walls). Evidence for a defect in cell wall synthesis among stable L-forms of *B. subtilis* and *B. licheniformis* comes from the work of Ward [21].

He isolated seven different L-forms that would grow on antibiotic-free minimal salts liquid medium containing 0.5 M sodium succinate for osmotic stabilization. No muramic acid or diaminopimelic acid was found in membrane hydrolysates of these L-forms. Uridine diphosphate (UDP) nucleotides were accumulated by all L-forms, but the length of the peptide chain associated with UDP-N-acetylmuramic acid was variable. Adding cloxacillin or D-cycloserine to these cultures did not alter these results. Ward measured several enzymes associated with cell wall biosynthesis and found that the L-forms were blocked at various stages of the cell wall synthesis. The most common block (six of the seven L-forms) was in the synthesis of cytoplasmic, cell wall nucleotide precursers. Ward placed the stable L-forms into three groups: two groups (six L-forms) were blocked at the cytoplasmic level (either diaminopimelic acid synthesis or L-alanine addition); the third group consisting of one L-form was blocked at the step where the cytoplasmic cell wall nucleotide precurser is incorporated into the membrane-bound lipid intermediate. Other stable L-forms isolated from *B. subtilis* are blocked at other locations, however. The *sal-1* L-form of *B. subtilis* BR151 does not accumulate any detectable nucleotide precursers even when penicillin G, vancomycin, or bacitracin are added to the culture [22]. A similar lack of accumulation results with D-cycloserine added to the *sal-1* cultures (S. Patterson and R. Gilpin, unpublished results). Although further proof is needed, there is support for the notion that the stable L-form phenotype may have a genetic basis.

III. *BACILLUS* L-FORM REPLICATION

Much of the theory on L-form division was developed during earlier work with mycoplasma and some species of L-forms [23] and will not be reviewed here. The findings from work with *Bacillus* L-forms are similar to previous reports on other L-forms. Most of the information has come from electron microscopic observations of thin sections [5,14,22,24]. Electron microscopic studies suggest that the L-forms are not always spherical [5] (S. Patterson and R. Gilpin, unpublished data). If this is not an artifact due to the fixation procedure, it would seem to imply that L-forms retain some mechanical rigidity on the cytoplasmic membrane, so that cytoplasm can be pinched off by closure of the membrane. Ryter and Landman [5] found that thin sections of small bodies (sometimes referred to as elementary bodies) 100-300 nm diameter did not contain nuclear material. The cytoplasm of large bodies 10-20 μm in diameter (sometimes called mother cells) resembled the density of lysed protoplasts. The authors concluded that the large bodies and small elementary bodies were not capable of replication. They suggested that L-forms replicated by constriction of the membrane. Cytoplasm and nuclear material seemed to be pinched off in a disorganized fashion, however, so that some of the L-forms were viable but others were nonviable. Burmeister and Hesseltine [8] supported the more established theory of L-form replication and suggested that small bodies at the limit of the resolving power of the light microscope were indeed viable units. Their support for this conclusion was based on cell counts of a bacillus L-form growing in liquid culture. Their colony-forming unit data were always 1000-fold greater than the number of large bodies that they counted by direct cell counts. Gilpin et al. [22], however, found that direct cell counts of *sal-1* L-form cultures increased in parallel with the colony-forming units. In addition, the direct counts were twofold greater than the viable counts. It is quite probable that discrepancies between results of direct cell counts and viable counts are related to the limitations of the techniques used to monitor the growth of L-forms [25] and not to major differences between modes of cell division among various L-form isolates. Wyrick and Rogers [14] examined ultrathin serial sections of an L-form large body and found that there were small, individual, elementary bodies within vacuoles. The authors felt these could not have resulted from portions of pinched off filaments or buds extending away from the large body that had fallen back into the large body during the fixation procedure.

The evaluation of cell division among such flexible microorganisms is difficult with electron microscopic techniques because membranes may change their position during the fixation steps. Using different cryoprotective agents and fixation methods, Higgins et al. [26] found that bacterial mesosome membranes appeared to change position and/or morphology depending on the preparation method used. However fixation of prechilled samples appears to preserve a close-to-life topology of the mesosomal membrane of bacterial cells and presumably will do the same for the membrane of L-forms [27]. Phase-contrast observations of samples from L-form batch cultures have resulted in various theories about L-form cell division. The only reproducible event that can usually be found is a progression from phase-dark, apparently viable L-forms, to large, phase-light spheres that eventually become membrane ghosts containing no phase-dark material (see Fig. 5 in Ref. 22; Fig. 2 in Ref. 28).

Gilpin and Patterson [29] were able to adapt the *sal-1* stable L-form of *B. subtilis* BR151 to growth in liquid medium without osmotic protection. This L-form was designated *sig-1*. No muramic acid, glucosamine, or diaminopimelic acid was detected by amino acid analysis of *sig-1* L-form membranes. In addition, no lysozyme-sensitive residue was found on membranes treated with chloroform: methanol (2:1, v/v), formamide, and trypsin. To obtain a clearer understanding of the mechanism of L-form cell division, a microscope slide culture chamber was designed that permitted continuous observation of *sig-1* multiplication in liquid medium for a period of several days [30]. Time-lapse photography was used to follow L-form growth in liquid medium [28]. The L-forms divided by a "budding-like" mechanism quite similar to the "disorganized constriction" described by Ryter and Landman [5]. It was possible to determine which L-forms were viable by looking for production of L-form daughter cells that would also produce progeny of a similar size class. It was concluded that the *sig-1* L-form had lost the ability to coordinate cell division because the membrane pinched off prematurely in many instances, creating small, nonviable vesicles that did not produce progeny. The *sig-1* L-forms began as individual cells (Fig. 2) which grew by pinching off progeny in linear chains [28] with no evidence of chain branching (S. Patterson and R. Gilpin, unpublished results). After a few days, the chains became quite long and drifted around in the liquid medium. Ultimately, a mass of intertwined L-form material was formed (Fig. 3). We believe that this type of growth may be common to other L-forms, and may explain the type of colony growth associated with L-forms. The chains of L-forms may grow into the agar and become entangled in the agar matrix so that removal of L-forms from the surface of the agar becomes quite difficult.

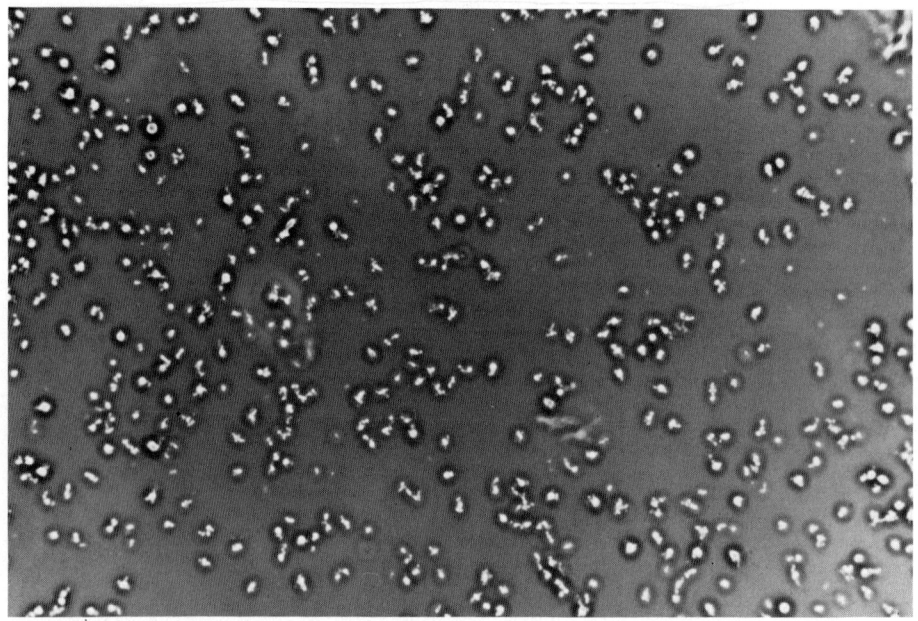

Figure 2 Phase-contrast photomicrograph of *sig-1* after incubation for 12 hr in a microculture chamber containing minimal salts liquid medium (see Ref. 28). The phase-dark L-forms were printed from a second negative and therefore appear phase-light for better contrast. Magnification approximately × 1000.

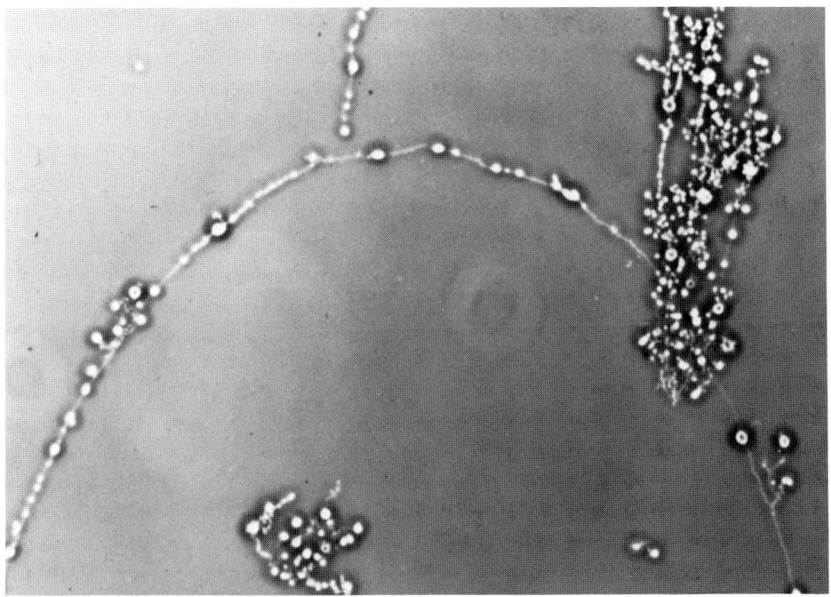

Figure 3 Phase-contrast photomicrograph of *sig-1* after incubation for 18 hr. (See Fig. 2 legend for details.)

Further circumstantial evidence against the involvement of large bodies and elementary bodies in L-form division came from our continuous culture study (S. Patterson and R. Gilpin, unpublished results). *Sig-1* L-forms maintained in the exponential phase of growth in a turbidostat for periods of up to 8 days ranged in size from 2 to 4 μm and showed no evidence of lysis or the formation of large bodies. If large bodies participated in the cell division process, they should have appeared during this relatively long period of observation. These experiments were performed with a small fermenter (Mini-Ferm, model M-1000, Fermentation Design, Inc., Allentown, Pennsylvania) with a 500-ml culture vessel connected to a pump that added minimal salts medium, supplemented with 0.01% gelatin to retard L-form growth up the walls, at the rate of 45 ml/hr. L-forms and medium were removed by gravity flow from an outlet at the surface of the culture. Viable counts remained constant during the 8-day period and the OD_{600} of the culture remained at 0.2 ± 0.02. This study did not preclude the possibility of large bodies or elementary bodies participating in the L-form division process, however, because it was not possible to prove that these morphological structures were physiologically inactive. This system was useful for obtaining large quantities of exponential-phase L-forms for other research projects.

IV. L-FORM MEMBRANE CHEMISTRY

Most research on *B. subtilis* L-form membrane composition and physiology has centered on the role of membrane components in the induction and reversion process discussed above. Other aspects have received some attention, however.

For example, how do stable L-forms survive and multiply in osmotically unprotected liquid culture medium that produces immediate lysis of protoplasts? Possible explanations include: (1) the presence of some new membrane polymer, which is unlikely; (2) a change in the relative amounts of one or more membrane polymers; or (3) an increased rate of membrane synthesis to compensate for expansion of the cytoplasmic volume produced by the influx of water. Several authors have characterized the chemical composition of *B. subtilis* protoplast and/or L-form membranes [29,31–39]. *Bacillus* L-forms may contain more of some phospholipids and less triglycerides than their protoplast counterparts (S. Horowitz, doctoral thesis, Univ. of Louisville, 1980), but there does not seem to be a direct correlation between lipid content and membrane turgor [40]. Membrane-bound protein has been implicated as an important factor in the mechanical strength of membranes, however [41–43].

To find out whether changes in L-form membrane protein composition accompanied an increase in osmotic stability, a stable L-form of *B. subtilis* strain BR151 (*sal-1*) was adapted to minimal salts medium without NaCl by serial transfers into medium containing decreasing amounts of NaCl [29]. The osmotically unprotected L-form (*sig-1*) was found to be at least twofold more resistant to osmotic shock by dilution in hypotonic buffer than the original *sal-1* L-form. Two additional L-forms of *B. subtilis* strain BR151 were isolated by mutagenesis or lysozyme treatment. After many transfers on minimal salts agar medium containing 1.0 M sucrose plus penicillin G or cycloserine, the two L-forms became stable and would not revert. Subsequently, these two L-forms (*sig-2* and *sig-3*) could also be adapted to growth in minimal salts medium without the osmotic protection provided by the sucrose (S. Patterson and R. Gilpin, unpublished results).

All of the *B. subtilis* BR151 L-forms could be adapted to growth in liquid medium at 50°C and in minimal salts medium containing 45 µg/ml of the ionic detergent, sodium dodecyl sulfate. Preliminary protein analysis of membranes isolated from L-forms grown with osmotic protection (1.2 M NaCl or 1.0 M sucrose) indicated that they contained less protein per milligram of membrane than the L-forms which had been adapted to hypotonic minimal salts medium (S. Patterson and R. Gilpin, unpublished observations). Although L-forms grown without osmotic protection seemed to be more osmotically stable, growth per se does not mean that their membranes were physically stronger. The twofold increase in susceptibility of *sig-1* to bacitracin and vancomycin, antibiotics known to bind membrane [44], lends circumstantial support to the idea that

L-FORMS OF BACILLUS 109

there was some change in membrane structure or permeability that was not present among *sal-1* membranes. *Sig-1* does not have the five membrane-associated proteins [45] that bind radioactive penicillin in *B. subtilis* (C. Buchanan, personal communication). The significance of this observation is not known.

Protoplast membranes from a variety of bacillus species when examined by the negative-stained smear technique often possess strikingly regular tiered strands on their outer surfaces. These are most prominent on the membranes of growing protoplasts (unstable L-forms). These protease resistant strands are made up of stacked rings, an appearance that has earned them the working name "monorails" [46]. They are resistant to lysozyme digestion and their formation seems resistant to penicillin but sensitive to novobiocin, bacitracin, and tunicamycin. When purified by mild procedures and concentrated, these monorails aggregate into longer strands and net-like structures and can be labeled with radioactive glycerol (P. Fitz-James, unpublished observation). They are suspected of being lipoteichoic acid (see Chaps. 4 and 6). Monorails have been found on the membranes of all gram-positive bacilli and several clostridia.

The surface of *sal-1* is well covered with monorails. In the lysed and protease-digested membrane residue, they can be seen both free and in a mat-like formation (Fig. 4a), which has also been observed on the surface of reverting unstable L-forms of *B. megatherium* KM (P. Fitz-James, unpublished observation). These structures can be separated from the membranes by the EDTA washing procedure of Hughes et al. [47] and when concentrated by ultrafiltration appear in the smears to be free or in varying degrees of aggregation (Fig. 4b).

Free monorails were also found in the lysed residues of *sig-1* but here they appear to be adherent to or running out of denser wall-like sheets (Fig. 4c). In the concentrates of the EDTA washes of *sig-1* membranes, matted monorails appeared to form sheets mixed with other materials and could be more clearly detected only in thinner areas (Fig. 4d, e).

These smear data suggest that monorails or lipoteichoic acid polymers may self-assemble or complex with other extracellular products to form a wall substitute on the surface of *sal-1* and *sig-1* L-forms. A careful thin-section comparison of the *sal-1* and *sig-1* surface with that of the protoplast of *B. subtilis* indicated surface material on the L-forms that was not evident on the protoplast. Faint strands of material occasionally were seen streaming from the surface of protoplasts of *B. subtilis*. Both the intact protoplast and its ghost showed the typical asymmetrical membrane profile, the outer leaflet being slightly wider than the inner (Fig. 5a).

Thin-section profiles of the surface of both *sal-1* and *sig-1* L-forms show varying amounts of accumulation on the membrane surface. On *sal-1* the accumulations were poorly organized and showed fibrous extensions and some

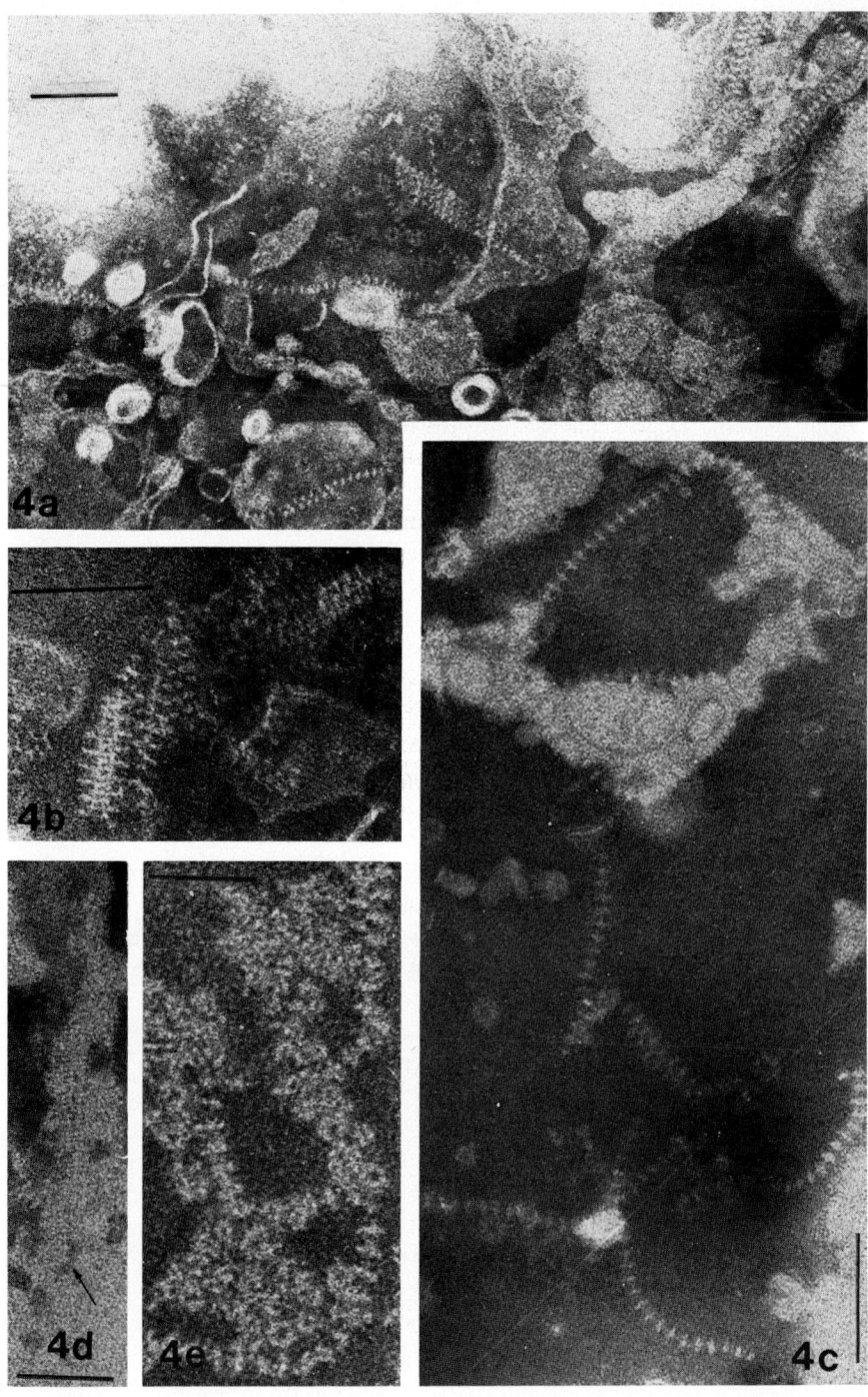

30-40 nm off the surface (Fig. 5b). The surface of *sig-1*, on the other hand, possessed a serrated profile of material organized into a well defined essentially continuous "wall." Unlike the typical peptidoglycan wall, this presumably teichoic acid-based wall was deposited directly on and seemed to be part of the outer membrane surface. This wall–membrane complex thus also formed the surface of the ghost forms present in the same sample (Fig. 5a).

Sal-1 does excrete large amounts of lipoteichoic acid-like material into the culture medium (A. Wicken, personal communication). So there is chemical evidence that this type of polymer is present, and if not all of it is excreted, it may play a role in the mechanical strength of these L-form membranes. It has become apparent that membranes of stable L-forms must undergo a variety of pleomorphic changes during the induction process and that these changes need to be studied further before any conclusions about osmotic stability can be reached.

Sodium dodecyl sulfate polyacrylamide gel electrophoresis (SDS-PAGE) can be used to study changes in L-form membrane protein composition. One disadvantage of the method is that SDS dissociates membrane proteins into polypeptides which may lack biological activity. One way to avoid this problem is to use a nonionic detergent such as Triton X-100, which permits isolation of membrane proteins with biological activity [49]. Polyacrylamide gel electrophoresis of acidified phenol extracts of intact L-forms and mycoplasma was used by Theodore et al. [50] to identify the parentage of L-forms by comparing their protein patterns with those derived from protoplasts of classical bacteria. A similar method was used to compare the proteins from the *sal-1* L-form with protoplasts of the parent bacillus [22]. Although the protein bands migrated to similar positions in the gels, there were large differences between the relative staining intensities (amounts of protein) of various bands (Fig. 6). The L-form protein bands showed a pronounced shift toward higher-molecular-weight,

---

Figure 4 *Sal-1* and *sig-1* surface structures in thin section. Negative-stained (1% phosphotungstic acid, pH 6.4 with KOH) electron micrographs of membrane fractions of *B. subtilis* stable L-forms; magnification markers are 100 nm, except Fig. 4d which is 50 nm. (*a*) Protease-digested membrane residue of *sal-1* showing single and aggregated monorails and membrane remnants. (*b*) Matted monorails typical of an ultrafiltration concentrate of an EDTA (0.003 *M*) wash of membranes of *sal-1*. (*c*) Protease-digested residue of *sig-1* membranes showing monorails free and apparently associated with wall-like sheets. (*d*) The monorails can be seen faintly (arrow) in the wall pieces that were separated from the membrane by EDTA extraction and ultrafiltrate concentrated. (*e*) In less well-organized pieces of residue, the monorail components were slightly more obvious.

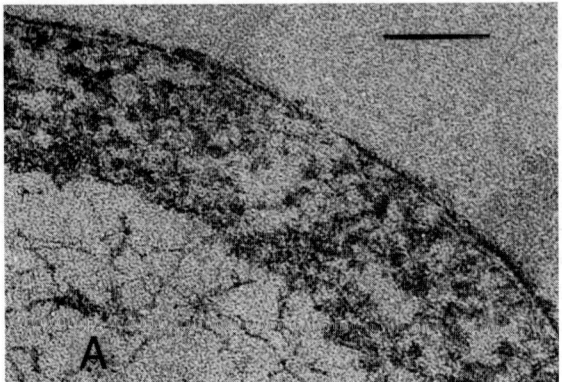

Figure 5 *Sal-1* and *sig-1* surface structures using negative staining. Electron micrographs of thin section of L-forms of *Bacillus subtilis*. The L-forms were fixed with glutaraldehyde, dehydrated in acetone, saturated with uranyl acetate, embedded in Vestopal and sectioned; sections were stained with lead citrate [48]. The bars denote 100 nm. (*A*) The membrane of a *B. subtilis* protoplast (unstable L-form) growing in *sig-1* minimal medium is relatively clear of surface accumulations. (*B*) The surface of *sal-1* L-forms growing in agar (or in fluid) medium is well endowed with surface accumulations forming a loose wall-like layer. (*C*) On *sig-1* L-forms the surface accumulations are well organized into a definite wall layer, closely applied, and often obscuring the outer surface of the membrane. The opposed arrows indicate the membrane layer in a ghost profile.

slower migrating bands. To compare membrane-associated proteins without interference by the quantitatively larger amounts of protein in the cytoplasm, we studied L-form membranes prepared by an osmotic shock method similar to that of Rottem et al. [51]. L-forms were sedimented at 10,000 g for 15 min, suspended with a Teflon pestle in buffer containing 2 M glycerol, and incubated for 10 min to allow time for the glycerol to diffuse into the L-forms. This was followed by rapid dilution in a large volume of ice-cold saline to rupture the membranes osmotically. After standing for 15 min, the L-form membranes were harvested by centrifugation at 30,000 g for 30 min. The membrane proteins were dissociated by the method of Fairbanks [52] and applied to gels prepared by the procedure of Weber and Osborn [53]. This procedure was used to compare SDS-PAGE membrane proteins of *B. subtilis* BR151 L-forms adapted to growth in minimal salts medium containing various concentrations of NaCl or 1% sucrose (Fig. 7). This illustrates a typical band pattern from samples that were run simultaneously and repeated several times on different days. Only one protein band, a high-molecular-weight band near the top of the gels (arrow), was

L-FORMS OF BACILLUS

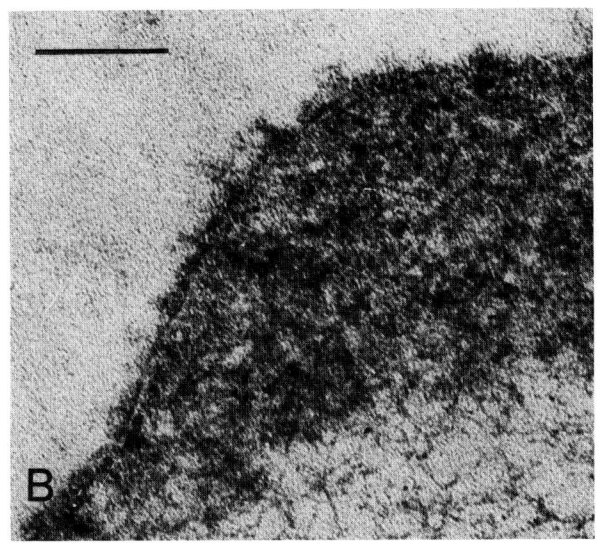

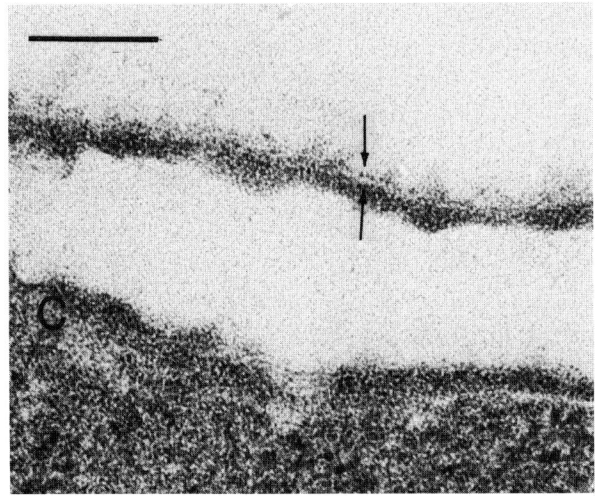

found at the same position on all of the gels. The band patterns obtained from samples of L-form cultures grown under the same conditions were quite reproducible, but the growth phase of a culture was found to affect the band pattern. The pattern from an exponential-phase culture of *sig-1* in minimal salts medium differs from the pattern of a 40-hr late stationary-phase culture (Fig. 7). Since

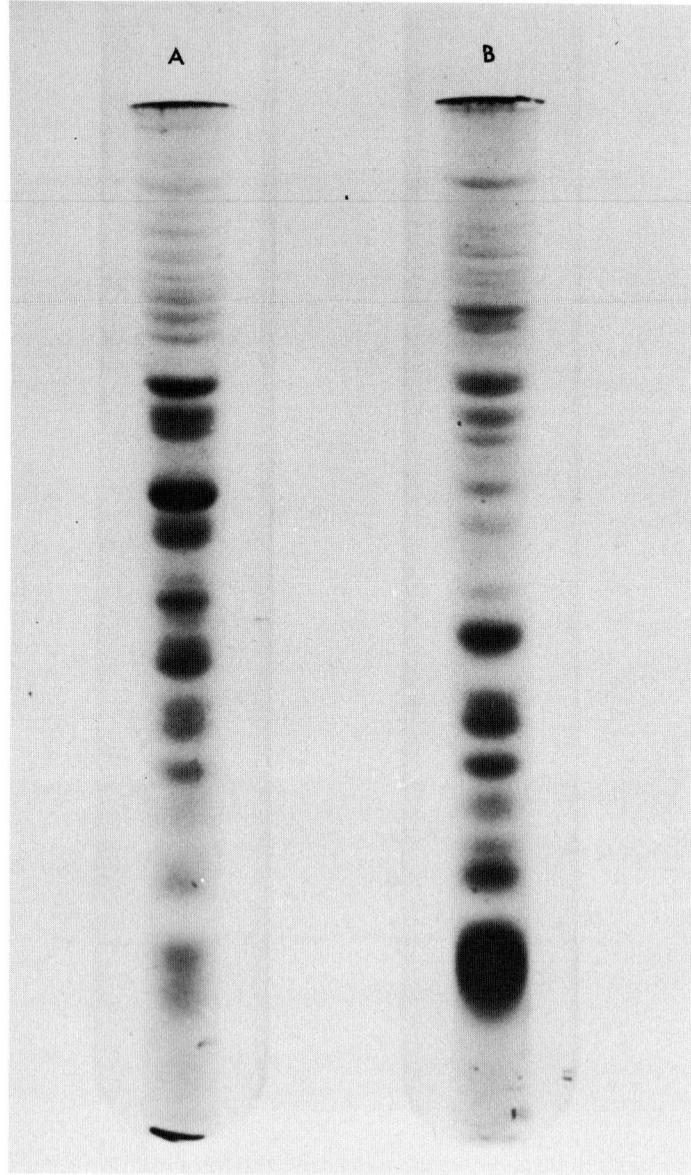

Figure 6 SDS-PAGE protein bands of intact *sal-1* forms (*A*) and bacillus protoplasts (*B*) grown in minimal salts medium containing 1.2 M NaCl or minimal salts medium alone, respectively.

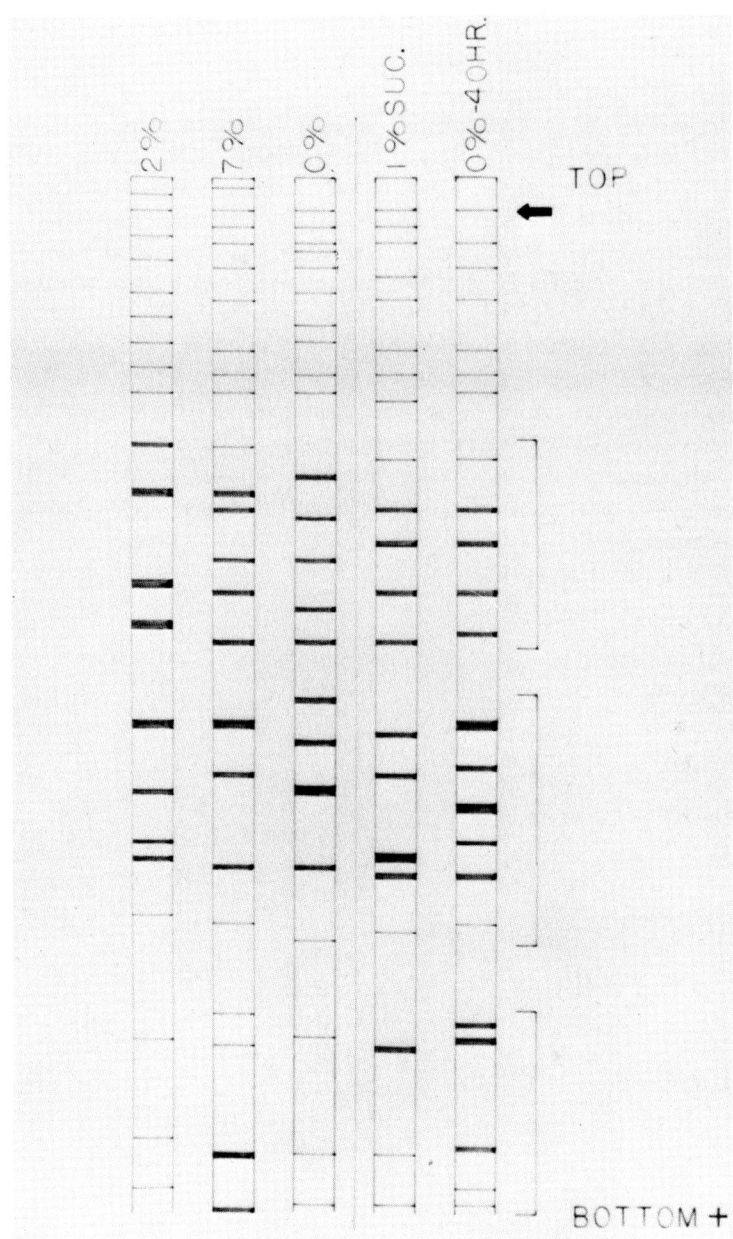

Figure 7 Line drawings of SDS-PAGE membrane protein bands of exponential-phase *sig-1* cultures grown in minimal salts medium containing 2, 7, or 0% NaCl, or 1% sucrose. The band pattern of a 40-hr late stationary-phase *sig-1* culture grown in minimal salts medium without NaCl is shown on the right-hand gel drawing.

membrane protein band patterns may reflect underlying changes in the physiology of L-forms, we also used this method to study the effects of antibiotics on membrane proteins. *Sig-1* L-forms were grown in minimal salts medium with experimentally determined sub-growth-inhibitory levels of two antibiotics, bacitracin (50 µg/ml) or vancomycin (200 µg/ml). Samples were removed at 2-hr intervals for analysis. Membranes from L-form cultures treated with bacitracin or vancomycin had a higher protein content than untreated, control cultures (Table 1). SDS-PAGE band densities and migration distances were the same in all samples except for the uppermost of the nine major bands located in the middle portion of the gels. This band was significantly larger ($p < 0.01$) in 9-hr samples of untreated L-form cultures and in samples taken at all times from vancomycin-treated cultures (Fig. 8). Bacitracin-treated cultures did not show any significant changes. The lack of major changes in either apparent molecular size (migration distance) or quantity (staining intensity), except for one band, was quite surprising. Mattingly et al. [54] found that vancomycin may specifically inhibit RNA and protein synthesis, so we suspect that our finding

Table 1 Protein Content of *sig-1* Membranes from Cultures Treated With Subinhibitory Antibiotics

Culture (hr)[a]	Growth rate[b]	OD_{600}	µg Protein/OD[c]
Control	3.0		
3		0.06	47
5		0.09	49
7		0.14	51
9		0.19	54
Bacitracin	2.3		
3		0.08	39
5		0.13	32
7		0.19	40
9		0.19	90
Vancomycin	2.7		
3		0.07	48
5		0.10	53
7		0.16	51
9		0.21	82

[a] Samples were removed from L-form cultures in minimal salts medium without antibiotic (control) or with 50 µg/ml of bacitracin or 200 µg/ml of vancomycin. The end of exponential-phase growth occurred at 7 hr.
[b] Doubling time in hours.
[c] L-forms were lysed by osmotic shock, membranes were isolated, and the amount of protein was determined. Membrane protein concentration was related to the OD_{600} of the culture sample.

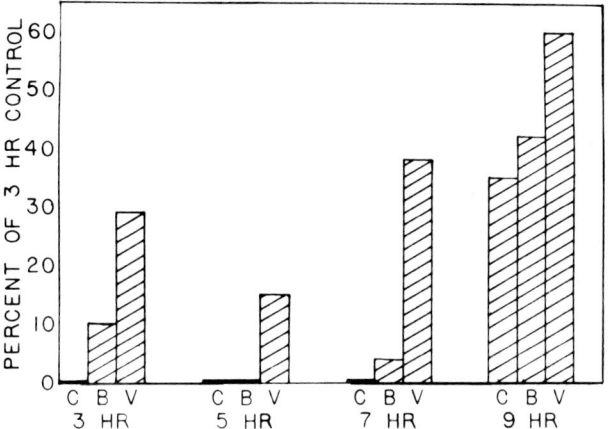

Figure 8 Histogram of the amounts (densitometric peak areas) of protein in SDS-PAGE band one (uppermost of the nine major membrane protein bands, center gel of Fig. 7) relative to the peak area of band one from a 3-hr culture sample of *sig-1* grown in minimal salts medium without NaCl. The percent change in band one peak area is shown for each of the sampling times (3, 5, 7, 9 hr) for untreated (C), bacitracin-treated (B), and vancomycin-treated (V) cultures of *sig-1*.

may be a reflection of this type of interaction. The SDS-PAGE method has several limitations, as discussed above, but it does provide a facile method to monitor changes among L-form membrane proteins. The use of more sophisticated techniques such as spin-labeling and specific labeling of inner and outer membrane proteins should greatly expand our knowledge of L-form membrane structure (see Chap. 4).

V. *BACILLUS* L-FORM GENETICS

In 1973, two groups of researchers, Wyrick et al. [55] and Bettinger and Young [56], described the use of DNA derived from L-forms as donor in DNA-mediated transformation of competent bacilli. Wyrick et al. [55] used purified DNA isolated from a *B. subtilis* 168 *trp* C2 stable L-form to transform two competent recipients derived from *B. subtilis* 168. Recombinants prototrophic for adenine and thymine were isolated on minimal salts medium containing 0.5 M succinate for osmotic protection, but without antibiotics. L-form colonies were isolated from about 10% of the total number of transformants on this medium. The L-form colonies retained the auxotrophic markers of the bacillary recipient from which they were derived. Recipient bacilli did not produce

L-form colonies on this medium unless transformed. The authors concluded that the stable L-form phenotype was transferred by the exogenous L-form DNA added during transformation. In a similar study, Levin and Landman [57] reported that competent *B. subtilis* recipients produced L-form colonies on osmotically stabilized media at a greater rate (26% vs. 3%) when exposed to purified DNA from L-forms during DNA-mediated transformation experiments. Therefore, they tentatively established a relationship between transformation and induction of L-forms.

Bettinger and Young [56] reported that DNA isolated by gentle lysis of the *sal-1* L-form resulted in transformation efficiencies for single markers that were 10–30 times higher than the efficiency obtained with DNA isolated by the usual phenol extraction method [58]. In addition, gently lysed L-form DNA transformed unlinked auxotrophic markers at a frequency greater than would be expected by congression (uptake of more than one strand of DNA by each recipient bacillus). Some transformants also had unusual colony morphologies resembling the cell division mutants isolated by Boylan et al. [59]. Streips and Young [60] constructed a strain of *B. subtilis* (RUB 758) *pur* A, *leu*, *met* B10 that could not be transformed by DNA excreted by several noncompetent mutants or by strain BR151. RUB 758 could be transformed, however, by phenol-extracted bacterial or phage DNA, and by DNA isolated by gentle lysis of *sal-1* L-forms. Bettinger and Young [61] extended their previous transformation results with DNA isolated from the *sal-1* L-form to also include DNA isolated by gentle lysis of lysozyme-induced protoplasts. The greater transforming efficiency for single markers and for previously unlinked markers was not affected by incubating the DNA for 30 min at 37°C with Pronase, trypsin, or ribonuclease. Only deoxyribonuclease significantly reduced the transformation frequency. In another series of experiments, incubation of phenol-extracted DNA with L-form lysate DNA did not produce an increase in the resultant transformation frequency for the *met* marker above that found when phenol-extracted DNA was used alone. It was also found that lysate DNA would bind more efficiently than phenol-extracted DNA to competent recipient bacilli, because lysate DNA would reduce the transforming frequency of markers on the phenol-extracted DNA by one-half, even when the lysate DNA was present at a sixfold lower concentration. Clearly, gentle lysis of L-forms or protoplasts provides a novel source of unfragmented, native DNA that can transform single or multiple markers with high efficiency, as predicted by Young et al. [11] in 1970.

An important new approach to the understanding of cell division in L-forms was reported in 1979 by Horowitz et al. [62]. These authors tested the idea that lack of coordinated cell division in L-forms is related to loss of one or more components of the cell division complex. The *sal-1* L-form of *B. subtilis* was grown in minimal salts medium containing 1.2 M NaCl plus radioactive thymidine to label the DNA. The parent bacillus, BR151 trp C2, *lys*-3, *met* B10, was changed to *met* B10 alone (BUL404) so that its genotype would be the same as that of *sal-1*. Protoplasts of BUL404 containing thymidine-labeled DNA were produced by lysozyme treatment. L-form or protoplast membranes were lysed and run on Renografin density gradients. Both the L-form and protoplast membranes had the same relative amounts of labeled DNA associated with their membranes. When the membrane-DNA complexes were analyzed for enrichment of auxotrophic markers usually associated with the replication origin and terminus in *B. subtilis* [63], it was discovered that only L-form membranes lacked markers associated with the chromosome terminus. Both the loss of the cell wall and growth in 1.2 M NaCl could have contributed to loss of terminus attachment in these cells [64]. The authors speculated that this loss could result in abnormal DNA segregation. Sargent [65] found that replication of a region at or close to the chromosome terminus was needed for the control of membrane synthesis. Lack of coordinated control over membrane synthesis may explain some of the unusual L-form morphologies that have been reported for many years. The nature of the membrane-associated component needed for binding of the chromosome terminus in this system has not been elucidated.

Another observation that may greatly expand our knowledge of L-form physiology was recently reported by White et al. [66]. These authors reported that the *sal-1* L-form can be transfected with DNA isolated from bacteriophages ϕ125, ϕ1, and ϕ29, if the reaction is performed in buffer containing 40% polyethylene glycol. This transfection process is sensitive to DNase up to 100 min following addition of the DNA. It has not been possible, however, to saturate the system with transfecting DNA, so there may either be some DNA binding to nonviable L-forms or degradation of DNA by nucleases from L-forms. Incoming DNA can be protected if cationic polypeptides are added to the DNA prior to transfection [67]. Transfection of the L-form is followed by phage replication, because samples of the phage DNA/L-form incubation mixture added to phage-sensitive bacilli produce plaques after 1 hr. There is a steady increase in plaque-forming units vs. time after the eclipse period. The indicator bacillus cannot be transfected by phage DNA, so the phage seems to have been produced in the cytoplasm of the L-form. *Sal-1* could also be infected by intact ϕ25 or ϕ29 phage in the presence of 40% polyethylene glycol, but only a single burst of phage was produced. We have found that batch cultures of *sal-1* in minimal salts medium may only produce two generations of progeny, so it is unlikely that a sustained production of phage could occur. This study provides the first evidence that exogenous DNA can be introduced into L-forms. Plasmid DNA can be introduced into L-forms by the same route (U. Streips, unpublished results). This may have important ramifications in the field of recombinant DNA, since gene products produced in the cytoplasm of L-forms could be readily isolated by lysing the L-forms. The lack of cell wall in these lysates facilitates the separation of wanted gene products and precludes the immunologic reactions associated with cell wall polymer.

In addition to the use of L-forms in genetic experiments, it is possible to introduce chromosomal or plasmid DNA into protoplasts of *B. subtilis* [68,69], followed by regeneration of the protoplasts through L-forms back to the bacillary form. Furthermore, protoplasts can be used directly to provide a mixing of genomes with subsequent regeneration to the bacillary form [70].

VI. CONCLUDING REMARKS

Research with L-forms of the *B. subtilis* genospecies is currently on the verge of a renaissance of renewed interest because of the many important findings that have been reported in the past few years. We have attempted to summarize much of this information in this chapter. It is apparent that N-acyl-muramyl-L-alanine amidase activity may influence the reversion of L-forms to the bacillary form. Formation of stable L-forms (unable to revert to bacilli) may in some cases have a genetic origin. The cell wall synthesis pathway may be blocked at the cytoplasmic or membrane-associated level. The mechanism of L-form division and the existence of a life cycle involving small elementary bodies and larger mother cells has not been completely resolved. The evidence, however, seems to point to binary fission with a lack of coordination between chromosome division and cytoplasmic division. This may be the result of, or accompanied by loss of, membrane attachment of the chromosome terminus. The ability of some stable L-forms to become adapted to medium without osmotic stabilizer may be related to their formation of a "substitute" cell wall. This may consist entirely or in part of lipoteichoic acid. Identification of the parentage of an L-form may be possible by comparing its SDS-PAGE whole-cell protein band patterns with those from protoplasts of suspected parent bacteria. The SDS-PAGE band patterns of L-form membrane-associated protein show more variation than the patterns from whole cells. Membrane protein patterns seem to be influenced by environmental conditions and the physiological state of the L-forms. The genetic manipulation of L-forms has progressed rapidly with the discovery that L-form lysate DNA serves as an excellent donor in DNA-mediated transformation of competent bacilli. The transfer of chromosomal and plasmid DNA into protoplasts of *Bacillus* indicates that such manipulations may be possible with L-form recipients. The successful transfection, plasmid transformation, and direct phage infection of a *Bacillus* L-form have laid the groundwork for such manipulations.

Future work with *Bacillus* L-forms is promising because of the broad background knowledge about genetic mapping and DNA transfer among members of this genospecies. L-forms may be used as propagators of recombinant DNA molecules, and they may be important to the study of chromosomal attachment and DNA replication. Studies of the excretion of extracellular enzymes, the mechanisms of cell wall synthesis, regulation of cell division, and membrane chemistry may be advanced by using genetic manipulation techniques on stable L-forms of the *B. subtilis* genospecies.

ACKNOWLEDGMENTS

The authors wish to thank Dr. Philip Fitz-James, Department of Microbiology and Immunology, University of Western Ontario Health Sciences Centre, London, Ontario, Canada, for his generous contribution to the L-form membrane chemistry section of this chapter. Portions of the works presented were supported in part by the Biomedical Research Support Grant Program and grants AI-10141, AI-10093, AI-07211, and GM-40845 from the Public Health Service, National Institutes of Health.

REFERENCES

1. Young, F. E. and Wilson, G. A. (1975). Chromosomal map of *Bacillus subtilis* in *Spores VI* (P. Gerhardt, R. N. Costilow, and H. L. Sadoff, eds.), Amer. Soc. for Microbiology, Washington, pp. 596–614.
2. Pierce, C. H. (1942). *Streptobacillus moniliformis*, its associated L form and other pleuropneumonia-like organisms. *J. Bacteriol. 43*:780.
3. Gooder, H. and Maxted, W. R. (1961). External factors influencing structure and activities of *Streptococcus pyogenes* in *Microbial Reaction to Environment* (G. G. Meynell and H. Gooder, eds.), Cambridge University Press, Cambridge, pp. 151–173.
4. Landman, O. E. and Halle, S. (1963). Enzymically and physically induced inheritance changes in *Bacillus subtilis. J. Mol. Biol. 7*:721–738.
5. Ryter, A. and Landman, O. E. (1964). Electron microscope study of the relationship between mesosome loss and the stable L state (or protoplast state) in *Bacillus subtilis. J. Bacteriol. 88*:457–467.
6. Fodor, M. and Rogers, H. J. (1966). Antagonism between vegetative cells and L-forms of *Bacillus licheniformis* strain 6346. *Nature 211*:658–659.
7. Miller, I. L., Zsigray, R. M., and Landman, O. E. (1967). The formation of protoplasts and quasi-spheroplasts in normal and chloramphenicol-pretreated *Bacillus subtilis. J. Gen. Microbiol. 49*:513–525.
8. Burmeister, H. R. and Hesseltine, C. W. (1968). Induction and propagation of a *Bacillus subtilis* L form in natural and synthetic media. *J. Bacteriol. 95*:1857–1861.
9. Lovett, P. S. and Young, F. E. (1969). Identification of *Bacillus subtilis* NRRLB-3275 as a strain of *Bacillus pumilus. J. Bacteriol. 100*:658–661.
10. Dienes, L. (1970). Alterations of the L-forms of a sporebearing bacillus. *J. Bacteriol. 104*:1378–1385.

11. Young, R. E., Haywood, P., and Pollock, M. (1970). Isolation of L-forms of *Bacillus subtilis* which grow in liquid medium. *J. Bacteriol.* 102:867–870.
12. Lovett, P. S. (1972). Spontaneous auxotrophic and pigmented mutants occurring at high frequency in *Bacillus pumilus* NRRLB-3275. *J. Bacteriol.* 112:977–985.
13. Forsberg, C. W. and Ward, J. B. (1972). N-acetylmuramyl-L-alanine amidase of *Bacillus licheniformis* and its L-form. *J. Bacteriol.* 110:878–888.
14. Wyrick, P. B. and Rogers, H. J. (1973). Isolation and characterization of cell wall-defective variants of *Bacillus subtilis* and *Bacillus licheniformis*. *J. Bacteriol* 116:456–465.
15. Elliott, T. S. J., Ward, J. B., and Rogers, H. J. (1975). Formation of cell wall polymers by reverting protoplasts of *Bacillus licheniformis*. *J. Bacteriol.* 124:623–632.
16. Elliott, T. S. J., Ward, J. B., Wyrick, P. B., and Rogers, H. J. (1975). Ultrastructural study of the reversion of protoplasts of *Bacillus licheniformis* to bacilli. *J. Bacteriol.* 124:905–917.
17. Landman, O. E. and Forman, A. (1969). Gelatin-induced reversion of protoplasts of *Bacillus subtilis* to the bacillary form: Biosynthesis of macromolecules and wall during successive steps. *J. Bacteriol.* 99:576–589.
18. Clive, D. and Landman, O. E. (1970). Reversion of *Bacillus subtilis* protoplasts to the bacillary form induced by exogenous cell wall, bacteria and by growth in membrane filters. *J. Gen. Microbiol.* 61:233–243.
19. Landman, O. E., DeCastro-Costa, M. R., and Bond, E. C. (1977). Mechanisms of stability and reversion of mass conversion stable L-forms of *Bacillus subtilis* in *Microbiology 1977* (D. Schlessinger, ed.), Amer. Soc. for Microbiology, Washington, pp. 35–43.
20. DeCastro-Costa, M. R. and Landman, O. E. (1977). Inhibitory protein controls the reversion of protoplasts and L-forms of *Bacillus subtilis* to the walled state. *J. Bacteriol.* 129:678–689.
21. Ward, J. B. (1975). Peptidoglycan synthesis in L-phase variants of *Bacillus licheniformis* and *Bacillus subtilis*. *J. Bacteriol.* 124:668–678.
22. Gilpin, R. W., Young, F. E., and Chatterjee, A. N. (1973). Characterization of a stable L-form of *Bacillus subtilis* 168. *J. Bacteriol.* 113:486–499.
23. Roux, J. (1960). La multiplication des formes L. *Annal. Inst. Pasteur* 99:286–296.
24. Bisset, K. A., Tallack, J., and Bartlett, R. (1979). Electron microscopy of the L-cycle in *Bacillus licheniformis* var. *endoparasiticus* (Benedek). *J. Med. Microbiol.* 12:469–472.
25. Gilpin, R. W., Patterson, S. K., and Knight, R. A. (1981). Quantitation of *Bacillus subtilis* L-form growth parameters in batch culture. *J. Bacteriol.* 145:651–653.
26. Higgins, M. L., Tsien, H. C., and Daneo-Moore, L. (1976). Organization of mesosomes in fixed and unfixed cells. *J. Bacteriol.* 127:1519–1523.

27. Fooke-Achterrath, M., Lickfield, K. G., Reusch, Jr., V. M., Aebi, U., Tschope, U., and Menge, B. (1974). Close-to-life preservation of *Staphylococcus aureus* mesosomes for transmission electron microscopy. *J. Ultrastruct. Res. 49*:270-285.
28. Gilpin, R. W. and Nagy, S. S. (1976). Time-lapse photography of *Bacillus subtilis* L-forms replicating in liquid medium. *J. Bacteriol. 127*:1018-1021.
29. Gilpin, R. W. and Patterson, S. K. (1976). Adaptation of a stable L-form of *Bacillus subtilis* to minimal salts medium without osmotic stabilizers. *J. Bacteriol. 125*:845-849.
30. Nagy, S. S. and Gilpin, R. W. (1976). Design of a microculture chamber to observe cell division of bacterial L-forms in liquid medium. *Appl. Environ. Microbiol. 31*:444-445.
31. Bishop, D. G., Rutberg, L., and Samuelsson, B. (1967). The chemical composition of the cytoplasmic membrane of *Bacillus subtilis*. *Eur. J. Biochem. 2*:448-453.
32. Ehrstrom, M., Eriksson, L. E. G., Israelachvili, J., and Ehrenburg, A. (1973). The effects of some cations and anions on spin labeled cytoplasmic membranes of *Bacillus subtilis*. *Biochem. Biophys. Res. Commun. 55*:396-402.
33. Ellwood, D. C., Turner, W. H., Hunter, J. R., and Moody, G. R. G. (1969). Changes in the cell-wall composition of a strain of *Bacillus subtilis* grown in a chemostat. *Biochem. J. 113*:27-28.
34. Kuska, I. (1974). Effect of glucose on the biosynthesis of the membranes of bacillus. *Biochim. Biophys. Acta 345*:62-73.
35. Lillich, T. T. and White, D. C. (1971). Phospholipid metabolism in the absence of net phospholipid synthesis in a glycerol-requiring mutant of *Bacillus subtilis*. *J. Bacteriol. 107*:790-797.
36. Minnikin, D. E. and Abdolrahimzadeh, H. (1974). Effect of pH on the properties of polar lipids, in chemostat cultures of *Bacillus subtilis*. *J. Bacteriol. 120*:999-1003.
37. Op den Kamp, J. A. F., Redai, I., and vanDeenen, L. L. M. (1972). Phospholipid composition of *Bacillus subtilis*. *J. Bacteriol. 99*:298-303.
38. Tria, E. and Scanu, A. M. (1969). Structural and functional aspects of lipoproteins in living systems in *Bacterial Phospholipids and Membranes* (J. A. F. Op den Kamp, L. L. M. vanDeenen, and V. Tomasi, eds.), Academic, New York, pp. 227-235.
39. van Iterson, W. and Op den Kamp, J. A. F. (1969). Bacteria-shaped gymnoplasts (protoplasts) of *Bacillus subtilis*. *J. Bacteriol. 99*:304-315.
40. Eisenberg, A. D. and Corner, T. R. (1973). Osmotic behavior of bacterial protoplasts: Temperature effects. *J. Bacteriol. 114*:1177-1183.
41. Corner, T. R. and Marquis, R. E. (1969). Why do bacterial protoplasts burst in hypotonic solutions? *Biochim. Biophys. Acta 183*:544-558.
42. Marquis, R. E., Porterfield, N., and Matsumura, P. (1973). Acid-base titration of streptococci and the physical states of intracellular ions. *J. Bacteriol. 114*:491-498.
43. Ruwort, M. J. and Haug, A. (1975). Membrane properties of *Thermoplasma acidophila*. *Biochemistry 14*:860-866.

44. Ward, J. B. (1974). The synthesis of peptidoglycan in an autolysin-deficient mutant of *Bacillus licheniformis* NCTC 6346 and the effect of β-lactam antibiotics, bacitracin and vancomycin. *Biochem. J. 141*:227–241.
45. Buchanan, C. E. and Strominger, J. L. (1976). Altered penicillin-binding components in penicillin-resistant mutants of *Bacillus subtilis. Proc. Natl. Acad. Sci. USA 73*:1816–1820.
46. Fitz-James, P. C. (1974). Discussion in *Mode of Action of Antibiotics on Microbial Walls and Membranes*, vol. 235 (M. R. J. Salton and A. Tomasz, eds.), Annals N.Y. Acad. of Sciences, New York, pp. 345–346.
47. Hughes, A. H., Hancock, I. C., and Baddiley, J. (1973). The function of teichoic acids in cation control in bacterial membranes. *Biochem. J. 132*: 83–93.
48. Maniloff, J. (1978). Molecular biology of mycoplasma in *Microbiology, 1978* (D. Schlessinger, ed.), Amer. Soc. for Microbiology, Washington, pp. 390–393.
49. Gulik-Krzywicki, T. (1975). Structural studies of the associations between biological membrane components. *Biochim. Biophys. Acta 415*:1–28.
50. Theodore, T. S., Tully, J. G., and Cole, R. M. (1971). Polyacrylamide gel identification of bacterial L-forms and *Mycoplasma* species of human origin. *Appl. Microbiol. 21*:272–277.
51. Rottem, S., Stein, O., and Razin, S. (1968). Reassembly of *Mycoplasma* membranes disaggregated by detergents. *Arch. Biochem. Biophys. 125*: 46–56.
52. Fairbanks, G., Steck, T., and Wallach, D. (1971). Electrophoretic analysis of the major polypeptides of the human erythrocyte membrane. *Biochemistry 10*:2606–2617.
53. Weber, K. and Osborn, M. (1969). The reliability of molecular weight determinations by dodecyl-sulfate polyacrylamide gel electrophoresis. *J. Biol. Chem. 244*:4406–4412.
54. Mattingly, S. J., Daneo-Moore, L., and Shockman, G. D. (1977). Factors regulating cell wall thickening and intracellular iodophilic polysaccharide storage in *Streptococcus mutans. Infect. Immun. 16*:967–973.
55. Wyrick, P. B., McConnell, M., and Rogers, H. J. (1973). Genetic transfer of the stable L-form state to intact bacterial cells. *Nature 244*:505–507.
56. Bettinger, G. E. and Young, F. E. (1973). Transformation of *Bacillus subtilis* using gently lysed L-forms; a new mapping technique. *Biochem. Biophys. Res. Commun. 55*:1105–1111.
57. Levin, B. C. and Landman, O. E. (1973). Relation between autolytic activity and transformation in *Bacillus subtilis*. Abstr. Ann. Meeting, Amer. Soc. for Microbiol., Abstr. #G192:58.
58. Yasbin, R. E. and Young, F. E. (1972). The influence of temperate bacteriophage φ105 on transformation and transfection in *Bacillus subtilis. Biochem. Biophys. Res. Commun. 47*:365–371.
59. Boylan, R. J., Mendelson, N. H., Brooks, D., and Young, F. E. (1972). Regulation of the bacterial cell wall: Analysis of a mutant of *Bacillus subtilis* defective in biosynthesis of teichoic acid. *J. Bacteriol. 110*:281–290.

60. Streips, U. N. and Young, F. E. (1974). Transformation in *Bacillus subtilis* using excreted DNA. *Mol. Gen. Genet. 133*:47–55.
61. Bettinger, G. E. and Young, F. E. (1975). Transformation of *Bacillus subtilis*: transforming ability of deoxyribonucleic acid in lysates of L-forms or protoplasts. *J. Bacteriol. 122*:987–993.
62. Horowitz, S., Doyle, R. J., Young, F. E., and Streips, U. N. (1979). Selective association of the chromosome with membrane in a stable L-form of *Bacillus subtilis. J. Bacteriol. 138*:915–922.
63. Hye, R. J., O'Sullivan, M. A., Howard, K., and Sueoka, N. (1976). Membrane association of origin, terminus and replication fork in *Bacillus subtilis* in *Microbiology 1976* (D. Schlessinger, ed.), Amer. Soc. Microbiol., Washington, pp. 83–90.
64. Streips, U. N., Horowitz, S., and Doyle, R. J. (1980). Genetic analysis of DNA-surface interactions in *Bacillus subtilis* in *Microbiology 1980* (D. Schlessinger, ed.), Amer. Soc. Microbiol., Washington, pp. 284–287.
65. Sargent, M. G. (1975). Control of membrane protein synthesis in *Bacillus subtilis. Biochim. Biophys. Acta 406*:564–574.
66. White, T. B., Doyle, R. J., and Streips, U. N. (1981). Transformation of an L-form form *Bacillus subtilis* with bacteriophage deoxyribonucleic acid. *J. Bacteriol. 145*:878–883.
67. White, T. B. and Streips, U. N. (1982). Parameters of transfection of an L-form from *Bacillus subtilis* in *Genetic Exchange* (U. N. Streips, S. H. Goodgal, W. R. Guild, and G. A. Wilson, eds.), Marcel Dekker, New York, pp. 153–162.
68. Chang, S. and Cohen, S. (1979). High frequency transformation of *Bacillus subtilis* protoplasts by plasmid DNA. *Mol. Gen. Genet. 168*:111–115.
69. Levi-Meyrueis, C., Fodor, K., and Schaeffer, P. (1980). Polyethyleneglycol-induced transformation of *Bacillus subtilis* protoplasts by bacterial chromosomal DNA. *Mol. Gen. Genet. 179*:589–594.
70. Gabor, M. H. and Hotchkins, R. D. (1982). Analysis of randomly picked genetic recombinants from *Bacillus subtilis* protoplast fusion in *Genetic Exchange* (U. N. Streips, S. H. Goodgal, W. R. Guild, and G. A. Wilson, eds.), Marcel Dekker, New York, pp. 283–292.
71. Domingue, G. J. (ed.) (1982). *Cell Wall-deficient Bacteria: Basic Principles and Clinical Significance*, Addison-Wesley, Reading, Massachusetts.

6
β-Lactam-Induced *Proteus* L-Forms

JEAN-MARIE GHUYSEN and MARTINE NGUYEN-DISTECHE
Department of Microbiology, University of Liège, Liège, Belgium

ANDRÉ ROUSSET*
Department of Bacteriology, University of Strasbourg, Strasbourg, France

I. Introduction: Mycoplasmatales and L-Forms	128
II. The Cell Envelope of the Gram-Negative Enterobacteria	129
A. Structure	129
B. DD-Peptidases	134
C. Penicillin Binding Proteins (PBPs)	138
III. The Cell Envelope of the Rod-Shaped *Proteus*	140
A. Peptidoglycan	140
B. Outer Membrane	141
C. PBPs and DD-Peptidases	142
IV. The Cell Envelope of β-Lactam-Induced L-Forms of *Proteus*	143
A. Conversion of *Proteus* to L-Form Growth	143
B. Unstable Spheroplast L-Forms of *P. mirabilis*	146
C. Stable Spheroplast L-Forms of *P. mirabilis*	150
D. Stable Protoplast L-Forms of *P. mirabilis* and *P. vulgaris*	151
V. Conclusions	156
References	158

---

*Present affiliation: Department of Bacteriology, University of Dijon, Dijon, France

I. INTRODUCTION: MYCOPLASMATALES AND L-FORMS

The mycoplasmatales, classified into the genera *Mycoplasma, Acholeplasma, Ureaplasma*, and *Spiroplasma*, form a large and heterogeneous group of wall-less prokaryotes. They occur widely in nature and have been isolated from humans, animals, plants, and insects.

The mycoplasmatales differ from the other prokaryotes not only by their complete lack of a cell wall but also by other profound cellular alterations. They are the smallest organisms capable of independent division; they have a genome of much reduced size; they lack several sequences in their 16S rRNAs and several proteins related to membrane functions; and most (but not all) species require cholesterol for growth.

The mycoplasmatales might form a separate phylogenetic class of eubacteria [1]. Thus, the extant representatives would be the surviving descendants of very primitive cells that existed before the development of a peptidoglycan-based cell wall. Alternatively, comparative enzyme immunological and other studies [2] suggest that the mycoplasmatales might have evolved from wall-containing gram-positive bacteria belonging in particular to the genera *Bacillus, Lactobacillus*, and *Streptococcus*. Mycoplasmatales are agents of (human, animal, and plant) diseases for which there are no counterpart bacterial diseases, suggesting that in their transition from wall-containing to wall-less eubacteria, their ancestors have gained new capacities for pathogenicity.

L-forms are "modern" wall-less or wall-deficient eubacteria. They can be produced from a large number of bacterial taxa through the action of wall peptidoglycan-degrading enzymes (glycosidases, peptidases and N-acetylmuramyl-L-alanine amidases) or antibiotics that inactivate the wall peptidoglycan-synthesizing enzyme machinery. The L-forms do not show those profound cellular alterations found in the mycoplasmatales. They resemble the normal bacteria from which they originate except for physical and chemical changes that permitted transition to life in the form of wall-less or wall-deficient bacteria (see Chap. 1).

Penicillins, whose original molecule stems back to Fleming's discovery in 1928, cephalosporins, and other β-lactams are wall peptidoglycan inhibitors that are massively used in medicine, stock farming, and the cultured fish industry. The ability of these antibiotics to induce conversion of penicillin-sensitive bacteria to penicillin-resistant wall-less or wall-deficient L-forms may have important, practical implications in chemotherapy.

The aim of this chapter is to review the various types of L-forms that proteus, a rod-shaped, gram-negative enterobacterium, produces in responses to the action of β-lactam antibiotics.

II. THE CELL ENVELOPE OF THE GRAM-NEGATIVE ENTEROBACTERIA

A. Structure

The cell envelope in all gram-negative bacteria is a multilayered structure in which the peptidoglycan is sandwiched between the inner plasma membrane and an outer membrane. There have been several reviews [3,4] and books [5,6] on these bacterial cell envelopes and the reader is referred to them for specific information. We will summarize their most relevant properties, using *Escherichia coli* as model.

1. Peptidoglycan

The peptidoglycan is a network structure (Fig. 1). Essentially, the glycan moiety consists of linear strands of alternate pyranoside residues of N-acetylglycosamine and N-acetylmuramic acid linked together by 1-4,β-bonds; the D-lactyl group of the N-acetylmuramic acid is substituted by a tetrapeptide L-Ala-γ-D-Glu(L)-meso-A_2pm-(L)-D-Ala; and tetrapeptides substituting adjacent glycan strands are covalently linked together by D-alanyl-(D)-meso-A_2pm linkages. The average glycan chain length is (depending on the authors) between 30 and 60 disaccharide

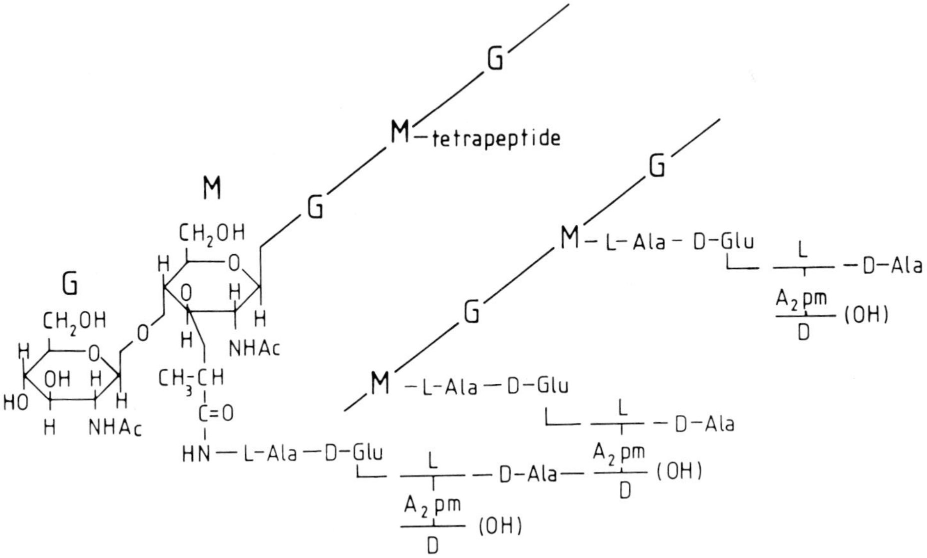

Figure 1 Structure of the peptidoglycan in gram-negative bacteria, showing sections of two glycan chains, a tetrapeptide unit, and a cross-linked peptide dimer. G = N-acetylglucosamine; M = N-acetylmuramic acid.

units and the chains are terminated by a nonreducible 1,6-anhydro-N-acetylmuramic acid residue (Fig. 2). The peptidoglycan is weakly peptide cross-linked. Approximately equal amounts of uncross-linked tetrapeptide units and the dimer of this unit make up the bulk of the peptide moiety. About 5% of the total peptide units occur as trimers and about 2-3% of the total N-acetylmuramic acid residues are substituted by truncated dipeptides L-Ala-γ-D-Glu.

2. Outer Membrane

The outer membrane is a phospholipid-lipopolysaccharide-protein structure stabilized by Mg^{2+} cations (Fig. 3). It contributes to the mechanical strength of the cell envelope and provides the bacteria with an additional permeability barrier.

The lipopolysaccharide molecules (Fig. 4) of the outer membrane are polysaccharide chains covalently linked to an unique lipid, known as lipid A. Typically, the polysaccharide moiety is composed of superficial O-antigen chains that cover the exterior of the cell, and a core that is characterized by the presence of two unique sugars in it, L- or D-glycero-D-mannoheptose and 2-keto-3-deoxyoctonate. The core is, in turn, linked to lipid A, the backbone of which is a disaccharide of D-glucosamine with the specific 3-D-hydroxymyristic acid in an amide linkage to the amino groups and with long-chain fatty acids in ester linkages to the hydroxyl groups.

The phospholipid molecules of the outer membrane are, in composition, qualitatively similar to those of the inner plasma membrane. Phosphatidylethanolamine and phosphatidylglycerol are the major constituents; small amounts

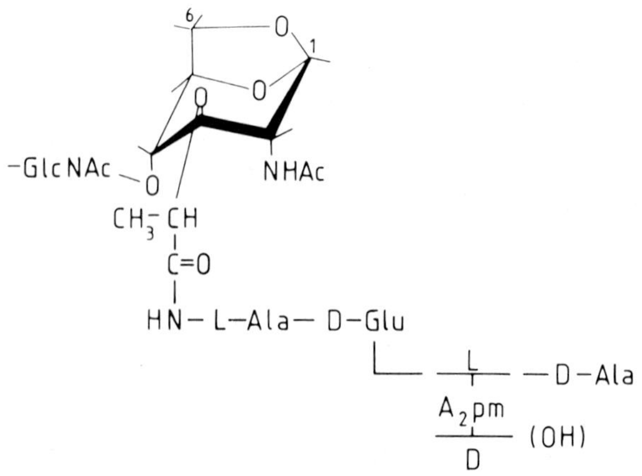

Figure 2 Tetrapeptide-substituted 1,6-anhydro-N-acetylmuramic acid occurring at the end of a glycan chain.

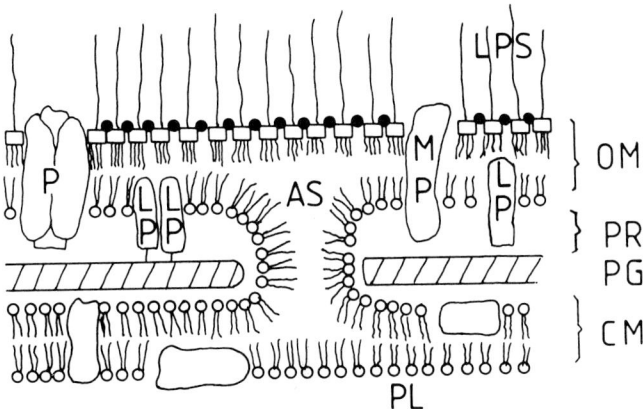

Figure 3 The cell envelope in gram-negative bacteria. OM = outer membrane; PR = periplasmic region; PG = peptidoglycan; CM = cytoplasmic membrane; P = porin (in the form of a trimer); LP = lipoprotein (either free or covalently linked to the peptidoglycan); MP = major protein; AS = adhesion site; PL = phospholipid; • = divalent cation (Mg^{2+} or Ca^{2+}); LPS = lipopolysaccharide.

of cardiolipin are also present. When compared with the plasma membrane, the outer membrane has a high ratio of protein to total phospholipid, resulting in a much decreased freedom of the membrane components for lateral diffusion.

The outer membrane is very unusual in that the lipopolysaccharide molecules are present only in the outer leaflet whereas the glycerolphospholipid molecules are present mainly, if not exclusively, in the inner leaflet of the bilayer (Fig. 3). This extremely asymmetric distribution of the component lipids makes the basic continuum of the outer membrane very poorly permeable to both hydrophobic and hydrophilic solutes. Passage of the nutrients (and other molecules such as the antibiotics) is made possible thanks to a special class of proteins, called porins. The porins so far examined usually have molecular weights in the range of 35,000–45,000, contain large amounts of β-sheet structure, and have a characteristic property to form water-filled, transmembrane, diffusion channels both in intact cells and in reconstituted liposome systems. *E. coli* possesses two different porins called OmpF and OmpC according to the names of the structural genes, with the OmpF porin producing somewhat larger pores than the OmpC porin.

Other major components of the outer membrane are specific proteins that contain ester- and amide-linked fatty acids and for this reason, are qualified as lipoproteins. *E. coli* possesses at least two lipoproteins with apparent molecular weights of about 7200 and 21,000, respectively. The 21,000 M_r lipoprotein is

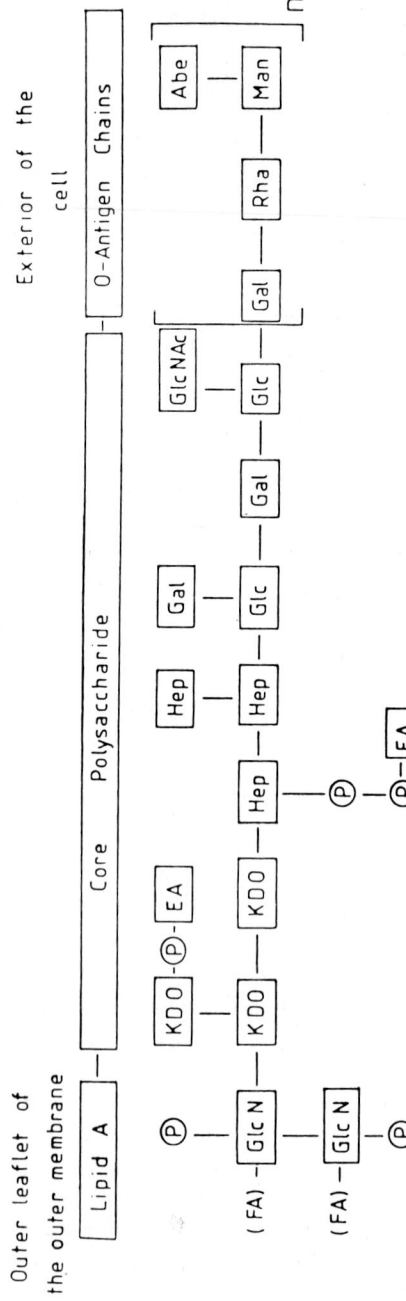

Figure 4 Structure of a complete lipopolysaccharide molecule showing the inner lipid A, the core polysaccharide, and the superficial O-antigens. FA = fatty acid; GlcN = glucosamine; KDO = 2-keto-3-deoxyoctonate; EA = ethanolamine; Hep = glycero-D-mannoheptose; Glc = glucose; Gal = galactose; GlcNAc = N-acetylglucosamine; Rha = rhamnose; Man = mannose; Abe = abequose. Incomplete lipopolysaccharides may occur with shorter polysaccharide chains.

tightly bound, but not covalently linked, to the peptidoglycan. The 7200 M_r lipoprotein occurs both in a free form and in covalent linkage with the underlying peptidoglycan (Fig. 5). The attachment site is at the carboxyl terminal of the protein where the ε-amino group of a lysine residue is bound to the carboxyl group at the L-center of meso-A_2pm of peptide units of the peptidoglycan (i.e., where a D-alanine residue occurs in a conventional tetrapeptide unit). The attachment site of the lipid moiety is at the amino terminal of the protein. One fatty acid is bound as an amide of the α-amino group of a cysteine and two other fatty acids occur as esters of the hydroxyl groups of S-glycerylcysteine.

Much has been written on the importance that, altogether, the peptidoglycan, the lipopolysaccharide, and the major proteins and lipoproteins play in the integrity of the cell envelope of the gram-negative bacteria. A mechanism has been proposed in which outer membrane vesicles, containing none of the covalently bound 7200 M_r lipoprotein and little free lipoprotein, are released from *E. coli* cells during normal growth when the outer membrane expands faster than the underlying peptidoglycan layer [7]. Outer membrane blebs are produced by *E. coli* mutants lacking the 7200 M_r lipoprotein (lpp⁻) [8]. Single *lpp* or *ompA* proteim mutants are rod-shaped (*ompA* is a major protein of the outer membrane playing a role in stabilization of mating aggregates in F-pilus-mediated conjugation), but double mutants of *lpp* and *ompA* grow as spheres.

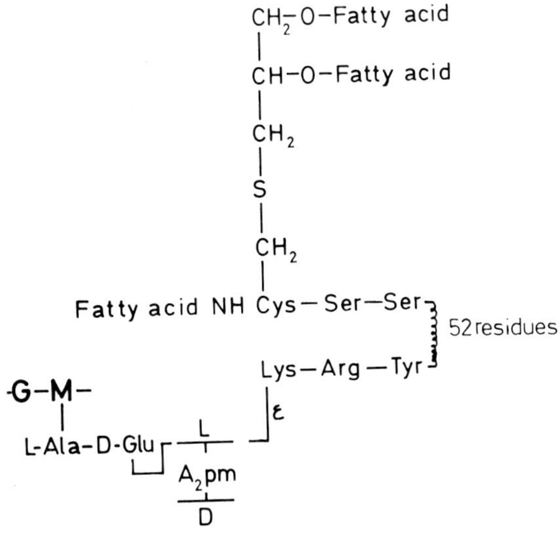

$$\begin{array}{l} CH_2-O-\text{Fatty acid} \\ | \\ CH-O-\text{Fatty acid} \\ | \\ CH_2 \\ | \\ S \\ | \\ CH_2 \\ | \\ \text{Fatty acid NH} - Cys-Ser-Ser \\ \quad\quad\quad\quad\quad\quad\quad Lys-Arg-Tyr \end{array}$$

Figure 5 Peptidoglycan-linked lipoprotein. In *E. coli*, the 7200-M_r lipoprotein contains 58 amino acid residues. G = N-acetylglucosamine; M = *N*-acetylmuramic acid.

Finally, there are many distinct areas in the cell envelope at which both outer and plasma membranes are physically attached to each other. About 200 to 400 such adhesion sites (Fig. 3) are seen in a growing cell of *E. coli*. They are considered as physical channels through which the outer membrane components, such as the lipopolysaccharide molecules, are translocated across the peptidoglycan layer once they have been synthesized at the plasma membrane.

B. DD-Peptidases

A discussion of the enzyme machinery responsible for the synthesis and assembly of the various components of the cell envelope of the gram-negative enterobacteria is beyond the scope of this article. But the DD-peptidases—which are the specific targets of the β-lactam antibiotics—deserve attention. For specific information, the reader is referred to Ref. 9-11.

Following the synthesis of the nucleotide precursors in the cytoplasm and the lipid-facilitated transfer of the disaccharide-pentapeptide units across the plasma membrane, peptidoglycan assembly requires the action of several membrane-bound enzymes (Fig. 6). Essentially, transglycosylases catalyze extension of the glycan strands and DD-transpeptidases catalyze insolubilization of the expanding network by peptide cross-linking. In combination, these two types of enzyme activities permit initial incorporation of newly synthesized disaccharide peptide units. Recent data [12] support the view that this material is incorporated directly in the preexisting peptidoglycan sacculus without first existing as a "soluble, nascent" intermediate. In turn, maturation of the peptidoglycan, wall remodelling throughout the bacterial life cycle and control of the extent of peptide cross-linking require additional DD-transpeptidase/carboxypeptidase/endopeptidase activities. Remarkably, β-lactam antibiotics are susceptible to inactivate (but with widely varying efficiency) all the DD-peptidases (but not the transglycosylases) involved in these various steps of peptidoglycan metabolism. Finally, modeling of the peptidoglycan within the bacterial cell envelope also involves covalent attachment of some appendages, such as lipoprotein molecules. It has been proposed, but never proved nor disproved, that lipoprotein attachment might be catalyzed by a cell envelope-associated, β-lactam-insensitive, LD-transpeptidase (Fig. 7). Whatever its nature, this enzyme does not discriminate between peptide monomers, dimers, and trimers [12].

Basically, the DD-peptidase active sites catalyze transfer of the electrophilic group L-Ala-γ-Glu-(L)-meso-A_2pm-(L)-D-Ala from pentapeptides L-Ala-γ-D-Glu-(L)-meso-A_2pm-(L)-D-Ala-D-Ala to a nucleophilic acceptor. They are specifically designed to attack peptide bonds that are located in α-position to a free carboxylate and extend between two carbon atoms having the D-configuration. The unique optical specificity of these enzymes justifies their qualification as DD-peptidases.

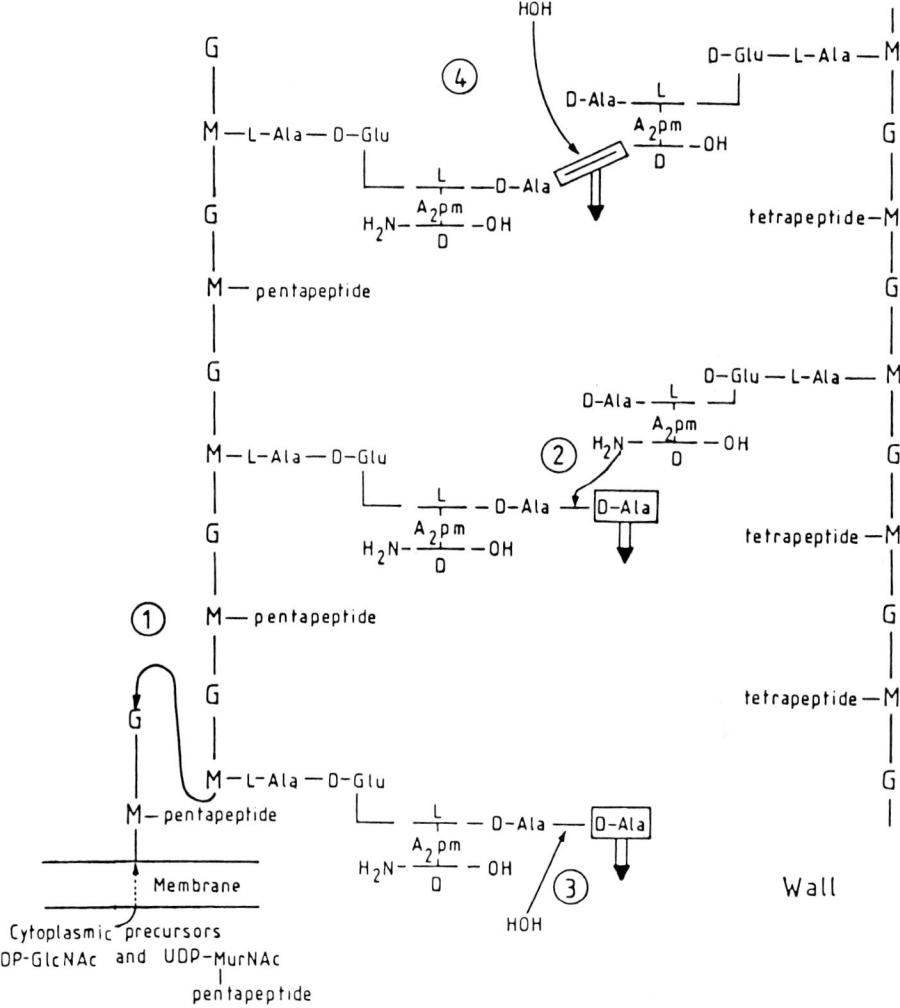

Figure 6 Enzyme activities involved in the last steps of peptidoglycan metabolism in gram-negative bacteria. 1 = transglycosylase activity; 2 = DD-transpeptidase activity; 3 = DD-carboxypeptidase activity; 4 = DD-endopeptidase activity.

The exact reaction catalyzed by the DD-peptidases depends on the nature of the acceptor which is effectively utilized in the transfer reaction (Fig. 6). If the acceptor is the amino group located on the D-center of meso-A_2pm of another peptide unit, transpeptidation occurs. If the acceptor is water, carboxypeptidation, i.e., hydrolysis, occurs. DD-carboxypeptidases also exist which can

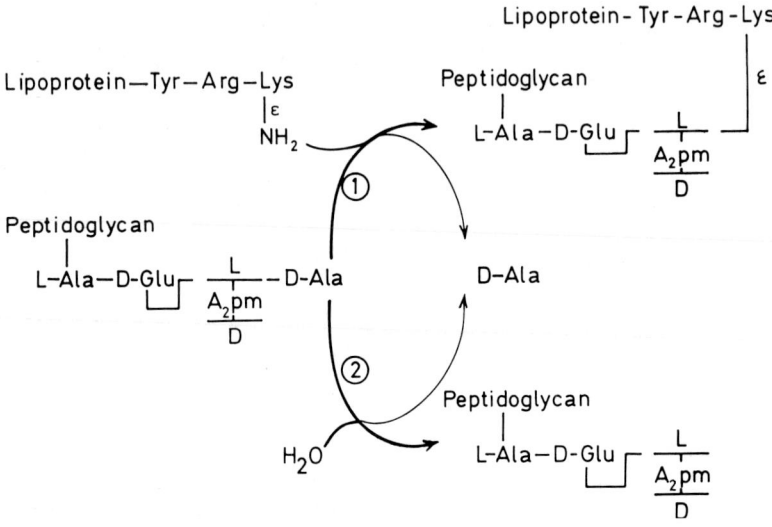

Figure 7 Possible mechanism of enzyme-catalyzed attachment of lipoprotein to peptidoglycan by LD-transpeptidase activity (1) and hydrolysis of tetrapeptide into tripeptide by LD-carboxypeptidase activity (2).

accommodate D-centers with very bulky side-chains at the carboxy-terminal position of the carbonyl donor peptide. Such enzymes can hydrolyze into tetrapeptide units, cross-linked peptide dimers or oligomers previously made by transpeptidation, thus performing peptidoglycan hydrolase activity (or "endopeptidase" activity).

Several serine DD-peptidases, isolated from gram-positive bacilli and actinomycetes, have been studied in detail. They operate by covalent catalysis through the transitory formation of a serine-ester-linked acyl enzyme intermediate. When in operation on D-Ala-D-Ala-terminated carbonyl donor substrates, the process is highly effective and the reaction flux is to reaction products (Fig. 8). When in operation on β-lactams (which are suicide substrates of the DD-peptidases), the reaction flux stops at the level of the acyl (penicilloyl, cephalosporoyl, etc.) enzyme intermediate (Fig. 9), thus conferring on the serine DD-peptidases the property to behave as "penicillin binding proteins" (PBPs). These adducts (i.e., acyl enzyme intermediates) are sufficiently stable to be submitted to gel electrophoresis in the presence of sodium dodecylsulfate. If [^{14}C] or [^{3}H]-benzylpenicillin (or another radioactive β-lactam) is used, fluorography of the gels permits visualization and quantitation of the DD-peptidases in the form of PBPs.

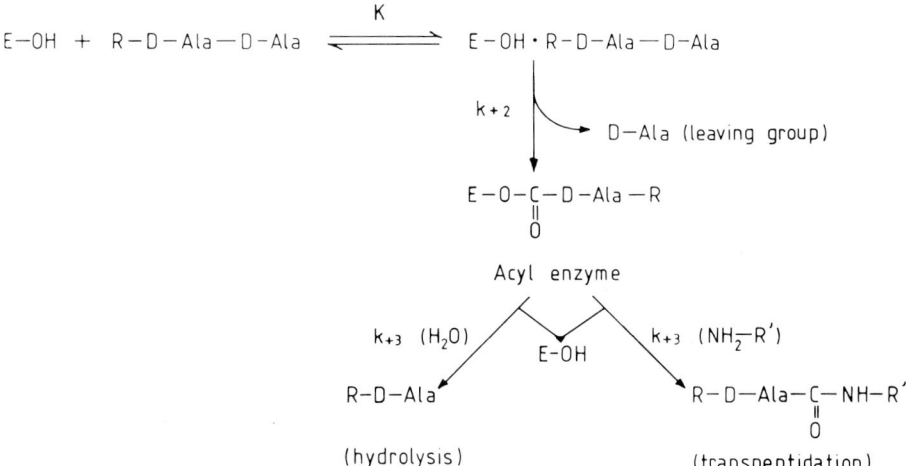

Figure 8 Mechanism of action of the serine DD-peptidases (E-OH) on D-Ala-D-Ala-terminated carbonyl donor peptides.

The reason for the abortive reaction between β-lactams and serine DD-peptidases is that the scissile amide bond of the β-lactam ring is endocyclic (Fig. 9). What should be regarded as the leaving group of the enzyme acylation step cannot leave the enzyme active site, which, therefore, remains occupied. Enzyme regeneration, however, may occur so that either the bound acyl moiety is released by transfer to water (in which case the DD-peptidase functions as a classical β-lactamase of very weak efficiency) or that the bound acyl moiety is first fragmented so that the "leaving group" can diffuse away and the active site can undergo deacylation. Whatever the case, enzyme regeneration is a slow or very slow process.

The above model of β-lactam action on the serine DD-peptidases can be represented schematically by the reaction

$$E + I \overset{K}{\rightleftharpoons} E \cdot I \xrightarrow{k_{+2}} E\text{-}I^* \xrightarrow{k_{+3}} E + \text{reaction products} \qquad [1]$$

where E = DD-peptidase; I = β-lactam; E-I* = acyl enzyme; K = dissociation constant; k_{+2} and k_{+3} = first-order reaction rates. Thus it follows that the higher the bimolecular rate constant of enzyme acylation (k_{+2}/K) and the smaller the rate constant of enzyme deacylation k_{+3} (whatever the underlying mechanism), the more potent a β-lactam as a DD-peptidase inactivator, or the higher the capacity of a β-lactam of immobilizing a DD-peptidase in the form of a PBP. Depending on both the DD-peptidase and the structure of the β-lactam, the

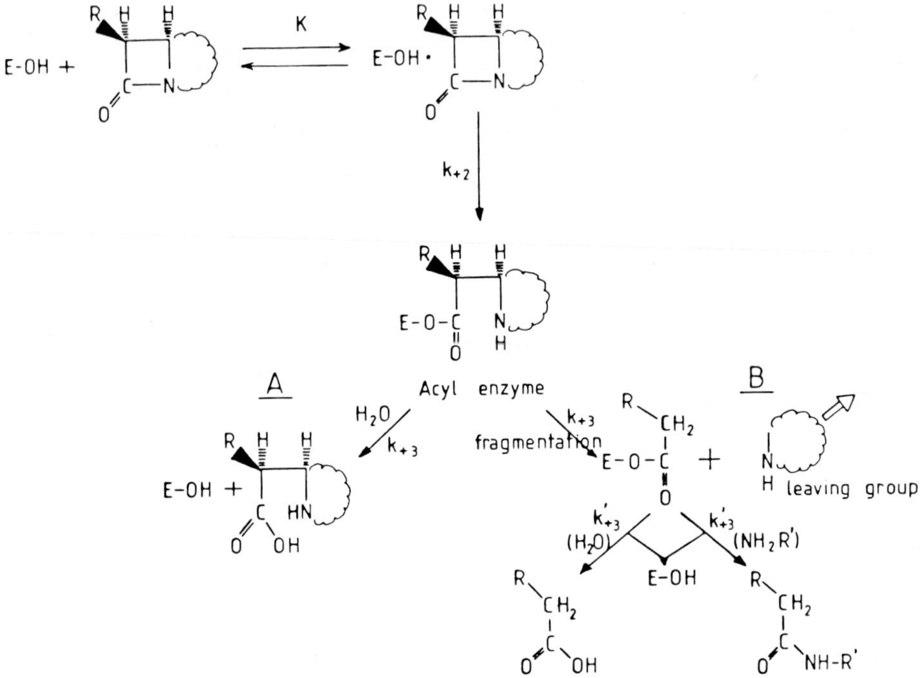

Figure 9 Mechanism of action of the serine DD-peptidases (E-OH) on β-lactams. (A) Acyl enzyme breakdown occurs by direct release of the acyl (penicilloyl, cephalosporoyl, etc.) moiety. (B) Acyl enzyme breakdown involves prior fragmentation of the acyl (penicilloyl, cephalosporoyl, etc.) moiety. In this pathway, fragmentation (k_{+3}) is rate-limiting.

values of these kinetic parameters vary widely. These observations suggest variations in the geometry and properties of the DD-peptidase active sites and multiple modes of binding of the β-lactams, leading to enzyme-ligand associations of highly varying complementarity and productiveness.

C. Penicillin Binding Proteins (PBPs)

Fluorography of the gels obtained by SDS electrophoresis of bacterial plasma membranes previously exposed to a radioactive β-lactam shows that all bacteria possess a set of membrane-bound proteins that bind penicillin and behave as PBPs [11,13]. Very few of these proteins have been characterized as serine DD-peptidases but, as an extension of these studies, it is assumed that, in all cases, penicillin binding is by acylation of a serine residue, implying that all PBPs are serine DD-peptidases (and function as shown in Figs. 8 and 9).

The interactions between PBPs and β-lactams have been studied at least superficially. Most often, the "affinity" of a radioactive β-lactam for a PBP is roughly expressed as the antibiotic concentration, which under given conditions of temperature, pH, and duration of the incubation, leads to 50% of maximal binding. If the β-lactam is not available in a radioactive form, the "affinity" relates to the concentration which is necessary to inhibit by 50% the binding of, most often, radioactive benzylpenicillin. With those PBPs that have been characterized as DD-peptidases, "sensitivity" to a β-lactam is expressed as the β-lactam concentration that causes 50% inhibition of the enzyme activity.

Using these techniques, the PBP patterns (number, apparent molecular weight, relative abundance, thermostability and protease sensitivity, "affinity" for β-lactams, stability of the adducts formed, sensitivity of enzymatic activity) have been determined for many bacterial species. However imprecise they may be, these studies have led to valuable conclusions. One of them is that the PBP pattern is highly species specific, and great variations are observed between taxonomically unrelated bacteria.

All the enterobacteria possess at least seven PBPs that are usually qualified as high-molecular-weight PBPs (PBPs 1A, 1Bs, 2, and 3) and low-molecular-weight PBPs (PBPs 4, 5, and 6) [14]. Because of the close similarity in the PBP patterns, it is thought that the individual corresponding PBPs in all enterobacteria catalyze similar reactions and perform similar physiological functions. In *E. coli*, detailed biochemical and genetic studies [13] have shown that the high-molecular-weight PBPs play specific functions in wall elongation (PBPs 1A and 1Bs), rod shape maintenance (PBP2), and initiation of cell septation (PBP3), respectively. PBPs 1A, 1Bs, and possibly PBPs 2 and 3 have been identified as bifunctional transglycosylase-DD-transpeptidase enzymes [15]. In contrast, PBPs 4, 5, and 6 are believed to be involved in processes related to maturation and remodelling of the wall peptidoglycan (see above). They have been identified as monofunctional DD-peptidases performing, to various extents, transpeptidase/carboxypeptidase/endopeptidase activities.

Characteristic features of the PBP pattern in the enterobacteria are the relatively high abundance of the low-molecular-weight PBPs 5 and 6, the high stability of PBP 1Bs to heat and detergent, and the highly specific targeted action of some β-lactams [14]. Thus, mecillinam binds exclusively to PBP2 over a wide range of concentrations (causing generation of osmotically stable round forms) while, in contrast, cefoxitin has an especially low affinity for this PBP2. Azthreonam and to a lesser extent, cefuroxim bind preferentially to PBP3 (and are effective in inhibiting cell division and causing cell filamentation). Cephaloridin has highest "affinity" for PBPs 1A/1B (and is effective in causing spheroplast formation and rapid cellular lysis). PBPs 4 and 5 show relatively high and low "sensitivity," respectively, to several penams such as benzylpenicillin, ampicillin, carbenicillin, and methicillin.

The first direct demonstration that penicillin inhibits peptide cross-linking during wall peptidoglycan metabolism stems from the work of Wise and Park [53] and Tipper and Strominger [16]. In particular [16], it was shown that *Staphylococcus aureus* grown in the presence of sublethal doses of benzylpenicillin accumulates the nucleotide precursor UDP-N-acetylmuramyl-pentapeptide in the cytoplasm and has a higher proportion of D-Ala-D-Ala-terminated peptide units and a lower extent of interpeptide cross-linking in the wall peptidoglycan than the control cells grown in the absence of the antibiotic. Since then, inhibition of transpeptidation has been regarded as the foundation stone of the mechanism of penicillin action.

In fact, the picture is much more complex. It is now well known (but not well understood) that PBP inactivation may have multiple effects on each of the bacterial cell envelope integuments, may affect both the peptide and the glycan moieties of the peptidoglycan, and does not necessarily nor always result in an overall decrease of peptide cross-linking. Thus, at those concentrations (30 µg/ml) that in *E. coli* inhibit cell division and induce cell filamentation by impairing septum initiation, benzylpenicillin both enhances the attachment of newly synthesized peptidoglycan units to the wall sacculus by transpeptidation, resulting in an increased degree of peptide cross-linking, and, subsequently, causes a sudden increase of incorporation of lipopolysaccharide in the outer membrane [17]. The same effects are seen with mecillinam at those concentrations (2 µg/ml) that induce conversion of *E. coli* into round cells. But (as estimated by measuring the amounts of anhydromuramic acid present), mecillinam, under these conditions, also reduces the average glycan chain length of the peptidoglycan to about half its normal value [17,18]. Alterations in the phospholipid composition of the plasma membrane in response to changes in the cell wall induced by β-lactams and other wall inhibitors [19-23] show the close interdependency that exists between the peptidoglycan and both the outer and inner membranes. Finally, complications in the interpretation of the observed phenomena also arise from the fact that, under partial PBP inactivation, PBPs left intact may compensate for the loss of other PBPs [13].

III. THE CELL ENVELOPE OF THE ROD-SHAPED *PROTEUS*

Basically, the above description of the cell envelope of the gram-negative enterobacteria applies to *Proteus* spp. But there are peculiarities.

A. Peptidoglycan

The peptidoglycan of proteus possesses a remarkable marker (Fig. 10) which is that more than half of the N-acetylmuramic acid residues are substituted by an ester-linked O-acetyl group on C6 [24]. Non-O-acetylated peptidoglycan

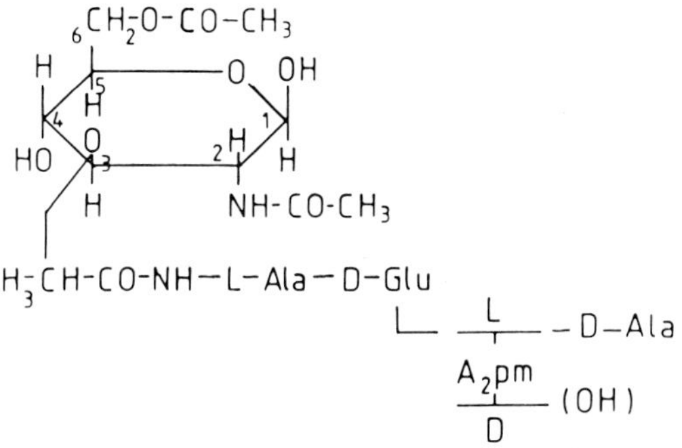

```
        CH₂-O-CO-CH₃
       6|
    H   |5──────O  OH
     \ H|      / \ /
    4 \ |     /   \1
   HO  \|3  2H    H
        |    |
        H    NH-CO-CH₃
        |
    CH₃-CH-CO-NH—L-Ala—D-Glu
                    |    |
                    L    L —D-Ala
                      A₂pm
                      ──── (OH)
                       D
```

Figure 10 Tetrapeptide-substituted di-O-acetylmuramic acid.

disaccharide peptide units are incorporated in the growing sacculus and it is at a later stage that part of them become O-acetylated. O-acetylation is accompanied by an increase in peptide cross-linking and there is suggestive evidence that a peptidoglycan strand (or strand section) has to be properly cross-linked before acetylation can occur. The presumed O-acetylase (which, so far, has not been characterized) seems not to discriminate between N-acetylmuramic acid residues on the basis of their peptide substituents. Enzymatic degradation of the glycan strands into disaccharide units yields all possible O-acetylated and non-O-acetylated disaccharide-L-Ala-D-Glu, disaccharide-tetrapeptide, bis-disaccharide peptide dimers and tris-disaccharide peptide trimers. O-acetylation, increased peptide cross-linking and generation of a limited amount of L-Ala-D-Glu dipeptides [25] are considered as "maturation" processes of the wall peptidoglycan.

B. Outer Membrane

The outer membrane of proteus also possesses one interesting marker, which is the occurrence, side by side, of two types of lipopolysaccharides. One of them has much shorter O-specific polysaccharide side-chains attached to the core-lipid A structure and thus is more hydrophobic than the other [26].

Another feature of the outer membrane in proteus is the complete absence in exponential-phase cultures of lipoprotein covalently linked to the peptidoglycan [27]. Stationary cells, however, contain a covalently linked lipoprotein of low molecular weight ($M_r \cong 7200$) in amounts similar to those found in *E. coli* where, irrespective of the growth phase, statistically one lipoprotein is covalently linked to about every tenth to twelfth peptidoglycan unit. The proteus 7200 M_r lipoprotein closely resembles that of *E. coli*. However, it lacks methionine and contains more acidic and fewer basic residues and has a somewhat different distribution of amide- and ester-linked fatty acids [28].

Proteus manufactures at least three other major proteins for export in the outer membrane. On the basis of their ability to form hydrophilic pores in reconstituted membranes, the 39,000 M_r protein and the peptidoglycan-associated 36,000 M_r protein appear to be porins [29]. (The term "peptidoglycan-associated protein" is meant to emphasize that separation of the protein from the peptidoglycan requires drastic treatments such as extraction with SDS at 100°C.) In turn, the peptidoglycan-associated, 15,000 M_r protein mediates little permeation of low-molecular-weight solutes and has been characterized as a second lipoprotein [30]. This latter lipoprotein might play an important role in outer membrane assembly. This suggestion seems to be especially pertinent since proteus, which lacks the covalently linked lipoprotein of low molecular weight in exponentially growing cultures, contains, when compared with *E. coli*, much larger quantities of the peptidoglycan-associated lipoprotein of high molecular weight. It has also been hypothesized that *O*-acetylation might confer increased hydrophobicity to the peptidoglycan, thus facilitating its association with the inner leaflet of the outer membrane [27].

C. PBPs and DD-Peptidases

The PBP pattern in *Proteus* spp. is very similar to that of *E. coli* [31] and the corresponding PBPs in these two organisms are thought to play similar functions. Using saturating concentrations of [^{14}C]benzylpenicillin, the relative abundance of the PBPs in *Proteus vulgaris* (Fig. 11) is about 14-15% for PBP1A and PBP1B, 3-5% for PBPs 2, 3, and 4, and 59% for PBPs 5/6 [32].

PBPs 4 and 5 have been isolated from both *P. mirabilis* [33] and *P. vulgaris* [32]. In vitro and on peptide substrate analogues, PBP4 ($M_r \cong 48,000$) functions as a carboxypeptidase and, to a lower extent, as a transpeptidase. It also performs endopeptidase activity. PBP4 shows high sensitivity to several penams. The half-inhibitory concentration of benzylpenicillin is about 0.01-0.05 μM and the penicilloyl enzyme "intermediate" has a long half-life of about 200-300 min (which corresponds to a k_{+3} value of Equation [1] of about $0.5 \times 10^{-4} s^{-1}$). Enzyme regeneration is by fragmentation of the bound penicilloyl moiety with formation of phenylacetylglycine (Fig. 9B).

Under similar conditions, PBP5 ($M_r \cong 43,000$) shows no endopeptidase activity, may perform low transpeptidase activity (at least the *P. mirabilis* enzyme) and functions essentially as a carboxypeptidase. It exhibits relatively low sensitivity to benzylpenicillin (half-inhibitory concentrations, 1-4 μM) and forms a short-lived benzylpenicilloyl enzyme "intermediate" (half-life, 7-10 min). Enzyme regneration proceeds through the direct release of penicilloate so that PBP5 behaves as a β-lactamase of very low efficacy (Fig. 9A).

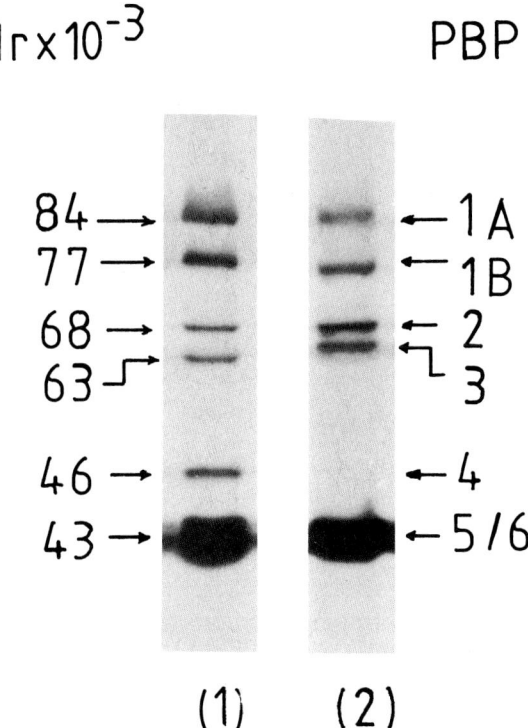

Figure 11 PBP patterns of *Proteus vulgaris* P18 (1) and the corresponding stable protoplast L-form (2).

IV. THE CELL ENVELOPE OF β-LACTAM-INDUCED L-FORMS OF *PROTEUS*

A. Conversion of *Proteus* to L-Form Growth

Benzylpenicillin converts the rod-shaped proteus cells into filaments at low antibiotic concentration (1 μM) and into osmotically fragile spheroplasts at higher antibiotic concentration (15 μM) (Fig. 12a-f). Prolonged treatment results in cell lysis. In spite of this, proteus is notable for its ability to escape, under certain conditions, the lethal consequences of benzylpenicillin action by making a transition to peculiar growth types called L-forms.

As defined by H. H. Martin [34], L-forms qualify as "all artificially induced or spontaneously arising aberrant growth states of previously normal bacteria, where multiplication occurs in the form of fragile, osmotically sensitive cells, mostly of spherical shape, but often also pleomorphic, resulting from the

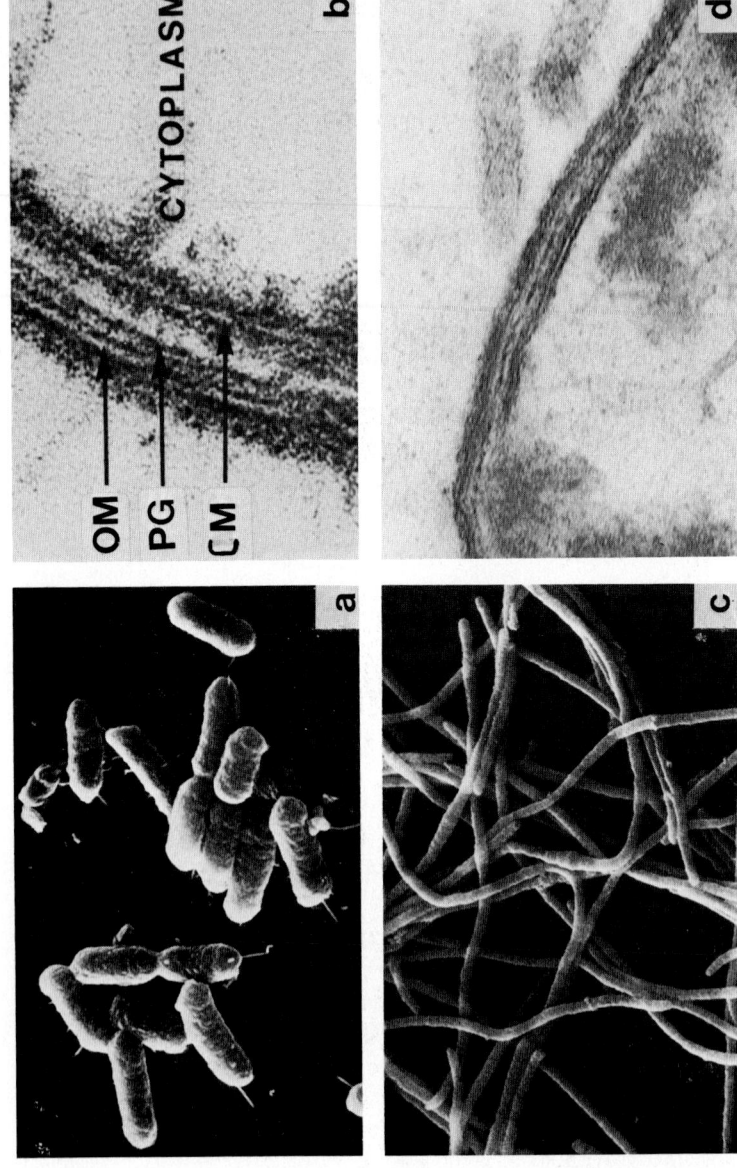

Figure 12 Morphology of *Proteus vulgaris* P18 and effects caused by growing the cells in the presence of benzylpenicillin and mecillinam. Scanning (*a,c,e,g*) and thin-layer (*b,d,f,h*) electron microscopy of: normal bacteria (*a* and *b*); filaments induced by $\cong 1\ \mu M$ benzylpenicillin (*c* and *d*); spheroplasts induced by $\cong 15\ \mu M$

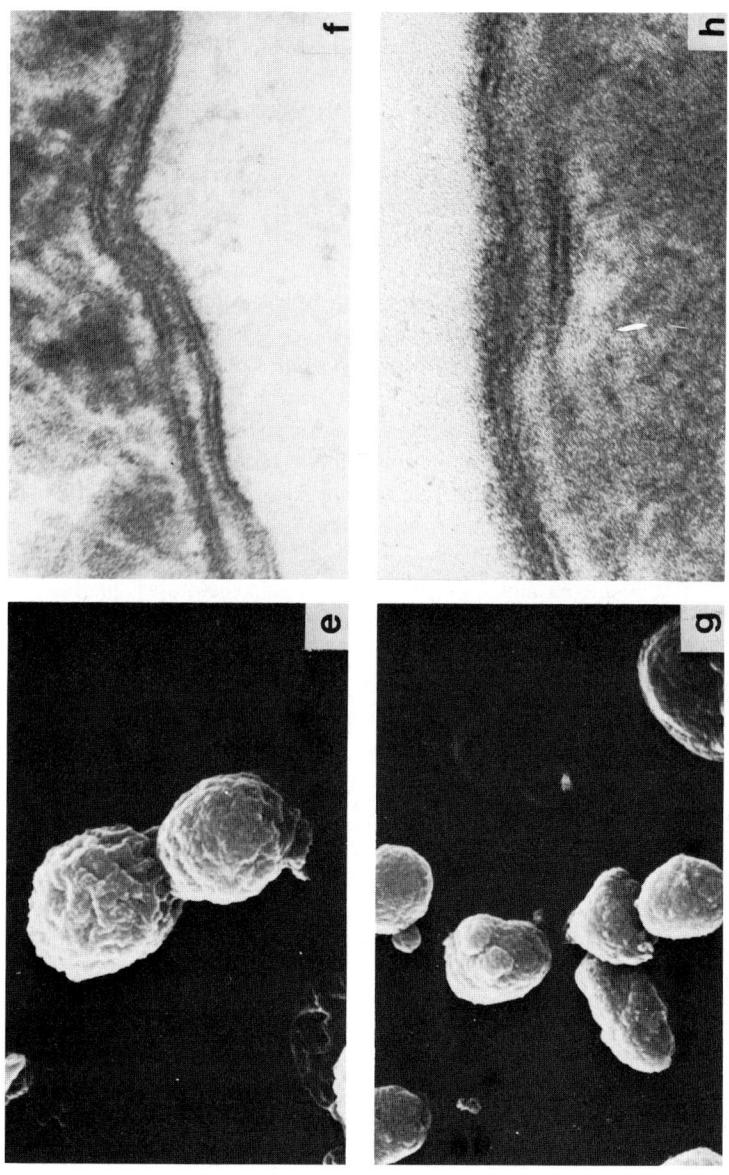

benzylpenicillin (e and f); ovoid cells induced by ≅ 15 μM mecillinam (g and h). Magnifications: ×1250 in c, ×10,000 in a,e, and g; ×181,200 in f; ×239,400 in d; ×350,000 in h; and ×400,000 in b. OM = outer membrane; PG = peptidoglycan; CM = cytoplasmic membrane.

response of a pliable cell surface to external forces." Osmotic fragility relates to high (although varying) sensitivity to mechanical stress (fragmentation can be achieved by simple freezing and thawing), osmotic shock (dilution of an L-form shake culture into distilled water causes rapid lysis), and to the dissolving action of anionic detergents such as SDS. Normal proteus cells are unimpaired by these treatments.

Proteus may give rise to two main types of L-form survivors to β-lactam action. The unstable spheroplast L-forms, on the one hand, retain portions of a defective cell wall and can revert to the normal, rod-shaped bacteria upon removal of the β-lactam from the culture medium. The stable protoplast L-forms, on the other, have the plasma membrane as sole cell integument and do not revert to normal bacteria under any conditions.

Experiments leading to the simultaneous appearance of these two types of L-forms involve, classically, exposure of proteus to a β-lactam in a rich complex agar medium supplemented with an osmotic stabilizer (0.5 M sucrose; 20% v/v NaCl or 4% w/v polyvinylpyrollidone) and 5-10 vol% of defibrinated horse serum. Colonies of protoplast L-forms are small (diameter, 0.2-0.3 mm), compact, and exhibit a granular appearance. Colonies of spheroplast L-forms are 5-10 times larger and have a typical "fried-egg" appearance. Subcultures on solid media and, eventually, liquid shake cultures, in the absence of serum and with only little osmotic stabilization, can then be achieved.

In principle, the above procedure applies to many gram-negative bacteria. But, the difficulty and percentage of failures greatly vary depending on the cases. There is no general rapid and simple way of obtaining β-lactam-induced spheroplasts and protoplast L-forms from these bacteria. *P. mirabilis*, however, is a remarkable exception at least when the goal pursued is only the exclusive preparation of homogeneous populations of unstable spheroplast L-forms. In this case, the presence of an osmotic stabilizer and of serum supplement in the primary cultures can be omitted. Furthermore, with some β-lactams including benzylpenicillin (but not with all of them), spheroplast L-form growth can be initiated by direct inoculation of *P. mirabilis* into liquid medium supplemented with the selected β-lactam. *P. vulgaris*, however, is much more restricted in this respect (for more information, see Ref. 34).

B. Unstable Spheroplast L-Forms of *P. mirabilis*

Established liquid shake cultures of unstable spheroplast L-forms of *P. mirabilis* can be obtained with almost every available β-lactam (although, in some cases, conversion to L-form growth is possible only on agar medium), with final titers, at the stationary phase, of 2×10^8 to 3×10^8 colony-forming units. The average doubling time during exponential growth varies depending on the β-lactam. Unstable L-forms grow with a generation time of 45 min with cefoxitin, 60 min with benzylpenicillin, and 90 min with amoxycillin and ampicillin (instead of 30 min for the original bacterial cells in the absence of β-lactam [34].

1. Benzylpenicillin-Induced Spheroplast L-Forms

One way to readily obtain such L-forms is, for example, to inoculate agar slants of suitable medium containing 120 μg of benzylpenicillin/ml with 2×10^8 stationary-phase cells of *P. mirabilis*. Heavy growth can be obtained after incubation for 2-3 days at 37°C; the harvested cells can then be transferred to liquid media containing 120 μg of benzylpenicillin/ml and final adaptation to growth in the presence of high antibiotic concentrations and with a generation time of about 60 min is usually obtained after a few serial transfers.

Morphologically, the benzylpenicillin-induced spheroplast L-forms appear as flagellated spherical cells covered with fimbriae and loosely attached superficial wall materials [35]. Their cell envelope contains both an outer membrane and a peptidoglycan layer; the latter can be isolated after extraction with phenol and further purified with trypsin (as it is done with the normal proteus cells). Hence, a full assortment of wall integuments is present but with defect(s) causing loss of both rod shape and mechanical strength. The induced lesion(s) is (are) unstable; upon removal of benzylpenicillin from the growth medium, reversion to the original rod-shaped bacteria occurs.

When compared with the normal bacteria, the benzylpenicillin-induced spheroplast L-forms have more than one alteration and both the outer membrane and the peptidoglycan layer are affected. The outer layer has reduced amounts of lipopolysaccharide [36], enterobacterial common antigen [37], and total proteins (but still possesses the 40,000 M_r and 36,000 M_r porins) [38]. In turn, the peptidoglycan layer has a slight decrease in the overall extent of peptide cross-linking [39], shows alterations in the tetrapeptide to tripeptide (L-Ala-γ-D-Glu-(L)-meso-A_2pm) pattern [39], and exhibits a large decrease in the degree of O-acetylation of the N-acetylmuramic acid residues [39].

While all the tripeptide units present in the peptidoglycan of stationary phase cells of proteus serve to anchor the lipoprotein molecules, an appreciable amount of free tripeptides occurs in the unstable spheroplast L-forms. If, as suggested above, covalent attachment of lipoprotein to peptidoglycan is catalyzed by a penicillin-insensitive LD-transpeptidase, then one indirect consequence of the benzylpenicillin-induced conversion of proteus to unstable spheroplast L-forms might be the conversion of this LD-transpeptidase into an LD-carboxypeptidase. As shown in Figure 7, utilization of water as acceptor of the transfer reaction causes hydrolysis of the tetrapeptides into tripeptides, preventing lipoprotein attachment. Note that a penicillin-insensitive LD-peptidase that effectively performs hydrolysis of the tetrapeptides can be readily isolated from the bacterial cells where, to all appearances, it is part of the periplasmic compartment [32].

The O-acetylation pattern of the peptidoglycan can be expressed by the ratio of non-O-acetylated to O-acetylated N-acetylmuramic acid residues. The ratio value is about 0.5 in the normal bacterial cells. It is much higher, about 1.3, in the peptidoglycan of the unstable spheroplast L-forms. On the basis of these observations, it has been suggested that in proteus, the peptidoglycan might be built up from different areas of the polymer differing in the O-acetyl content and that, in the unstable spheroplast L-forms grown in the presence of benzylpenicillin, the synthesis of the O-acetyl-rich peptidoglycan is selectively depressed whereas the synthesis of the O-acetyl-low peptidoglycan remains virtually unaffected [39].

2. Effects of Pairs of β-Lactams

The continued synthesis of a peptide cross-linked (but defective) peptidoglycan by the unstable spheroplast L-forms in the presence of benzylpenicillin can be attributed either to some unknown penicillin-insensitive DD-peptidase enzyme system or to the functioning of one or several PBPs that escape complete inactivation by benzylpenicillin. In this latter case, the unstable spheroplast L-forms should possess a reduce assortment of PBPs left in a free form (and thus capable of subsequently binding [^{14}C]benzylpenicillin) and, moreover, complete L-form growth inhibition should be made possible by the addition of a second β-lactam able to complement benzylpenicillin action. As shown below, experimental evidence supports this latter view.

In the continuous presence of a β-lactam, as it occurs during β-lactam-induced spheroplast L-form growth, the percentage of a given PBP which remains constantly present in a free active form is given by

$$\text{PBP}_{\text{free}} = \text{PBP}_{\text{total}} - \text{PBP}_{\text{bound}}$$

with

$$\text{PBP}_{\text{bound}} = \text{PBP}_{\text{total}} \frac{1}{1 + \dfrac{k_{+3}}{k_{+2}}\left(1 + \dfrac{K}{[I]}\right)} \quad [2]$$

where K, k_{+2}, and k_{+3} are the constants of Reaction [1] and [I] is the β-lactam concentration which is actually accessible to the PBP. This latter value depends on both the ease with which the β-lactam permeates through the outer membrane and the competition between the various PBPs present for the amount of β-lactam available. Assuming [I] = 100 μM; K = 10 mM; k_{+2} = 1 s^{-1} and k_{+3} = 3 × 10^{-3} s^{-1} (which corresponds to a half-life of the bound PBP of about 5 min), then 22% of the PBP under consideration remains in a free form all the time. Under identical conditions but with k_{+3} = 3 × 10^{-4} s^{-1} (half-life = 38 min), only 3% of the PBP remains free.

Many β-lactams other than benzylpenicillin induce good spheroplast L-form growth but, unfortunately, the exact resulting biochemical lesions are not known in most cases and the available data do not permit quantitation of the PBPs left in a free form on the basis of Equation [2]. Nevertheless, with, for example, the pair benzylpenicillin-cefoxitin, it is known [40] that PBP4 forms an adduct (i.e., PBP_{bound}) that is very stable in the case of benzylpenicillin (half-life, 300 min) but short-lived in the case of cefoxitin (half-life, 14 min). Conversely, PBPs 5/6 form adducts that are very stable in the case of cefoxitin (half-life, 900 min) but short-lived in the case of benzylpenicillin (half-life, 7 min). It is therefore not surprising (as the experience shows) that benzylpenicillin-induced L-forms contain no free PBP4 but appreciable amounts of free PBPs 5/6, together with free PBP2. Similarly, the cefoxitin-induced L-forms (which also contain a normally cross-linked peptidoglycan) grow and divide with appreciable amounts of free PBPs 4 and 2 but vastly reduced quantities of free PBPs 5/6 and some high-molecular-weight PBPs.

Benzylpenicillin and cefoxitin complement each other at the level of the PBPs. Most likely, they also complement each other at the level of the lesions that each of them induces in the cells. Following this expectation, benzylpenicillin and cefoxitin, in combination, effectively inhibit spheroplast L-form growth, and, remarkably, cause a 50% decrease of peptide cross-linking in the peptidoglycan [40].

Following the above approach, many β-lactams were tested to find other suitable pairs of compounds that would complement each other to achieve complete and permanent inactivation of all essential targets in *P. mirabilis*. Most of the β-lactams did not show complementation. However, the pair ampicillin-cefoxitin was found to be very effective (H. H. Martin, personal communication), and the pair benzylpenicillin-mecillinam deserves special attention.

The amidinopenicillin, mecillinam, binds exclusively to PBP2 over a wide range of concentrations. When exposed to mecillinam, *Proteus* is massively converted into large spherical cells [39]. These cells remain resistant to osmotic shock (and thus cannot be regarded as L-forms), exhibit a multilayered cell envelope (Fig. 12.g–h), and possess a peptidoglycan that has virtually the same extent of peptide cross-linking and the same degree of O-acetylation as those found in the normal bacteria [39]. By analogy with similar studies carried out on *E. coli* [17], one may assume that the peptidoglycan has glycan strands of reduced length. No growth inhibition or cell death occurs at mecillinam concentrations up to 100 μg/ml, and shake cultures of spherical cells grown in the presence of 15 μg/ml divide with a generation time of 54 min. The mecillinam-induced spherical cells are unstable. Upon removal of mecillinam from the medium, reversion to rod-shaped normal bacteria occurs.

Mecillinam action results in profound morphological alterations of the cells but does not produce any apparent striking biochemical lesions. In particular, it does not cause the extensive shift in the O-acetylation pattern observed with benzylpenicillin. Nevertheless, mecillinam stops growth of benzylpenicillin-induced spheroplast L-forms (presumably by inactivating the PBP2 left in free form in these organisms) in a rather spectacular manner. Upon addition of 15 μg of mecillinam/ml to a shake culture of spheroplast L-forms growing logarithmically in the presence of 120 μg benzylpenicillin/ml, one observes a further two- to fourfold increase in cell density, conversion of the L-forms into nongrowing, gigantic spherical cells with a diameter of 20 μm, and (as observed with the pair benzylpenicillin-cefoxitin) a drastic decrease of peptide cross-linking in the peptidoglycan [39].

Study of the effects of suitable pairs of β-lactams shows that the O-acetyl groups in proteus are important markers of peptidoglycan synthesis. O-acetylation is also a crucial event in other gram-negative and gram-positive bacteria. Thus, similar to the situation found in proteus, *Neisseria gonorrhoeae* (which has only three major PBPs and where acquisition of intrinsic resistance to β-lactams is accompanied by stepwise decreases in the penicillin "affinity" of PBPs 1 and 2) possesses O-acetyl groups in its peptidoglycan [41]. Examination of isogenic sensitive and resistant strains shows that the primary effects of benzylpenicillin at the corresponding growth inhibitory concentrations differ strikingly depending on the strains. The effect is only a slight change in peptide cross-linking but a sharp decline in the degree of O-acetylation in the penicillin-sensitive gonococcus. In marked contrast, it is a very moderate change in O-acetylation but a substantial decline in cross-linking in the penicillin-resistant gonococcus. On the basis of the extent of saturation of the individual PBPs found under these conditions, it has been suggested that (1) PBP2 has a role in controlling (directly or indirectly) the degree of *O*-acetylation; (2) PBP1 is probably implicated in the transpeptidation reaction of the peptidoglycan; and (3) PBP3 probably fulfils a "maturation" function (analogous to the *E. coli* low-molecular-weight PBPs). Mention should also be made of more recent investigations revealing the presence of a secondary transpeptidase in gonococci that appears to be insensitive to penicillin action [41]. The possible function of this enzyme system during prolonged exposure to penicillin has not yet been reported.

C. Stable Spheroplast L-Forms of *P. mirabilis*

Prolonged maintenance of the benzylpenicillin-induced, unstable spheroplast L-forms in a growing state is probably not feasible. Indeed, the longer the subcultivation period in the presence of benzylpenicillin, the higher the proportion of spheroplast L-forms that lose their ability to revert to normal bacteria and, concomitantly, acquire resistance to the combined action of benzylpenicillin and mecillinam. On the basis of this double resistance to benzylpenicillin and mecillinam, stable spheroplast L-forms can be detected in freshly prepared cultures of unstable spheroplast L-forms already after three or four transfers [39].

When compared with the unstable spheroplast L-forms, the stable spheroplast L-forms exhibit a much more sharply defined surface which is sparsely covered with slender fimbriae (but without any loosely attached material) [35]. They also show a classical multilayered cell envelope from which a normally peptide cross-linked peptidoglycan can be isolated as a defined entity but they contain higher amounts of both lipopolysaccharide and proteins (although in lesser amounts than in the normal bacteria). These properties suggest a tighter organization of the outer membrane. In spite of this, the stable spheroplast L-forms remain mechanically and osmotically sensitive.

How the originally reversible lesions present in the unstable spheroplast L-forms are perpetuated as hereditary defects, with concomitant acquisition of mecillinam resistance, in the stable spheroplast L-forms is a question that remains to be explored. The process is best explained as the spontaneous appearance in the benzylpenicillin-induced spheroplast L-forms population of mutants that rapidly accumulate by a still unknown selective mechanism [39]. Chemically induced and frequently appearing spontaneous mutants of *E. coli* have been described showing mecillinam resistance and, depending on the cases, spherical or rod cell shape.

D. Stable Protoplast L-Forms of *P. mirabilis* and *P. vulgaris*

Conversion to stable protoplast L-form growth is the ultimate response of proteus to penicillin action. The stable protoplast L-forms are wall-less, ovoid organisms (Fig. 13). They grow in the absence of extensive osmotic stabilization or other protective measures, do not reverse to normal bacteria under any conditions, and show complete resistance to β-lactams, including mecillinam, alone or in combination. Their cell envelope consists of one single membrane that, in thin sections, appears as two layers of irregular thickness. They exhibit a smooth surface and possess multiple flagella. The protoplast L-forms do not divide at regular intervals (perhaps because of the missing wall) so that the resulting unbalanced growth yields cells of different sizes (0.1–10 μm in diameter), including the so-called small bodies (0.1–0.4 μm). Vigorous growth in liquid shake culture can be obtained with generation times of about 2 hr but propagation of individual protoplasts is erratic and often abortive.

The first stable protoplast L-form was isolated by Tulasne in 1949 as a benzylpenicillin-resistant organism originated from *P. vulgaris* [42]. Since then, these organisms have been subcultured twice a week in suitable growth medium in the absence of penicillin. Soon after Tulasne, Kandler and Kandler [43] isolated similar stable protoplast L-forms from strains of *P. mirabilis*. Propagation

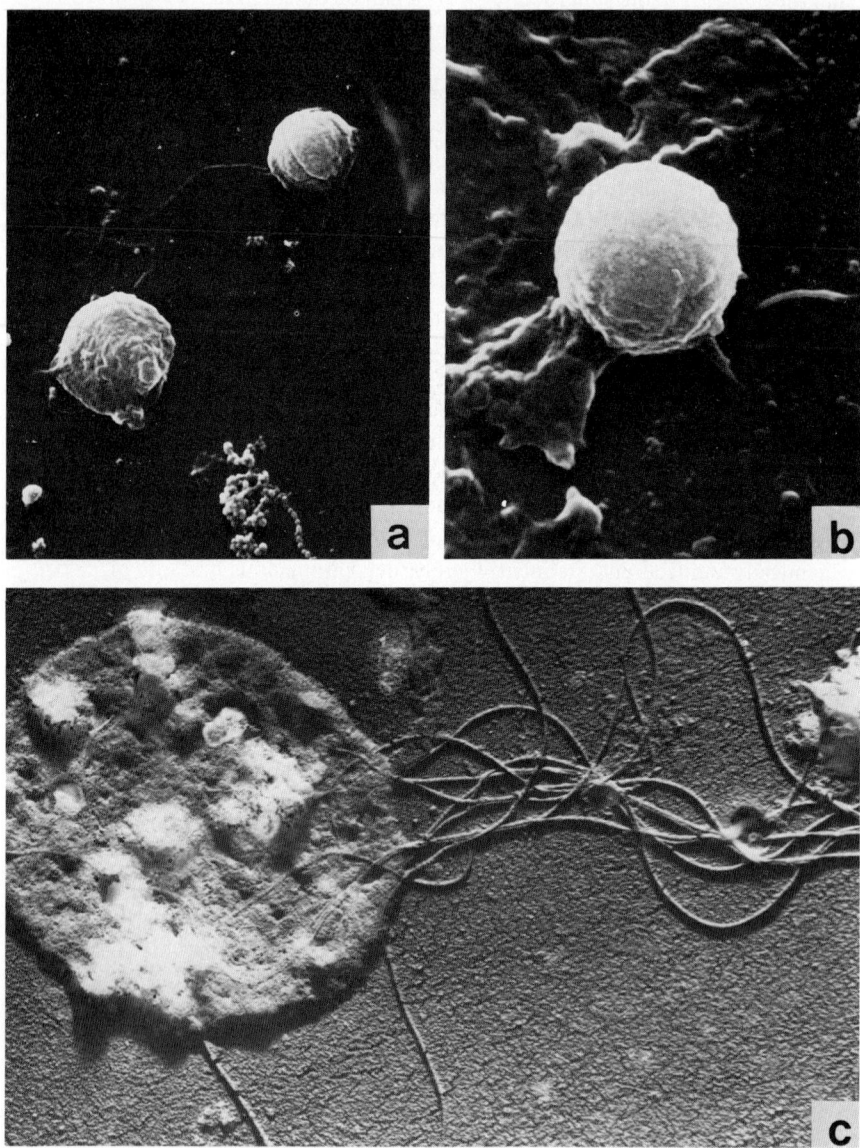

Figure 13 Morphology of the stable protoplast L-forms derived from *Proteus vulgaris* P18. Scanning (a,b), metal shadowing (c), and thin-layer (d,e) electron microscopy. Magnifications: ×10,000 in a; ×20,000 in b; ×24,000 in c; ×60,000 in e; ×400,000 in d.

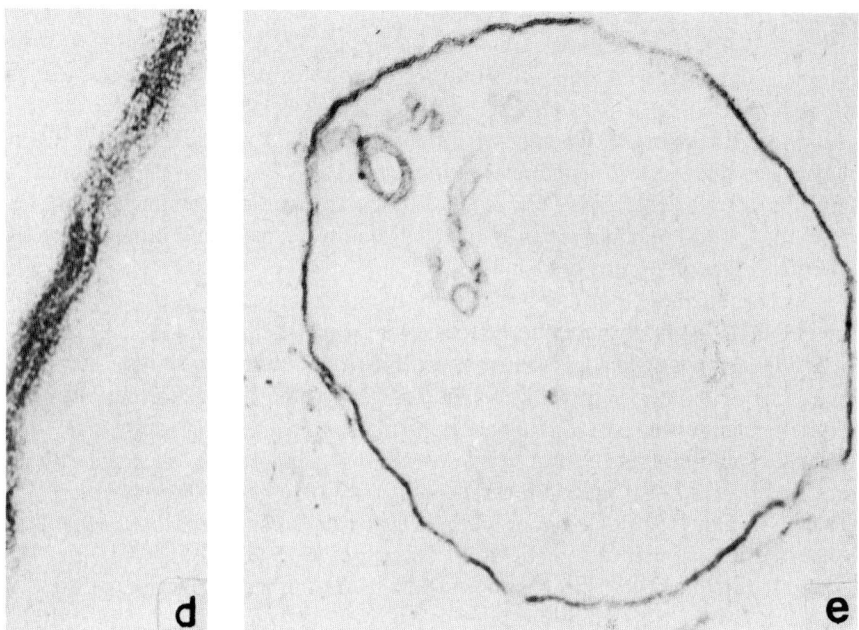

Figure 13 (Continued)

of a freshly induced protoplast L-form requires the addition of an unknown growth factor in the form of 5-10% horse serum to the culture medium. Established protoplast L-forms can then be adapted to life without serum.

1. Heterogeneity of the Membranous Structures

Thin sections of the stable protoplast L-forms reveal a great variety of different membranous structures [38] and this heterogeneity is also reflected in the complex pattern obtained when the membranes are fractionated by density gradient centrifugation [38] according to the technique of Osborn et al. [44]. The reason for this heterogeneity is not known. Separation into cells of different sizes and analysis of the isolated fractions might clarify the situation.

When submitted to fractionation by density gradient centrifugation, the membranes of the protoplast L-forms (of *P. mirabilis*) do not yield predominant banding at that low density where a cytoplasmic membrane is expected. Instead, they give rise to a multiple-banded pattern of "heavy" and "light" fractions, similar to that obtained with the cell envelopes of normal proteus or the unstable spheroplast L-forms (in which cases, the heavy band essentially contains the outer membrane with the typical major proteins, lipoproteins and lipopolysaccharide, while the lighter bands are considerably enriched in the cytoplasmic membrane). In spite of this unexpected behavior, all heavy and light bands generated by the membranes of the protoplast L-forms have protein and enzyme patterns that essentially are those of a cytoplasmic membrane [38]. Yet, the 15,000 M_r lipoprotein is found in the heavy band and lipopolysaccharide is present in the light bands.

Outer membrane (and periplasmic) proteins are known to be produced in membrane-bound polysomes in the form of a precursor that contains a characteristic signal peptide. This signal peptide is processed during or shortly after synthesis of the polypeptide. Depending on the proteins, evidence has been presented suggesting cotranslational or posttranslational transfer across the cytoplasmic membrane, and, in the case of the 7200 M_r lipoprotein, the possibility has been evoked that maturation can occur only on a glyceride-containing prolipoprotein [45]. Why among all the major proteins and lipoproteins that are exported to the outer membrane in *Proteus* only the 15,000 M_r lipoprotein is found sequestered (perhaps in a nonprocessed form) in the membranes of the stable protoplast L-forms, is not known.

In the gram-negative enterobacteria, the O-side chains of the lipopolysaccharide are synthesized in the plasma membrane independently of the other portions of the polymer. This synthesis involves the same C55 undecaprenyl–phosphate lipid carrier as that involved in peptidoglycan synthesis and the reactions sequence is analogous to that leading to the formation of the peptidoglycan disaccharide peptide units. Transfer of the polymerized O-side chains to the preformed core-lipid A then takes place within the plasma membrane itself. After the two components are joined, the resulted complete lipopolysaccharide molecules are translocated into the outer membrane through the adhesion sites mentioned above and distributed over the entire surface of the cell within the outer leaflet of the outer membrane [6]. In the protoplast L-forms, the above synthesis and assembly reactions are still in operation but with defects so that incomplete lipopolysaccharide molecules with short side chains largely predominate. In addition, these molecules can no longer be exported and necessarily remain associated at their site of assembly. Their exact location is unknown, but they apparently do not give the membrane an asymmetrical character similar to that found in the outer membrane of the normal bacteria.

2. Physical Stability and Fluidity

Central to the problem of the protoplast L-forms is how the membrane has enough physical stability to permit vigorous growth under conditions of minimal osmotic stabilization and, at the same time, has a sufficient degree of fluidity in order to maintain normal "plasma membrane" functions [46].

It is known that lipopolysaccharide exerts a stabilizing action on phospholipid model membranes. Lipopolysaccharide thus may also exert a protective function in the membranes of the protoplast L-forms (and impart to them an increased viscosity). In addition, preferential synthesis of the more hydrophobic lipopolysaccharide molecules with short O-side chains may also provide for increased stability of the membrane.

In turn, membrane fluidity probably occurs by a shortening of the saturated fatty acids in both the lipopolysaccharide and phospholipid molecules (and not by an increased incorporation of unsaturated fatty acids, which would be the alternative for gaining more fluidity). Thus, while in the lipopolysaccharide of the normal bacteria, tetradecanoic, hexadecanoic, and 3-hydroxytetradecanoic acids occur in the molar ratio of 5:1:6, the same fatty acids in the lipopolysaccharide of the protoplast L-forms occur in the ratio 5:0.1:6 [46]. Similarly, while the quantitative and qualitative composition of the phospholipids is very similar in the normal bacteria and the protoplast L-forms (the range of mole percentages of phospholipid species is 76-80 for phosphatidylethanolamine, 10-13 for phosphatidylglycerol, 4-5.5 for diphosphatidylglycerol, and 1-2 for lysophospholipid), all phospholipid species in the L-form differ from those of the normal bacteria by a lower content of long-chain fatty acids and a higher content of short-chain fatty acids [46].

The effect of horse serum as a "growth factor" in the early propagation of freshly induced protoplast L-forms is not understood. Short fatty acids occur to a lesser extent in the lipids of the protoplast L-forms grown in the presence of serum than in its absence and lipids present in the serum appear in the membranes of the protoplast L-forms [46]. Cholesterol, for example, is taken up from the serum and incorporated in the membranes. However, it is unlikely that the incorporated cholesterol fulfils any essential role since cholesterol-containing protoplast L-forms do not show any increased sensitivity to amphotericin B or digitonin [46]. It may be that some of the serum lipids are temporarily needed for the initial conversion of the bacteria to the L-form life. However, none of them is essential for the maintenance of established protoplast L-forms.

3. PBPs and Inability to Revert to Normal

It has been reported (W. Hammes; cited in Ref. 34) that proteus protoplast L-forms synthesize the peptidoglycan cytoplasmic precursors UDP-GlcNAc and UDP-MurNAc-pentapeptide. In addition, their membranes are known to possess a normal PBP pattern [32,47] (Fig. 11) except for the lack of PBP4 which (as shown with *P. vulgaris*) is excreted in the culture medium during growth. Finally, PBP4 and PBP5 have been isolated and shown to perform the same enzyme activities and to exhibit the same sensitivities to β-lactams as the corresponding PBPs of the normal bacteria [32,33,48,49].

We have seen that the benzylpenicillin-induced unstable spheroplast L-forms continue to manufacture a cross-linked wall peptidoglycan although they lack free PBP4. In addition, mutants of *E. coli* lacking PBP4 grow normally under a wide range of laboratory conditions. It thus follows that the defect for the hereditary and permanent inability of the proteus stable protoplast L-forms to reverse to walled bacteria is unlikely to be the lack of integration of PBP4 in the plasma membrane.

These protoplast L-forms might have all the enzymes required for peptidoglycan synthesis but, because of lack of wall "primer," glycan strands with uncross-linked peptide substituents might be excreted into the culture medium. This situation would be similar to that found with glycosidase (lysozyme)-induced protoplasts of gram-positive bacteria. Alternatively, the proteus protoplast L-forms might be unable to manufacture the disaccharide peptide units from the nucleotide precursors because of defects at the level of the membrane lipid cycle. In support to this view, one should bear in mind that preferential synthesis of incomplete lipopolysaccharide molecules with short side-chains in these organisms might be due (among other possibilities) to defects in the functioning of the undecaprenyl phosphate carrier and that the same carrier is involved in peptidoglycan synthesis. One may also note that defects in the synthesis of the nucleotide precursors and translocation into the plasma membrane have been reported [50] in the case of some stable L-forms of gram-positive bacteria.

Assuming that the observations made with proteus apply to other bacterial species, then the presence of defined PBP patterns in the stable protoplast L-forms may have important, practical applications. It may help to identify the parental bacterial species. In addition, it may help to distinguish the L-forms from the mycoplasmatales (see Sect. I) since, as shown with *Acholeplasma laidlawii* and several *Mycoplasma* species, these organisms do not contain, even in trace amounts, any protein having the ability to bind penicillin with high affinity [47].

V. CONCLUSIONS

Bacteria have developed several mechanisms to withstand β-lactam antibiotic therapy by raising the antibiotic concentration necessary for killing beyond the level that can be achieved clinically (for recent information, see Ref. 51).

Plasmid-mediated and chromosomally determined β-lactamases very effectively degrade susceptible β-lactams into biologically inactive metabolites by hydrolyzing the β-lactam amide bond.

In the gram-negative bacteria, the β-lactamase molecules are "concentrated" in the periplasmic region. Diminishing the rate of penetration of the β-lactams through the porin channels of the outer membrane is an important mechanism of resistance, at least against those β-lactams that show high susceptibility to β-lactamase. Indeed, their extremely rapid degradation must be counteracted by bringing in new molecules at a very rapid rate.

Alterations of the PBPs is another mechanism of resistance. The case of *Neisseria gonorrhoeae* has already been mentioned. In *Streptococcus pneumoniae*, the shift in PBP pattern involves loss of some PBPs and acquisition of others. Methicillin-resistant staphylococci, when compared with sensitive ones, show, depending on the cases, either a major decrease in the affinity of PBPs 1, 2, and 3, or an affinity change of only PBP3. Changes in PBPs have also been shown in β-lactam-resistant strains of *Pseudomonas aeruginosa*.

The above mechanisms result, in one way or another, in a decreased effectiveness of β-lactam action at the level of the primary targets, the PBPs. However, there is also very strong experimental evidence for "an indirect mode of β-lactam action" in which PBP inactivation is not lethal per se but initiates a chain of secondary events that abolish protein (and RNA/DNA) synthesis and affect the specific activity and/or cellular control of peptidoglycan hydrolases (autolytic enzymes). Alterations at the level of presumed "effector molecules" that normally link the synthesis of the wall peptidoglycan and the synthesis and/or functioning of other essential biopolymers may result to tolerance to β-lactams. Tolerance, as first seen in pneumococci, can be defined as diminished and/or delayed killing by growth-inhibiting concentrations of the antibiotic.

Persistence, a widespread phenomenon among penicillin- and ampicillin-sensitive bacteria including *E. coli*, relates to the survival of a small fraction (about 1 in 10^6 cells) of bacteria that remain viable despite prolonged exposure to bacteriocidal doses of β-lactams. Neither resistance, tolerance, impaired growth, nor reversion of spheroplasts account for persistence. The recent recognition of a gene (*hipA*) in *E. coli* that affects the frequency of persistence after inhibition of peptidoglycan synthesis may shed light on the underlying mechanism [52].

Finally, as shown in the present article, environmental conditions are susceptible to influence profoundly survival of bacteria from β-lactam action. *Proteus* is able to survive in the presence of high β-lactam antibiotic concentrations in the form of wall-deficient spheroplast L-forms if it finds an environment of suitable osmolality. Life under these conditions may not be practicable forever, but these L-forms keep the capacity of reverting to normal bacteria once the inducing β-lactam is removed from the medium. Alternatively, *Proteus* can shift to a permanent life in the form of wall-less protoplast L-forms (whether the β-lactam remains present or not) providing that it finds appropriate lipids in the environment until it can redirect its own lipopolysaccharide and lipid syntheses to manufacture a plasma membrane with both sufficient physical stability and fluidity.

Studies on these *Proteus* L-forms (remarkably conducted by H. H. Martin, J. Gmeiner, and their colleagues at the Technische Hochschule of Darmstadt) have also greatly contributed to the establishment of important (and "nonorthodox") concepts with respect to β-lactam action. Thus, peptidoglycan exhibiting a correct average extent of peptide cross-linking, but with defects in physical strength, can be synthesized by bacteria possessing only a minor proportion of PBPs left in a free form. Sharp decrease in peptide cross-linking by β-lactam action may be achieved only through the combined action of "complementing" β-lactams. PBP inactivation can induce (directly or indirectly) lesions in components of the bacterial cell envelope other than the peptide moiety of the peptidoglycan. Simple chemical substituents in the peptidoglycan, as the O-acetyl groups in proteus, may be markers of great physiological significance.

ACKNOWLEDGMENTS

This work has been supported by the Fonds de la Recherche Scientifique Médicale, Brussels (contract 3.4501.79) and an Action concertée financed by the Belgian State (convention 79/84-I1). We thank Dr. H. H. Martin and Dr. J. Gmeiner for discussion and critical reading of the manuscript. The electron micrographs shown in Figures 12 and 13 were taken at the Département de Bactériologie (Professeur R. Minck), Université de Strasbourg, France.

REFERENCES

1. Razin, S. (1978). The mycoplasmas. *Microbiol. Rev. 42*:414–470.
2. Neimark, H. and London, J. (1982). Origins of the mycoplasmas: Sterol-nonrequiring mycoplasmas involved from Streptococci. *J. Bacteriol. 150*: 1259–1265.
3. Ghuysen, J. M. (1968). Use of bacteriolytic enzymes in determination of wall structure and their role in cell metabolism. *Bacteriol. Rev. 32*:425–464.
4. Lugtenberg, B. and Van Alphen, L. (1983). Molecular architecture and functioning of the outer membrane of *Escherichia coli* and other gram-negative bacteria. *Biochim. Biophys. Acta 737*:51–115.
5. Rogers, H. J., Perkins, H. R., and Ward, J. B. (1980). *Microbial Cell Walls and Membranes*, Chapman and Hall, London, New York.
6. Inouye, M. (1979). *Bacterial Outer Membranes. Biogenesis and Functions*, Wiley, New York.
7. Wensink, J. and Witholt, B. (1981). Outer membrane vesicles released by normally growing *Escherichia coli* contain very little protein. *Eur. J. Biochem. 116*:331–335.

8. Lugtenberg, B. (1981). Composition and function of the outer membrane of *Escherichia coli. Trends Biochem. Sci. 6*:262-266.
9. Ghuysen, J. M., Frère, J. M., Leyh-Bouille, M., Dideberg, O., Lamotte-Brasseur, J., Perkins, H. R., and De Coen, J. L. (1981). Penicillins and Δ^3-cephalosporins as inhibitors and mechanism-based inactivators of D-alanyl-D-Ala peptidases in *Topics in Molecular Pharmacology* (A. S. V. Burgen and G. C. K. Roberts, eds.), Elsevier/North-Holland Biomedical Press, pp. 63-97.
10. Charlier, P., Dideberg, O., Dive, G., Dusart, J., Frère, J. M., Ghuysen, J. M., Joris, B., Lamotte-Brasseur, J., Leyh-Bouille, M., and Nguyen-Distèche, M. (1983). The active sites of the D-alanyl-D-alanine-cleaving peptidases in *The Murein Sacculus of Bacterial Cell Walls. Architecture and Growth* (R. Hakenbeck, J. V. Höltje and H. Labischinski, ed.), International FEMS Symposium. March 13-18, 1983 (Berlin West). Walter de Gruyter and Co., Berlin, New York.
11. Waxman, D. J. and Strominger, J. L. (1983). Penicillin binding proteins and the mechanism of action of β-lactam antibiotics. *Ann. Rev. Biochem. 52*: 825-869.
12. Burman, L. G. and Park, J. T. (1983). Change in the composition of *Escherichia coli* murein as it ages during exponential growth. *J. Bacteriol. 155*:447-453.
13. Spratt, B. G. (1983). Penicillin binding proteins and the future of β-lactam antibiotics. *J. Gen. Microbiol. 129*:1247-1260.
14. Curtis, N. A. C., Orr, D., Ross, G. W., and Boulton, M. G. (1979). Competition of β-lactam antibiotics for the penicillin binding proteins of *Pseudomonas aeruginosa, Enterobacter cloacae, Klebsiella aerogenes, Proteus rettgeri,* and *Escherichia coli.* Comparison with antibacterial activity and effects upon bacterial morphology. *Antimicrob. Ag. Chemother. 16*:325-328.
15. Matsuhashi, M., Nakagawa, J., Ishino, F., Nakajima-Iijima, S., Tomioka, S., Doi, M., and Tamaki, S. (1981). Penicillin binding proteins: Their nature and functions in the cellular duplication and mechanism of action of β-lactam antibiotics in *Escherichia coli*, in *β-Lactam Antibiotics* (S. Mitsuhashi, ed.), Japan Scientific Societies Press, Tokyo, and Springer-Verlag, pp. 203-223.
16. Tipper, D. J. and Strominger, J. L. (1965). Mechanism of action of penicillins: a proposal based on their structural similarity to acyl-D-alanyl-D-alanine. *Proc. Natl. Acad. Sci. USA 54*:1133-1141.
17. Essig, P., Martin, H. H., and Gmeiner, J. (1982). Murein and lipopolysaccharide biosynthesis in synchronized cells of *Escherichia coli* K12 and the effect of penicillin G, mecillinam and nalidixic acid. *Arch. Microbiol. 132*: 245-250.
18. Gmeiner, J., Essig, P., and Martin, H. H. (1982). Characterization of minor fragments after digestion of *Escherichia coli* murein with endo-N,O-diacetylmuramidase from *Chalaropsis*, and determination of glycan chain length. *FEBS Lett. 138*:109-112.

19. Kariyama, R. (1982). Increase of cardiolipin content in *Staphylococcus aureus* by the use of antibiotics affecting the cell wall. *J. Antibiotics 35*: 1700–1704.
20. Rozgonyi, F., Kiss, J., Jékel, P., and Vaczi, L. (1980). Effect of methicillin on the phospholipid content of methicillin sensitive *Staphylococcus aureus*. *Acta Microbiol. Acad. Sci. Hung. 27*:31–40.
21. Zickler, W. (1967). Phagenrezeptorsynthese durch die stabile L-form in *Proteus mirabilis* VI. *Z. Allg. Mikrobiol. 7*:283–285.
22. Starka, J. and Moravova, J. (1970). Phospholipids and cellular division of *Escherichia coli. J. Gen. Microbiol. 60*:251–257.
23. Fleck, J. and Mock, M. (1972). Etude de la forme filamenteuse de *Proteus vulgaris* P18 induite par la pénicilline. *Annales de l'Institut Pasteur 123*: 319–332.
24. Gmeiner, J. and Kroll, H. P. (1981). Murein biosynthesis and O-acetylation of N-acetylmuramic acid during the cell division cycle of *Proteus mirabilis*. *Eur. J. Biochem. 117*:171–177.
25. Gmeiner, J. and Kroll, H. P. (1981). N-acetylglycosaminyl-N-acetylmuramyl-dipeptide. A novel murein building block formed during the cell division cycle of *Proteus mirabilis*. *FEBS Lett. 129*:142–144.
26. Gmeiner, J. (1975). The isolation of two different lipopolysaccharide fractions from various *Proteus mirabilis* strains. *Eur. J. Biochem. 58*:621–626.
27. Gmeiner, J. (1979). Covalent linkage of lipoprotein to peptidoglycan is not essential for outer membrane stability in *Proteus mirabilis*. *Arch. Microb. 121*:177–180.
28. Gmeiner, J., Kroll, H. P., and Martin, H. H. (1978). The covalent rigid-layer lipoprotein in cell walls of *Proteus mirabilis*. *Eur. J. Biochem. 83*:227–233.
29. Nixdorff, K., Fitzer, H., Gmeiner, J., and Martin, H. H. (1977). Reconstitution of model membranes from phospholipid and outer membrane proteins of *Proteus mirabilis*. *Eur. J. Biochem. 81*:63–69.
30. Gmeiner, J. (1981). Characterization of a new murein-associated lipoprotein in the outer membrane of *Proteus mirabilis*. *Arch. Microbiol. 128*:299–302.
31. Ohya, S., Yamazaki, M., Sugawara, S., and Matsuhashi, M. (1979). Penicillin binding proteins in *Proteus* species. *J. Bacteriol. 137*:474–479.
32. Rousset, A., Nguyen-Distèche, M., Minck, R., and Ghuysen, J. M. (1982). Penicillin binding protein and carboxypeptidase activities in *Proteus vulgaris* P18 and its penicillin-induced stable L-forms. *J. Bacteriol. 152*:1042–1048.
33. Schilf, W. and Martin, H. H. (1980). Purification of two DD-carboxypeptidases-transpeptidases with different penicillin sensitivities from *Proteus mirabilis*. *Eur. J. Biochem. 105*:361–370.
34. Martin, H. H. (1983). Protoplasts and spheroplasts of gram-negative bacteria—with special emphasis on *Proteus mirabilis* in *Protoplasts 1983*, Lecture Proceedings, 6th International Protoplast Symposium, Basel, August 12–16, 1983 (I. Potrykus, C. T. Harms, A. Hinnen, R. Hütter, P. J. King, R. D. Shillito, eds.), Publ. Birkhäuser Verlag, Basel, Boston, Stuttgart, pp. 213–225.

35. Martin, H. H. (1964). Composition of the mucopolymer in cell walls of the unstable and stable L-form of *Proteus mirabilis. J. Gen. Microbiol. 36*:441–450.
36. Hofschneider, P. H. and Martin, H. H. (1968). Diversity of surface layers in L-forms of *Proteus mirabilis. J. Gen. Microbiol. 51*:23–33.
37. Rinno, J., Golecki, J. R., and Mayer, H. (1980). Localization of enterobacterial common antigen: Immunogenic and nonimmunogenic enterobacterial common antigen-containing *Escherichia coli. J. Bacteriol. 141*:814–821.
38. Kroll, H. P., Gmeiner, J., and Martin (1980). Membranes of the protoplast L-form of *Proteus mirabilis. Arch. Microbiol. 127*:223–229.
39. Martin, H. H. and Gmeiner, J. (1979). Modification of peptidoglycan structure by penicillin action in cell walls of *Proteus mirabilis. Eur. J. Biochem. 95*:487–497.
40. Martin, H. H., Tonn-Ehlers, M., and Schilf, W. (1980). Cooperation of benzyl-penicillin and cefoxitin in bacterial growth inhibition. *Phil. Trans. R. Soc. Lond. B 289*:365–367.
41. Dougherty, T. H. (1983). Peptidoglycan biosynthesis in *Neisseria gonorrhoeae* strains sensitive and intrinsically resistant to β-lactam antibiotics. *J. Bacteriol. 153*:429–435.
42. Tulasne, R. (1949). Existence of L-forms in common bacteria and their possible importance. *Nature 164*:876–877.
43. Kandler, O. and Kandler, G. (1956). Trennung and Charakterisierung verschiedener L-Phasen-Typen von *Proteus mirabilis. Z. Naturforsch. 11*: 252–259.
44. Osborn, M. J., Gander, E., Parisi, E., and Carson, J. (1972). Mechanism of assembly of the outer membrane of *Salmonella typhimurium*. Isolation and characterization of cytoplasmic and outer membrane. *J. Biol. Chem. 247*: 3962–3972.
45. Hussain, M., Ichihara, S., and Mizushima, S. (1980). Accumulation of glyceride-containing precursor of the outer membrane lipoprotein in the cytoplasmic membrane of *Escherichia coli* treated with globomycin. *J. Biol. Chem. 255*:3707–3712.
46. Gmeiner, J. and Martin, H. H. (1976). Phospholipid and lipopolysaccharide in *Proteus mirabilis* and its stable protoplast L-form. *Eur. J. Biochem. 67*: 448–494.
47. Martin, H. H., Schilf, W., and Schiefer, H. G. (1980). Differentiation of mycoplasmatales from bacterial protoplast L-forms by assay for penicillin binding proteins. *Arch. Microbiol. 127*:297–299.
48. Martin, H. H., Schilf, W., and Maskos, Ch. (1976). Purification of membrane-bound DD-carboxypeptidase of the unstable spheroplast L-form of *Proteus mirabilis* by affinity chromatography. *Eur. J. Biochem. 71*:585–593.
49. Schilf, W., Frère, Ph., Frère, J. M., Martin, H. H., Ghuysen, J. M., Adriaens, P., and Meeschaert, B. (1978). Interaction between penicillin and the DD-carboxypeptidase EC.3.4.12.6 of the unstable L-form of *Proteus mirabilis* strain 19. *Eur. J. Biochem. 85*:325–330.

50. Ward, J. B. (1975). Peptidoglycan synthesis in L-phase variants of *Bacillus licheniformis* and *Bacillus subtilis. J. Bacteriol. 124*:668–678.
51. Wiedemann, B. and Ghuysen, J. M. (1983). Symposium: Mechanisms of resistance to β-lactam antibiotics in *13th International Congress of Chemotherapy*, Vienna, 28th August–2nd September 1983, Proceedings (K. H. Spitzy and K. Karrer, eds.), pp. 12/1–12/42.
52. Moyed, H. S. and Bertrand, K. P. (1983). *Hip*A, a newly recognized gene of *Escherichia coli* K-12 that affects frequency of persistence after inhibition of murein synthesis. *J. Bacteriol. 155*:768–775.
53. Wise, E. M., Jr., and Park, J. T. (1965). Penicillin: Its basic site of action as an inhibitor of a peptide cross-linking reaction in cell wall mucopeptide synthesis. *Proc. Natl. Acad. Sci. USA 54*:75–81.

7
Brucella L-Forms—Their Occurrence and Characteristics

BETTY A. HATTEN
Department of Clinical Laboratory Sciences, Oklahoma University Health Sciences Center, Oklahoma City, Oklahoma

JANINE SCHMITT-SLOMSKA
U.65 INSERM: National Institute of Health and Medical Research, Department of Microbiology, Faculty of Medicine, Nimes, France

I. Occurrence and Characteristics of *Brucella* L-Forms from Natural and Experimental Infections	163
II. In Vitro Studies in Cell Cultures	169
III. Characteristics of *Brucella* L-Forms in Artificial Media	170
IV. Antigenic Properties of *Brucella* L-Forms	171
V. Summary	181
References	181

I. OCCURRENCE AND CHARACTERISTICS OF *BRUCELLA* L-FORMS FROM NATURAL AND EXPERIMENTAL INFECTIONS

In 1951, Nelson and Pickett [1] observed L-forms after primary plates of broth cultures of human blood had been subcultured to thioglycollate medium. Subcultures of the same blood cultures to *Brucella* broth or *Brucella* agar plates did not grow. The L-form growth appeared in thioglycollate medium immediately below the zone of diffused oxygen. *Brucella* broth medium containing 5% peptic digest of blood and 100 μg/ml thiamine and nicotinamide (BTN medium) also supported L-form growth, giving rise to a slightly turbid and occasionally granular sediment. After several passages in this medium, precipitin tests performed between the supernatant broths from such cultures and antismooth *Brucella* serum gave positive reactions. On 5% peptic digest BTN plates containing 0.7% agar, typical L-form colonies were observed. In addition, a secondary growth of large, opaque, white colonies was often present that obscured the L-type growth soon after their appearance. Microscopically, the L-forms were described to be a mixture of rods, chains, branching forms, ghost cells, and large bodies.

Carrere and Roux [2] also reported the isolation of L-forms in primary subcultures from sheep blood. The organisms were initially grown in peptone broth containing penicillin and human plasma and subsequently in peptone and Albimi broth without penicillin. The L-forms were described as small, round bodies of 5-6 μm which increased in number until about 20 hr. After 48 hr, the broth cultures were opaque and contained a flocculent suspension which consisted of conglomerated bodies varying in size from 5 to 50 μm.

An interesting aspect of these early investigations on isolating organisms in blood cultures from patients with brucellosis concerned the repeated observation of plaques that developed in the confluent growth of organisms on agar plates [1,3]. The plaques were inhibited by acriflavine and increased in titer when inoculated into broth cultures of brucellae. This bacteriophage was considered to be weakly lytic since smooth strains often became lysogenic. Infected cells had a prolonged lag period, however, and frequently no growth occurred on agar plates inoculated with very turbid broth cultures. When citrated human bloods from patients whose cultures had previously been negative were washed prior to culturing, microorganisms antigenically typical of brucellae were recovered. Most of these isolates were nonsmooth variants rather than smooth strains typically associated with infection. It was concluded that phage present in the blood, if not removed before culturing, lysed the smooth bacteria under the cultural conditions used for isolation. An additional observation made upon microscopic examination of clear areas on the agar plates was the occurrence of L-forms within the plaques. The authors therefore speculated that L-forms may be essential to survival of this bacterial species, since they appeared to be resistant to the lytic activity of the bacteriophage. These workers also suggested that such forms, as well as the bacteriophage, are present in vivo.

Evidence confirming the lysogenic state of *Brucella* isolates from various animals has been provided [4]. Of 60 isolates examined, all were found to carry phage. Plaques produced in cultures of these strains were of several types and were best observed when broth cultures were pipetted onto the plates. None were seen when the culture was applied with a cotton swab. Smooth isolates were sensitive to the phage and either lysed or, in some cases, transformed into sticky, white forms with a characteristic butyrous odor. The latter were designated as "porteuse colonies" and were shown to carry active phage. When subcultured, such colonies gave rise to phage-free smooth and smooth-intermediate colonies, as well as lysogenic colonies. The role of brucellaphage upon brucellae in vivo, therefore, was again conjectured, but no comments were made regarding the presence or absence of L-forms in these cultures. Evidence was later provided to suggest that brucellaphage can infect and lyse intracellular brucellae [5].

In an unpublished preliminary study, Hatten and co-workers obtained no conclusive evidence that L-forms of a virulent *Brucella abortus* strain could infect or kill chick embryos, since bacterial forms were always present. Results of studies by Schmitt-Slomska et al. [6,7] with *Brucella suis* strain 1330, however, provided evidence that L-forms may be induced and persist in vivo for extended periods of time. In these studies, gnotobiotic mice were inoculated with 0.2 ml of a suspension containing approximately 10^9 bacterial cells per ml. Intramuscular injections, each containing 50,000 U of penicillin G were subsequently given to the animals at 6, 24, and 48 hr postinoculation. Minced spleens from groups of animals sacrificed at different time intervals after infection were cultured on *Brucella* broth containing 1% purified Difco agar (Br-a medium) for bacterial growth; Br-a medium supplemented with 1% yeast extract (Difco), 0.3 M sucrose and 15% horse serum (L-a medium), for bacterial and L-form growth; and L-a medium containing 2500 U/ml penicillin (Special) for L-form growth. Results of such an experiment are shown in Table 1. While no L-forms were recovered from animals sacrificed at 6 and 24 hr after infection, cultures from two animals in each group sacrificed at 2, 7, and 14 days initially contained only L-form growth on penicillin-free medium. Isolation of L-type growth and

Table 1 Recovery of L-forms from the Spleens of Mice Inoculated (i.p.) with *B. suis* 1330 Strain and Treated (i.m.) with Penicillin

	Mice (gnotobiotic 20–22 g)				
				Number with positive cultures on penicillin-free media	
Group	Number infected with $\geq 10^8$ CFU	Penicillin $\times 10^3$ U	Sacrificed after	Bacterial overgrowth	L-forms only
I	8	50	6 hr	8	0
II	8	100	1 day	6	0
III	8	150	2 days	4[a]	2[a]
IV	8	150	7 days	6	2
V	8	250	14 days	6	2

[a]No growth in two cases; atypical, L-like growth, lost in subcultures, from the other two mice.
Control mice: for each group of mice, 6 animals were used as controls (2 inoculated, not treated; 2 not inoculated, not treated; and 2 not inoculated, penicillin-treated in a manner similar to the experimental groups); total = 30 control animals. i.p. = intraperitoneal; i.m. = intramuscular.

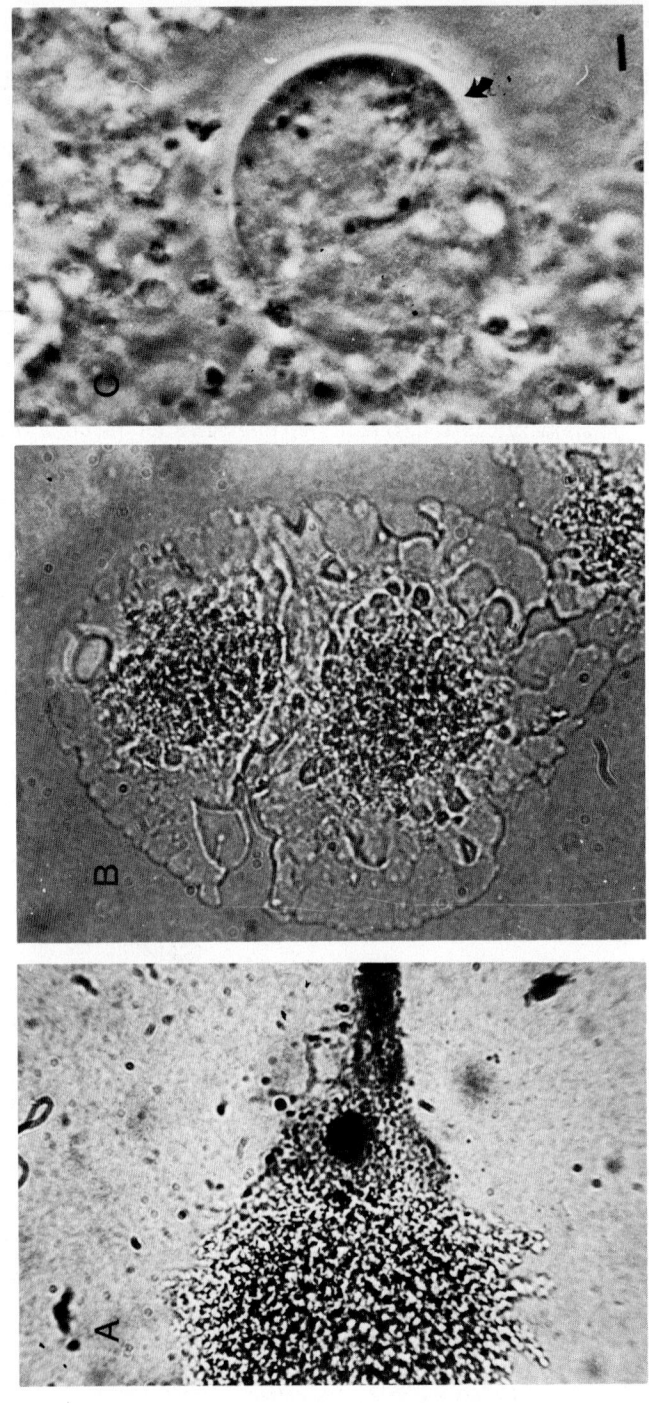

Figure 1 (*A–C*) Morphological appearance of *B. suis* L-form growth from spleens of mice experimentally infected with *B. suis* bacterial strain 1330. (*A*) "L-form like" microcolony associated with tissue remnants on L-a antibiotic-free medium (×500). (*B*) Tissue-free L-form colony obtained after six subcultures on penicillin-containing L-a medium. (*C*) Periphery of L-form 1330/Y

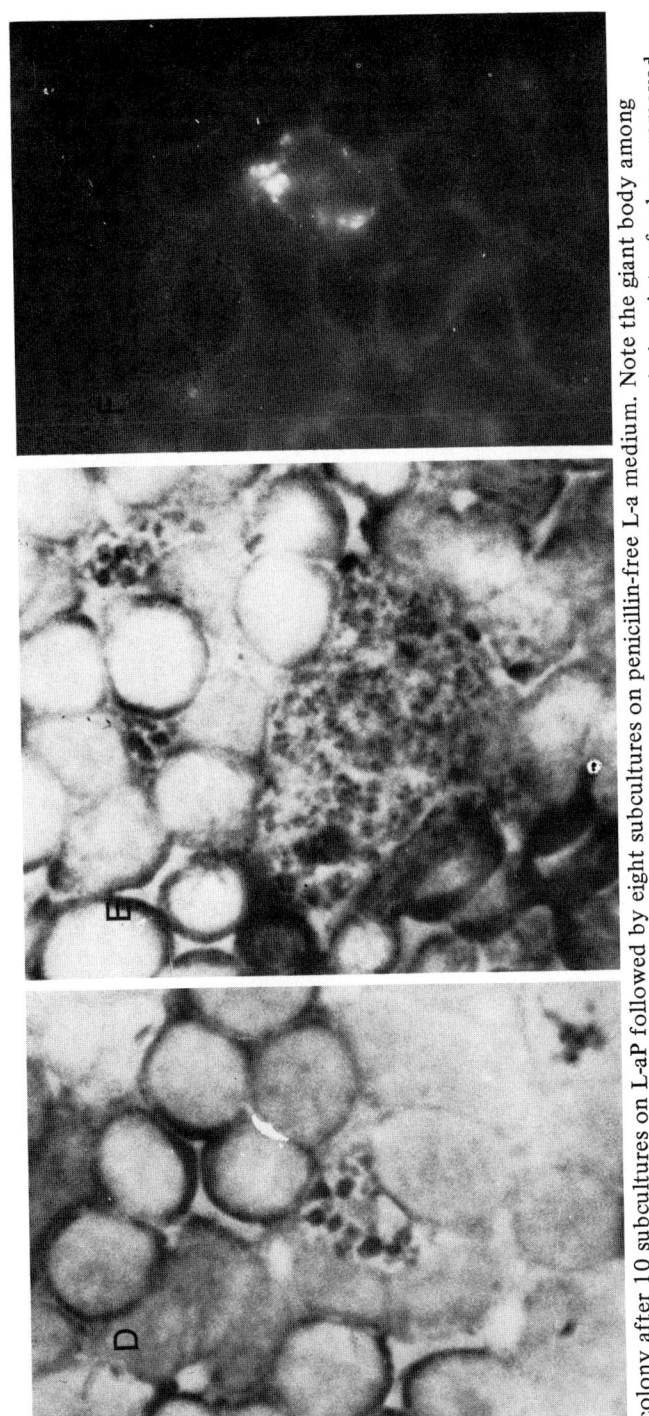

colony after 10 subcultures on L-aP followed by eight subcultures on penicillin-free L-a medium. Note the giant body among numerous globular elements. (Phase contrast; bar = 5 μm). (*D–E*) Show globular L-form elements in imprints of spleens removed after various periods of time from mice inoculated with L-form 1330/Y. (*D*) Mouse sacrificed 24 hr after inoculation (hot Giemsa stain, ×1200). (*E*) Mouse sacrificed 96 hr after inoculation (hot Giemsa stain, ×1200).(*F*) Identification of globular splenic L-form elements by indirect immunofluorescence staining with *B. suis* antiserum (UV, ×1200).(*G*) Splenic imprint from mouse sacrificed

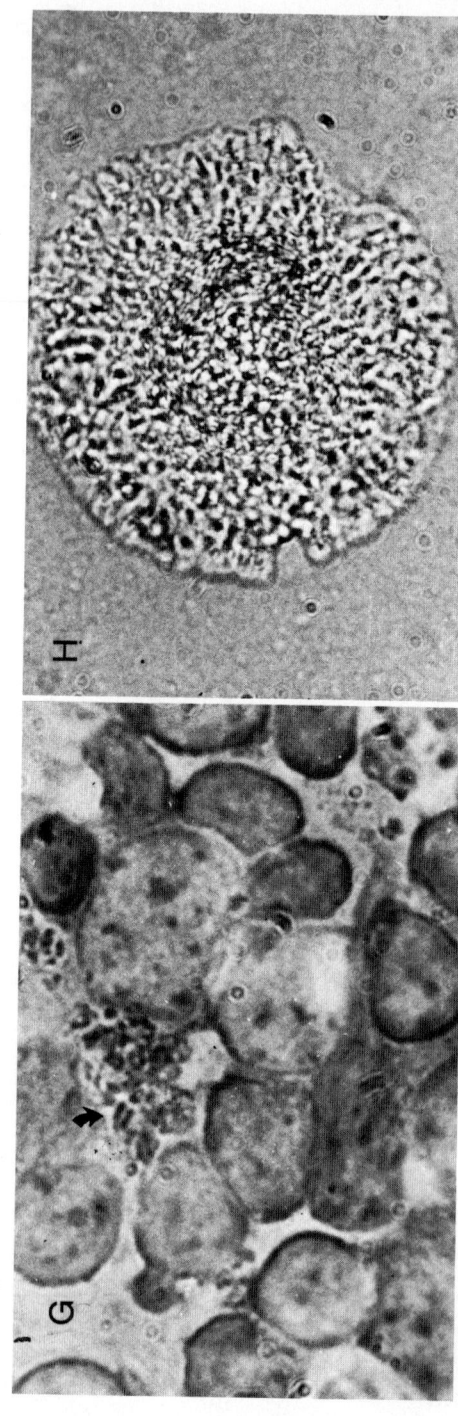

Figure 1 (Continued)

96 hr after inoculation showing occasional in vivo reversion to bacillary forms (arrow) which were subsequently identified as *B. suis* biotype I (hot Giemsa, ×1200). (*H*) Shows appearance of *B. suis* L-form colony after a total of 100 subcultures on artificial media, the last 12 of which were made on osmotically unprotected Br-agar (direct examination, ×500).

initial absence of bacterial growth in primary cultures on penicillin-free media was interpreted by these investigators to be evidence of induction and persistence of L-forms in vivo. Visual evidence of the presence of in vivo organisms resembling L-forms was obtained by a hot Giemsa staining technique [8] and similar in vivo forms were specifically stained by the indirect fluorescent staining technique (Fig. 1D-G). Similar studies showed that the duration of L-form recovery and observation by the methods described above was dependent upon the number of organisms inoculated, and in some cases they were found to persist for as long as 21 days after infection and treatment.

II. IN VITRO STUDIES IN CELL CULTURES

In 1964, Freeman and Rumack [9] demonstrated that mononuclear cells collected from the peritoneal cavity of guinea pigs were destroyed by short periods of exposure to *B. suis* spheroplasts that had been induced by treatment of bacterial cultures with 2% glycine or penicillin. Later, McGhee and Freeman [10] reported on the production of spheroplasts in immune guinea pig macrophages infected with *B. suis*. The spheroplasts required $0.3 M$ sucrose for survival and reversion to bacteria, and infected cells began to show evidence or cytopathic effects (CPE) shortly after their induction. No CPE was noted in infected cells from normal (nonimmune) animals, although the bacterial cells had multiplied 200-fold, and no osmotically sensitive forms were recovered from these cell cultures. Addition of rabbit anti-guinea pig sera stimulated rapid destruction of infected immune cells and reduced the number of osmotically sensitive forms. On the basis of these findings, the authors suggested that while immune macrophages were better equipped to cope with infection, surviving bacteria and spheroplasts might be important in the pathogenesis of the disease, because they had developed a physiological steady state making them more resistant to humoral responses of the host as well as to antibiotic therapy. This statement is somewhat controversial since development of CPE in tissue cultures infected with intact brucellae had been shown to be a characteristic of avirulent rather than virulent strains of *Brucella* [11]. Thus, occurrence of CPE in cells containing spheroplasts of the strain of *B. suis* used by McGhee and Freeman may actually imply that they were avirulent forms.

Hatten and Sulkin [12] found no evidence to suggest that L-forms induced by treatment of a virulent strain of *B. abortus* with penicillin were cytopathogenic for hamster kidney cells. Neither did these forms require immune cells for induction intracellularly nor increased osmolarity for their survivial. Results obtained in which L-forms were recovered in antibiotic-free media from tissue cultures for several days after inhibition of bacterial growth did suggest, however, that L-forms might survive and perpetuate an infection when intracellular conditions were adverse for bacterial growth [13]. Visual evidence that the majority or organisms had been altered by penicillin-treatment of cultures of this particular strain of *B. abortus* was later provided by electron microscopy studies [14]. Organisms in the treated cultures were structurally similar to other cell wall-defective forms, generally referred to as unstable L-forms. Those in untreated cultures were typical of gram-negative bacterial cells. In an extension of this study, infected monolayers were also examined by electron microscopy to determine if L-forms recovered from the cells by cultural methods were actually present in the tissue cultures or had been induced during recovery procedures [15]. Structures resembling L-forms were found in cytoplasmic vacuoles after short periods of infection but not after extended periods of time, although they persisted extracellularly and were most frequent in those cell cultures that had been treated with penicillin. Since the environment of tissue culture cells simulates conditions encountered by intracellular organisms in vivo, it was concluded that if *Brucella* L-forms are related to in vivo infections, they probably exist predominantly as extracellular forms. If this supposition is true, then the ability of such forms to perpetuate an infection would rely on their ability to survive in the presence of humoral factors, e.g., antibodies and complement. Their potential relationship to pathogenesis of brucellosis might also be dependent upon their ability to revert to bacteria under favorable conditions.

III. CHARACTERISTICS OF *BRUCELLA* L-FORMS IN ARTIFICIAL MEDIA

Difficulties encountered in controlling reversions to bacteria by unstable L-forms induced after penicillin treatment of *B. abortus* eventually led to a more in-depth study of the growth characteristics of such forms [16]. The results obtained by subculture of penicillin-treated broth cultures to agar plates containing penicillin indicated that microorganisms capable of producing L-colonies were present throughout a 7-day incubation period. Isolation of comparable numbers of bacterial colonies when the same cultures were subcultured to antibiotic-free agar plates also confirmed previous conclusions that most if not all organisms capable of producing L-colonies were also capable of reverting to bacteria. Nevertheless, results from repeated subculturing in penicillin-containing medium did not suggest that these microorganisms were capable of reproducing themselves in the L-state for prolonged periods of time. These results thus agree with those of Hines et al. [17] who induced osmotically stable spheroplasts with limited reproductive capabilities by treatment of *B. suis* with penicillin. The results of these two studies differ with respect to reverting ability of the forms induced, however, since only a few of the *B. suis* spheroplasts were found to be able to revert to bacteria. Persistence of occasional *B. abortus* organisms was indicated by recovery of bacterial colonies on the surface of filters, following transfer of those filters with no detectable growth from the surface of penicillin-containing agar plates to plates containing no antibiotics. Another observation concerned the increased incidence and magnitude of penicillin resistance among bacterial isolates of *B. abortus* that were recovered after reversion from the L-state. Resistance to carbenicillin by revertant bacteria of *Pseudomonas aeruginosa* has also been demonstrated [18]. The exact mechanism involved in either case is not clear, but the revertant strains of *Ps. aeruginosa* showed no differences in β-lactamase activity from the parent strains.

L-forms recovered by Schmitt-Slomska et al. [6,7,8] from mice experimentally infected with *B. suis* strain 1330 also had retained the ability to revert to bacteria. While such forms often showed marked pleomorphism and atypical colonial morphology, typical L-type colonies were observed in one case among the tissue remnants on primary isolation plates (Fig. 1A). After five or six subcultures, tissue-free L-type microcolonies were consistently obtained on penicillin-containing L-ap P medium (Fig. 1B). Revertant bacteria obtained when penicillin was removed from the medium had the same characteristics as the parent *B. suis* strain 1330, biotype 1. One L-form designated L-1330/4 was selected for further study. After 15 passages of the L-form, reversions to bacteria were no longer obtained. The small microcolonies on penicillin-free L-a medium had features common to L-forms including giant protoplasmic bodies at the periphery of the colonies (Fig. 1C). Proof of the origin from the parent *B. suis* strain was provided by immunofluorescence with specific antiserum. Serial passage of this strain eventually resulted in development of L-forms capable of growth on osmotically unprotected media. A microcolony typical of those produced by such forms after 100 subcultures is shown in Figure 1H.

L-forms of *B. suis* strain 1330, which retained the ability to revert to bacteria, were shown by electron microscopy to have structures typically found in unstable forms [7]. The ultrastructure of stable L-1330 forms seen in Figure 2A-D was observed and described through the courtesy of R. M. Cole. These forms from early transfers varied in size and structure but generally appear to have retained features associated with unstable L-forms or spheroplasts. After many passages over a 2-year period and adaptation to growth on osmotically unprotected media, structures in the microcolonies, as shown in Figure 3, were less variable in size and were now enclosed by a single unit membrane [19].

IV. ANTIGENIC PROPERTIES OF *BRUCELLA* L-FORMS

Speculation that cell wall components of brucella species are important to virulence and immogenicity make studies on the antigenic nature of brucella L-forms of particular interest. An immunoelectrophoretic study by Baughn and Freeman [20] of *B. suis* spheroplasts revealed that several components presumed to be surface antigens were absent in preparations of spheroplast antigens.

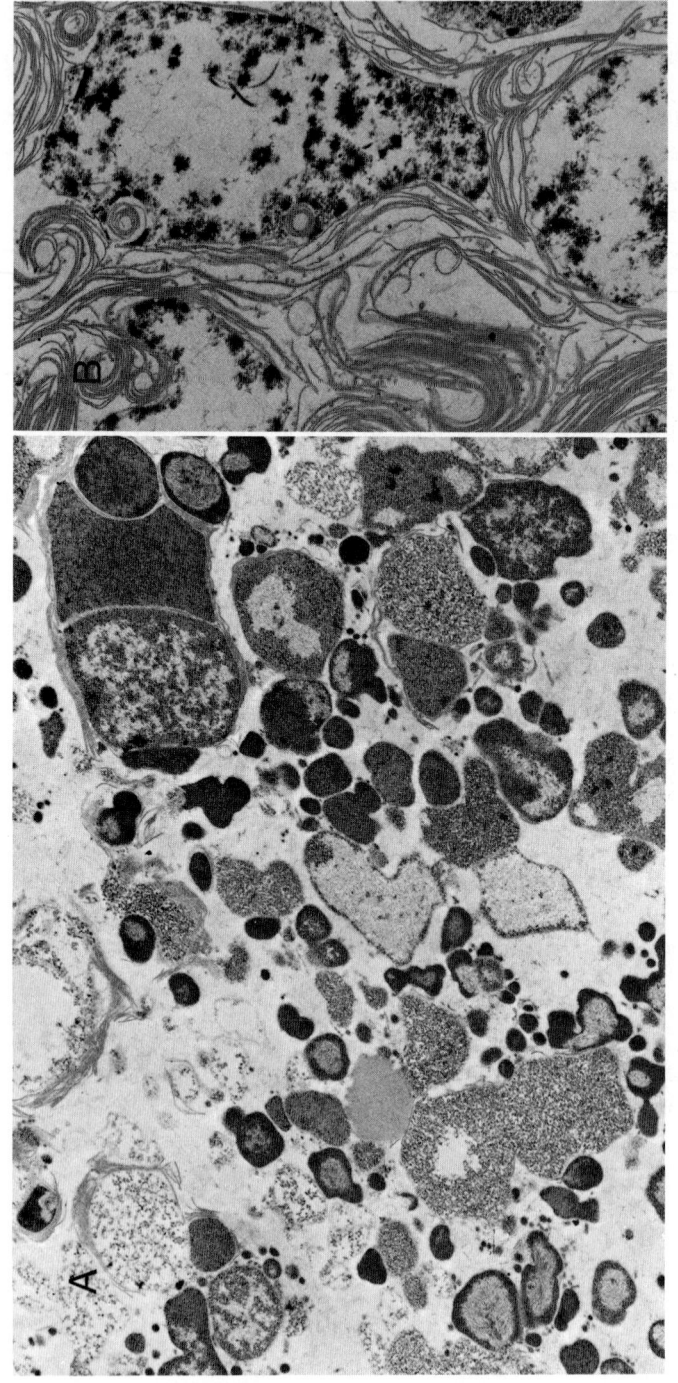

Figure 2 Electron micrographs of *B. suis* L-forms present in 5- to 6-day-old colonies grown on L-form agar with or without penicillin which show: (1) variability in general appearance, size, and shape typical of L-type organisms; (2) unusual multilayered membranes, often in whorls, surrounding many bodies; (3) frequent dispersion of the cytoplasm, or parts of it, into small

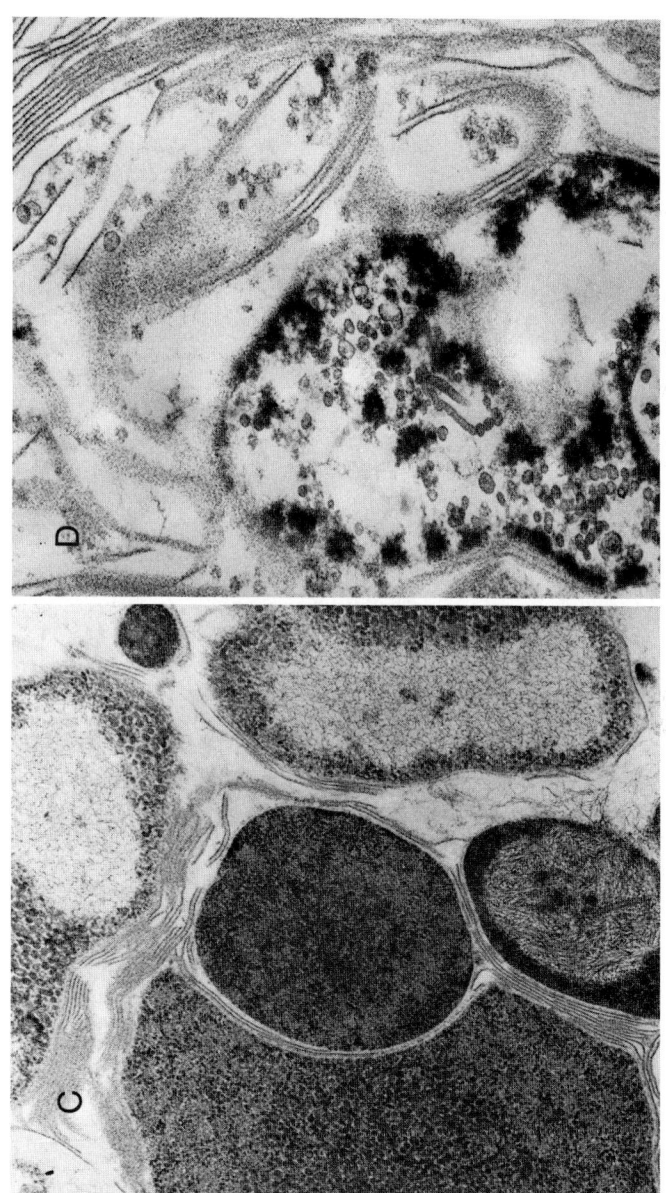

membrane-bounded vesicles; (4) absence of single membranes of classic structure and size enclosing the "protoplast-like" bodies. (Normal or expected width is 7–9 nm whereas those single and multiple membrane structures of the *B. suis* L-forms are much wider, ranging from 17 to 19 nm). (*A*) × 21,000; (*B*) × 30,000; (*C*) × 69,000; (*D*) × 117,000. (Courtesy of Roger M. Cole.)

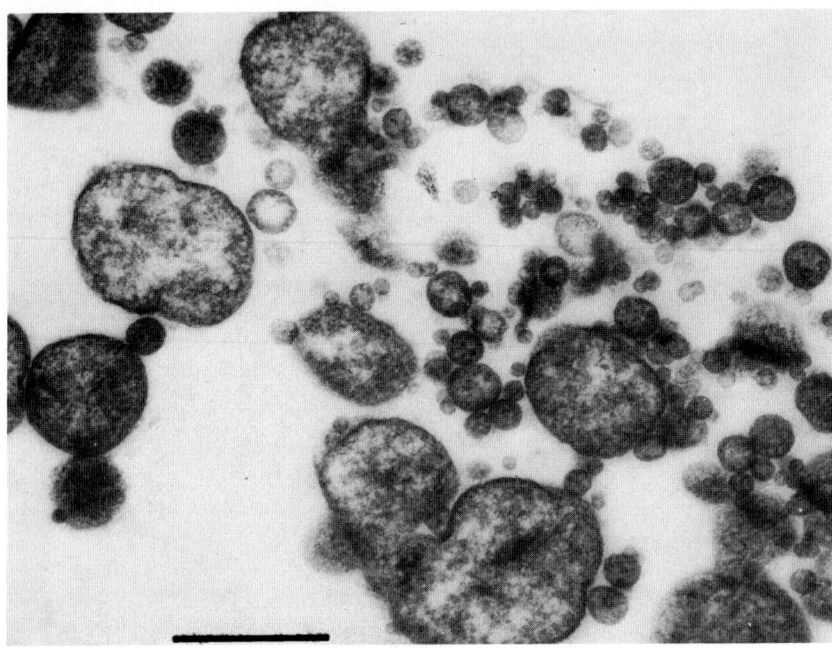

Figure 3 *B. suis* L-1330 forms adapted to growth on normal osmotically unprotected *Brucella* agar, without antibiotic and serum. L-colony grown on the 35th transfer: numerous small dense bodies limited by unit membrane; absence of giant bodies and multilayer membranes. (Reproduced by permission from J. Schmitt-Slomska, R. Caravano, P. Thomas, and J. Roux, Essai de caractérisation ultrastructurale et biochimique de Brucella à paroi déficiente (formes L). *Ann. Microbiol.* (*Inst. Pasteur*) *133 A*:377–386.)

Quantitative differences in those components present in both bacterial and spheroplast antigens were also noted. Although the spheroplasts displayed no endotoxic activity, retention of some cell wall material was demonstrated by CF tests utilizing antisera prepared against whole cells and against cell wall components. Work by B. Hatten and co-workers (unpublished data) compared soluble extracts of a virulent strain of *B. abortus* (3183B), an L-form derived from 3183B (3183L7), and an attenuated vaccine strain (S19). Electrophoretic patterns revealed subtle differences between each of the extracts analyzed, but suggested that components from the virulent bacterial strain and its L-form were more similar to one another than to components of the attenuated bacterial strain. Chromatographic patterns obtained by optical density readings at 260 and 280 of fractions eluted from DEAE-cellulose columns supported this finding and indicated that each extract consisted of varying amounts of two major components and numerous minor components. The distribution of antigenic activity in the separated fractions was measured by microhemagglutination inhibition and precipitin reactions. The latter tests revealed, as might be expected, that the number of reactive fractions obtained from the virulent bacterial extract was greater than for corresponding fractions obtained from the L-form extract. The complexity of the L-form extract again appeared to be more similar, however, to that of its virulent parent than to the extract of the attenuated strain of bacteria. Components of the attenuated S19 strain of *B. abortus* have also been shown to differ somewhat from several virulent strains representing biotypes in a similar study [21].

Chemical analysis of stable *B. suis* strain 1330 L-forms performed by Schmitt-Slomska et al. [19] showed that these forms lacked diaminopimelic acid, thus confirming the lack of peptidoglycan. These forms also lacked sodium 2-keto-3-deoxy-octonate. Biological assays, however, suggested that outer membrane components, such as lipopolysaccharides (LPS) and receptors for phage Weybridge (Figure 4) remained in the L-forms, albeit in reduced amount as compared to the parent brucellae. Figure 5 shows the electrophoretic distribution

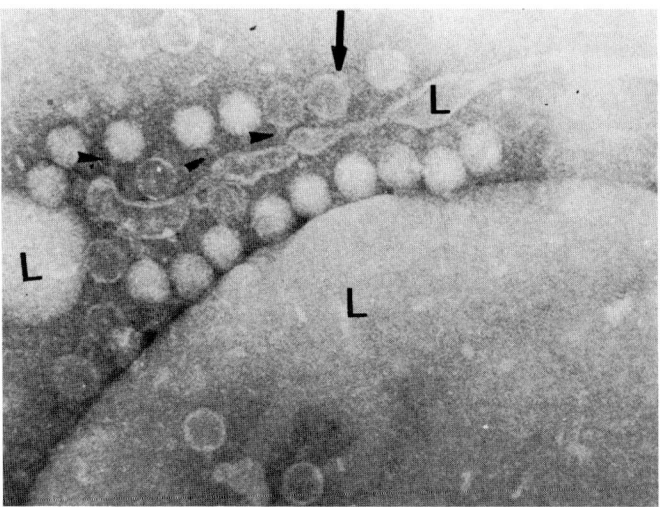

Figure 4 Electron micrograph of fixation of phage Weibridge on the membranes of *B. suis* stable L-1330 forms. (Reproduced by permission from J. Schmitt-Slomska, R. Caravano, P. Thomas, and J. Roux, Essai de caractérisation ultrastructurale et biochimique de Brucella à paroi déficiente (formes L). *Ann. Microbiol.* (*Inst. Pasteur*) *133 A*:377–386.

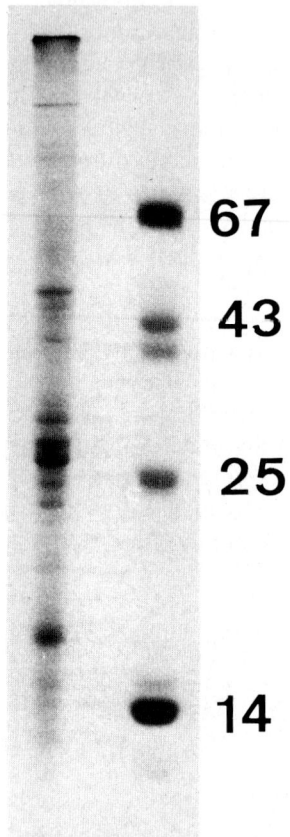

Figure 5 Gel polyacrylamide electrophoresis of proteins extracted from the membrane fraction of *B. suis* L-1330 forms; on the right, protein standard in kilodaltons. (Unpublished data, courtesy of G. Starka, Physiologie Microbienne, University Marseille-Luminy, France.)

of components extracted from L-form membranes by freeze-thawing and ultrasonic techniques.

Additional studies were designed to compare the antigenic properties of the stable L-forms with those of the parent bacteria [22-24]. In serological studies on mice inoculated with parent bacteria, stable L-forms, or membrane extracts, only those animals inoculated with the parent brucellae developed agglutinating antibodies (1:32-1:128). Some evidence of a specific antibody response to the L-forms was obtained, however, by the indirect fluorescent antibody technique.

Histological examination of lymphoid tissues of animals inoculated with similar preparations also showed a minimal response to the stable L-forms (i.e., granulomas and cell necrosis were observed only in those animals inoculated with bacteria). The L-forms characteristically produced marked stimulation of the paracortical regions of the lymph nodes and thymus-dependent zones of the spleen. Attempts were made to induce delayed hypersensitivity (DH) by inoculation of 12-week-old C3H and Balb/c mice with stable L-forms. In this study, the animals were sensitized by inoculation of a microbial suspension containing 100 µg of protein into the front foot pads. Some animals also received an equal volume of complete Freund's adjuvant (CFA) and some were pretreated with an intraperitoneal injection of 200 mg/kg body weight of cyclophosphamide monohydrate (Cy). Challenges were carried out over a period of 5-30 days after sensitization by injection of a 0.05-ml suspension containing 400 µg/ml protein into one paw. Differences in the thicknesses of the injected and uninjected paws were measured at 20 min and 1, 3, 6, and 24 hr after the injection. A delayed hypersensitive reaction, as seen in Figure 6, was observed in mice pretreated with Cy and sensitized 5-7 days before challenge with L-form suspensions either with or without CFA. Mice challenged 15-20 days after the sensitizing dose had swelling of the paws within 1-3 hr, but did not develop DH. Specificity of the DH response was shown by lack of DH responses to challenge with streptococcol L-forms. Mice pretreated with Cy and sensitized with L-forms which were subsequently challenged with either parent cell wall fractions, brucellin (suin), or L-form membrane extract also had responses that were specific for the sensitizing antigens (Figure 7). Some cross-reactivity between the parent extracts and L-form fractions were noted. These were characterized by early swelling of the paws (maximum at 3 hr) which disappeared at 24 hr in animals sensitized with parent brucellae and challenged with L-forms 7 days later.

Induction of macrophage inhibition factor (MIF) by the *B. suis* strain 1330 L-forms was investigated by an indirect, two-stage test on normal mouse pertineal exudates according to the method of McCoy and Ames [25]. Presence or absence of MIF induction was determined on supernates of spleen cells from DBA mice 20 days after immunization with a standard inoculum of live L-forms. Decrease in macrophage migration was observed after exposure to either undiluted or diluted (1:10) supernatant fluids from cells of sensitized animals.

These results suggest that L-1330 antigen induced the production of an MIF in mouse spleen cell suspensions and that this inhibitory factor was clearly amplified by the previous sensitization of the animals with live *Brucella* L-forms. Therefore attempts were made to confirm and clarify this ability by studying the mitogenic responses to various *Brucella* L-form antigens. The technique used was the measurement of [^{3}H]thymidine incorporation into microcultures [24]. The antigens used were L-1330 Ag and three factions of the parent brucellae:

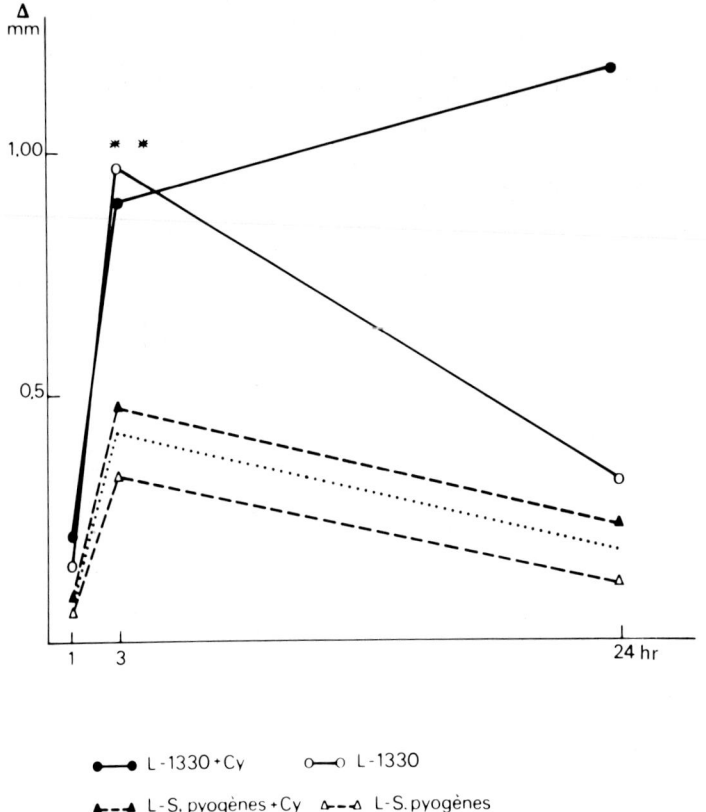

Figure 6 Swelling of paws in Balb/c mice immunized with *B. suis* L-1330 and tested 7 days after with L-1330 or heterologous L-forms. **Significant result.

membranes, murein + lipoprotein, and a cytoplasmic "soluble fraction." They were assayed in spleen cell suspensions of DBA/2 mice, either normal or sensitized by live *Brucella* L-forms, as described. The results shown in Table 2 demonstrated that L-1330 increased the mitogenic response of cells from sensitized animals.

Finally, the ability of stable *B. suis* strain 1330 L-forms to provide protective immunity to mice was explored. DBA/2 mice were inoculated i.p. with either 10^6 live parent B-1330 bacteria (in 1 ml of saline), or 1 ml of a suspension of live L-1330 forms. Control mice received 1 ml of saline. From the 20th to the 25th day, the mice were treated with a combination of streptomycin and tetracycline. On day 30, all of the groups were challenged with an i.p. injection

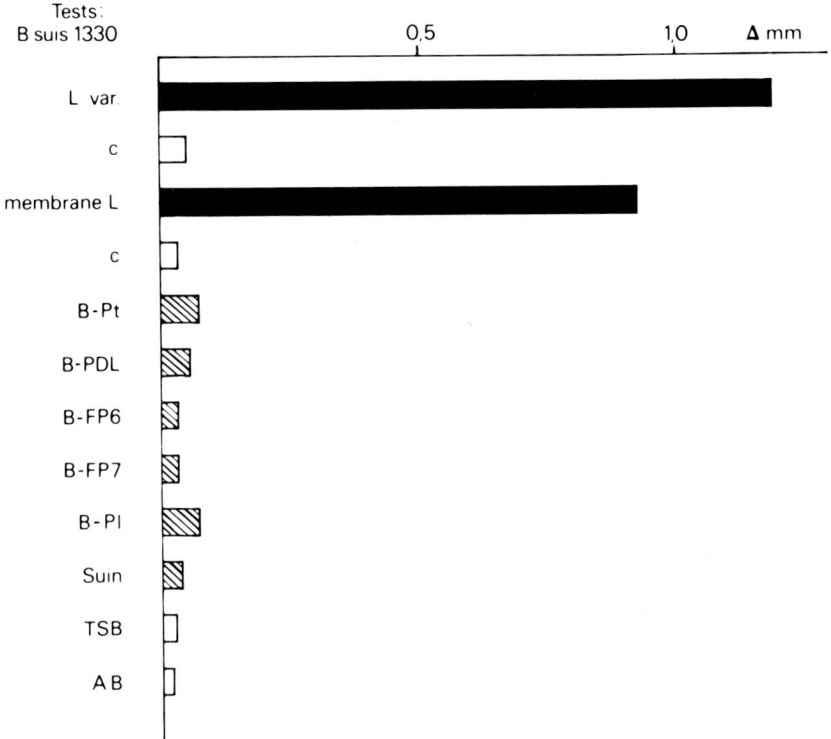

Figure 7 Response of mice to various *Brucella* antigens. Swelling of paws 24 hr after challenge. All mice were Cy-treated and immunized with L-forms L-1330 + CFA. Tests: L var., L-1330 forms; c, control nonimmunized; membrane fraction of L-1330; B-Pt, total cell wall; B-FP6, murein + lipoprotein fraction; B-FP7, murein; B-PI, peptidoglycan phenol-insoluble fraction; Suin, brucellin; TSB, trypticase soy broth (control); AB, bovine albumin (control).

of 1×10^6 live parent *B. suis* in 0.2 ml of saline. Five days after the challenge, the animals were sacrificed and their spleens were removed and homogenized. The tissue supernatants were diluted and plated for the determination of CFU. *Brucella* L-forms showed little, if any, protective effect. In contrast a significant difference was observed with the group of mice immunized with the parent brucella [24].

The difficulties encountered in obtaining *Brucella* L-forms have also been confirmed by Soviet Union investigators. Numerous attempts to convert brucella strains to stable L-forms in vitro using various antibiotics, lysozyme and immune sera were unsuccessful [26,27]. In a semiliquid, enriched penicillin-containing

Table 2 Mitogenic Activity of *Brucella* and *Brucella* L-forms (1330)

Antigen	Mice[a]	Mitogenic index
L-1330 Ag[b]	C	2.2
	E	8.1
B-1330 membranes[c]	C	1.9
	E	1.7
B-1330 murein + lipoprotein	C	1.6
	E	1.2
B-1330 "soluble" antigen	C	0.6
	E	1.1

[a] C, control; E, experimental.
[b] L-form antigen
[c] B-parental *Brucella* fraction.

medium, L-forms were obtained from only 2 of 11 strains of brucella tested; their growth in this medium was slow and poor, and most of the L-forms obtained were lost after 10–15 subcultures. In the absence of penicillin, reversion to the parent bacterium was rapid. The ultrastructure of L-forms obtained was characterized by marked polymorphism and tendency to budding; the granular and globular elements have two membranes on the cell surface and an extensively developed system of intracytoplasmic membranes [28,29]. As the L-forms reproduced only in a semiliquid medium, the colonial morphology typical for L-form growth was not established.

When inoculated into the inguinal region of guinea pigs, L-forms were less virulent than the parent *Brucella* but could persist in animals as atypical globular forms or revertant forms [30–32]. The index of dissemination for L-forms was 7.5% against 75% for parent *Brucella* inoculated into control animals. Determined by different immunological methods, the humoral and cellular responses of guinea pigs to L-forms were weak [31,33].

The development of *Brucella* L-form-like bodies in vivo was reported by Tsybin et al. [34]. Globular bodies were isolated from organs of mice that were inoculated in the inguinal region with *B. abortus* or *B. suis* strains and then treated with benzyl-penicillin. Globular bodies grew poorly (25-day incubation) and only in a semiliquid medium; no description of their colonial morphology or other characteristics of L-type structures was given. When inoculated with penicillin into the mice, the globular elements persisted for a long time in penicillin-treated mice and reverted rapidly, either in vivo or in vitro, upon the withdrawal of penicillin. Thus it was concluded that they were penicillin-dependent L-forms.

V. SUMMARY

Studies reviewed in this chapter describe the isolation of *Brucella* L-forms from both naturally occurring and experimental infections. In most cases, a direct relationship of L-forms to the disease processes in vivo was not established, because reversions to bacteria were present on primary isolation in the absence of penicillin. In one study, however, L-forms of *B. suis* strain 1330 were recovered, in the absence of bacterial growth, on penicillin-free primary isolation plates from a few experimentally infected gnotobiotic mice. The conclusion that such results were evidence of L-form induction and persistence in vivo was supported by the presence of organisms in tissues from infected animals that resembled L-forms microscopically. The primary *B. suis* strain 1330 isolates were also unstable L-forms becaue they eventually reverted to bacteria in the absence of penicillin. An early report suggesting that brucellaphage may be important in induction of brucella L-forms has not been verified, although demonstrations of brucellaphage in bacteria or materials from in vivo sources are not uncommon.

Several in vitro studies tend to agree that L-forms and other cell wall-defective forms of brucellae can be induced in tissue cell cultures. Differences observed in the properties of these forms and in their effect upon infected cells may reflect differences in experimental conditions and bacterial strains used in these studies. Most of the forms described had retained the ability to revert to the parent bacteria and persisted for limited periods of time in the absence of bacterial growth.

L-forms of *Brucella* spp. induced in artificial media by various methods were characteristically unstable forms. Attempts to convert those forms to stable L-forms were, for the most part, unsuccessful. In one instance, unstable L-forms of *B. suis* strain 1330 isolated from infected mice were converted to stable L-forms after many passages in artificial media.

Development of a stable brucella L-form allowed extension of other studies on L-form antigens to include an investigation of immune responses evoked in mice by the stable L-form. Under the experimental conditions employed, the L-forms induced little or no antibody responses or pathological lesions in these animals. On the other hand, evidence of delayed hypersensitivity specific for L-form antigens, as well as migration inhibition factor and mitogenic factor production, was shown. Immunization of mice with viable L-forms, however, provided no substantial immunity to mice subsequently challenged with the parent bacteria.

REFERENCES

1. Nelson, E. and Pickett, J. (1951). The recovery of L Forms of *Brucella* and their relationship to brucellaphage. *J. Infect. Dis.* 89:226–233.

2. Carrere, L. and Roux, J. (1953). Obtaining L Forms of *Brucella melitensis*. *Ann. Inst. Pasteur 84*:796-798.
3. Pickett, J. and Nelson, E. (1950). *Brucella* bacteriophage. *J. Hyg. 48*:500-503.
4. Renoux, G. and Suire, A. (1963). Spontaneous lysis and phage carrier state in *Brucella* cultures. *J. Bacteriol. 65*:642-647.
5. Kessel, R., Aronson, M., and Braun, W. (1960). Effects of brucellaphage on extracellular and intracellular *Brucella abortus. Proc. Soc. Exp. Biol. Med. 105*:447-450.
6. Schmitt-Slomska, J., Caravano, R., Anoal, M., Gay, B., and Roux, J. (1981). Isolation of L-forms from the spleens of *Brucella suis*-infected, penicillin-treated mice. *Ann. Microbiol. (Inst. Pasteur) 132 A*:253-265.
7. Schmitt-Slomska, J. and Lucel-Varnier, Y. (1969). Essai d'isolement de bactéries en phase L chez des souris inoculées avec des streptocoques du groupe A et traitées par la pénicilline. *Ann. Inst. Pasteur 117*:347-363.
8. Schmitt-Slomska, J., Boué, A., and Caravano, R. (1972). Induction of L-variants in human diploid cells infected by Group A Streptococci. *Infect. Immun. 5*:389-399.
9. Freeman, B. and Rumack, H. (1964). Cytopathogenic effect of *Brucella* spheroplasts on monocytes in tissue culture. *J. Bacteriol. 88*: 1310-1315.
10. McGhee, J. R. and Freeman, B. A. (1970). Separation of soluble *Brucella* antigens by gel-filtration chromatography. *Infect. Immun. 2*: 48-53.
11. Braun, W., Pomales-Lebron, A., and Stinebring, W. R. (1958). Interaction between mononuclear phagocytes and *Brucella abortus* strains of different virulence. *Proc. Soc. Exp. Biol. Med. 97*:395-397.
12. Hatten, B. A. and Sulkin, S. E. (1966). Intracellular production of *Brucella* L Forms I. Recovery of L Forms from tissue culture cells infected with *Brucella abortus. J. Bacteriol. 91*:285-296.
13. Hatten, B. A. and Sulkin, S. E. (1966). Intracellular production of *Brucella* L Forms II. Induction and survival of *Brucella abortus* L Forms in tissue culture. *J. Bacteriol. 91*:14-20.
14. Hatten, B. A., Schulze, M. L., Huang, S. Y., and Sulkin, S. E. (1969). Ultrastructure of *Brucella abortus* L Forms induced by penicillin in a liquid and in a semisolid medium. *J. Bacteriol. 99*:611-618.
15. Hatten, B. A., Huang, S. Y., Schulze, M. L., and Sulkin, S. E. (1971). Electron microscopy of tissue culture cells infected with *Brucella abortus. J. Bacteriol. 108*:535-544.
16. Hatten, B. A. (1973). Growth characteristics of microorganisms in penicillin-treated *Brucella abortus* cultures. *Proc. Soc. Exp. Biol. Med. 143*: 909-914.
17. Hines, W. D., Freeman, B. A., and Pearson, G. R. (1964). Production and characterization of *Brucella* spheroplasts. *J. Bacteriol. 87*:138-141.

18. Watanakunakorn, C., Phair, J. P., and Hamburger, M. (1970). Increased resistance to carbenicillin after reversion from spheroplast to rod form. *Infect. Immun.* 1:427-430.
19. Schmitt-Slomska, J., Caravano, R., Thomas, P., and Roux, J. (1982). Essai de caractérisation ultrastructurale et biochimique de Brucella à paroi déficiente (formes L). *Ann. Microbiol. (Inst. Pasteur) 133 A*:377-386.
20. Baughn, R. E. and Freeman, B. A. (1966). Antigenic structure of *Brucella suis* spheroplasts. *J. Bacteriol.* 92:1298-1303.
21. Hatten, B. A. and Brodeur, R. D. (1978). Soluble antigens of virulent and attenuated biotypes of *Brucella abortus*. *Infect. Immun.* 22:956-962.
22. Mauss, H., Schmitt-Slomska, J., and Caravano, R. (1981). Stimulation des organes lymphoides de souris par *Brucella suis* et ses variants à paroi déficiente (formes L). *Ann. Immunol. (Inst. Pasteur) 132 D*:291-298.
23. Schmitt-Slomska, J., Drach, G., and Mauss, H. (1981). Exploration des réponses immunitaires de la souris aux variants à paroi déficiente de *Brucella suis* Abstr. Coll. Soc. Franç. Microbiol. "Bactéries à multiplication intracellulaire," Paris, p. 24.
24. Schmitt-Slomska, J., Caravano, R., Starka, G., Mauss, H., Drach, G., and Lemaire, J. (1983). Immunogenic properties of the mouse, of cell wall-deficient Brucella (L Forms). Edit. 3rd International Congress of Brucellosis, 1983, Alger. *Rev. Biol. Std.* 56:187-197.
25. McCoy, J. L. and Ames, R. S. (1980). Production and analysis of macrophage and leucocyte inhibitory factors in *Manual of Macrophage Methodology* (H. B. Herscowitz, H. T. Holden, J. A. Bellanti, and Abdul Ghaffar, eds.), Marcel Dekker, New York, pp. 417-422.
26. Ostrovskaya, N. N., Vershilova, P. A., and Tolmacheva, T. A. (1972). L-transformation of Brucella in artificial media. *ZMEI N.* 4:108-111.
27. Tolmacheva, T. A. (1976). Study of L-transforming effect on Brucella cells of tetracycline, streptomycin, reifampicin or their combinations with penicillin *in vitro*. *Zh. Mikrobiol. Epidemiol. Immunobiol.* 9:771-774.
28. Tolmacheva, T. A. and Katz, L. N. (1974). Biological properties and ultrastructure of brucellae in the process of L-transformation and reversion. *Zh. Mikrobiol. Epidemiol. Immunobiol.* 1:90-93.
29. Katz, L. N., Konstantinova, N. D., Shulga, M. A., and Kagan, G. Ya. (1977). Intracytoplasmic membrane system in bacterial L-forms. *Seria Biologiczeskaja N.* 1:140-144.
30. Ostrovskaya, N. N. and Tolmacheva, T. A. (1972). Virulence of L-forms of *Brucella abortus* for guinea pigs. *Zh. Mikrobiol. Epidemiol. Immunobiol.* 6:146-147.
31. Schuvalov, L. P. and Tolmacheva, T. A. (1976). Characteristic of the immunological answer of guinea pigs inoculated with L-form of Brucella. *Zh. Mikrobiol. Epidemiol. Immunobiol.* 7:135-136.
32. Grekova, N. A., Tolmacheva, T. A., and Vershilova, P. A. (1979). On the pathogenicity of nonstable Brucella L-forms and their revertants. *J. Hyg. Epidemiol. Microbiol. Immunol.* (Prague) 23:129-134.

33. Tolmacheva, T. A. and Dranovskaja, E. A. (1980). Description of the antigenic and chemical composition of *Brucella* in the course of L-transformation and reversion in "Extracts from the report for the year 1978 of the WHO collaborating centre for research and reference of brucellosis." *WHO/Bruc. 80*:349.
34. Tsybin, B. P., Taran, I. F., and Krylova, A. A. (1979). Comparative evaluation of methods used for the induction of L-forms of *Brucella* and study of their adaptation to the body of animals. *Zh. Mikrobiol. Epidemiol. Immunobiol. 4*:66–70.

8
L-Forms of *Neisseria*

JOHN W. LAWSON*
Department of Microbiology, Clemson University, Clemson, South Carolina

I. L-Forms of *Neisseria gonorrhoeae*	185
A. In Vitro Induction	185
B. Effects of Antibiotics	188
C. In Vivo Isolation	189
II. L-Forms of *Neisseria meningitidis*	190
A. Growth and Development	190
B. In Vivo Isolation	191
III. Conclusions	192
References	192

I. L-FORMS OF *NEISSERIA GONORRHOEAE*

A. In Vitro Induction

In reports spanning more than 20 years, Dienes and his co-workers [1,2] described the isolation of L-forms of *Neisseria gonorrhoeae* on media stabilized osmotically with 2% NaCl. The L-forms were either induced spontaneously from "large bodies" produced by autolyzing gonococci or after exposure to penicillin or high concentrations of lysine. These isolates could not be continually subcultured. Barile et al. [3] also reported the observation of L-form-like colonies from *N. gonorrhoeae*, but they were unable to subculture them. However, in 1966 Roberts [4] successfully induced L-forms of the gonococci on medium osmotically stabilized with sucrose by using a penicillin gradient plate technique and succeeded in propagating the isolates as L-forms on sucrose media

---
*Present affiliation: Department of Medical Microbiology, University of Birmingham, Birmingham, England

containing penicillin. The stabilized gonococcal L-forms were found to be more resistant to penicillin and its derivatives than the parent organism. Reversion to the parent form was accomplished by serial passage on penicillin-free medium. Some of the revertant strains were subsequently able to produce L-forms in the absence of penicillin on osmotically stabilized media containing inactivated horse serum.

In 1973 Lawson and Douglas [5] reported that by incorporating 7% polyvinyl-pyrrolidone (PVP) into induction medium containing penicillin, highly efficient conversion of all tested strains of gonococci to the L-form could be achieved. They found pronounced strain variation in induction frequencies on sucrose or on unstabilized L-media. L-forms induced on PVP L-media could be transferred to fresh PVP L-media or to media stabilized with sucrose or NaCl by the agar-block technique. Surprisingly, growth on subculture to NaCl L-medium was possible even though no gonococcal growth or L-form induction occurred on this medium. Reversion was achieved by subculturing the L-form on medium without penicillin. Interestingly, colonial type 1, as described by Kellogg et al. [6], was retained during passage as the L-form. Perhaps less pressure is exerted for change to other colonial types during growth as L-form rather than as parent. In a subsequent paper Bacigalupi and Lawson [7] defined the physiological conditions for the induction of the L-forms of *N. gonorrhoeae*. Gonococci were cultured on a synthetic medium consisting of tissue culture medium 199 and a supplemental mixture of cysteine, glucose, and various salts. The addition of bicarbonate or CO_2 enrichment was not required. For solidification, only agarose allowed growth of all strains while glutamic acid stimulated growth of some strains and inhibited others. The addition of 7% PVP, 2% albumin, and penicillin resulted in induction to the L-form of all strains tested with frequencies up to 0.3%. L-form induction did occur on sucrose L-medium but at significantly lower frequencies. The colonies appeared 1 week later than those on PVP L-medium and remained very small and poorly developed. Geary and Watkins [8] tried to explain the difference in induction frequencies by comparing the effects of both stabilizers on the developing L-forms. On PVP L-medium large bodies were found to form and to develop granules that spread and ultimately became large bodies. On sucrose, on the other hand, growth consisted mainly of large bodies and colonies were found to develop much more slowly. They suggested that on sucrose the large bodies remained intact and granules were not released. They postulated that sucrose may prevent spontaneous lysis of the large bodies.

More recent work by Gooder [9] led to the adaptation of L-forms of *N. gonorrhoeae* to fluid medium preparatory to biochemical characterization. He found that sucrose was not useful as an osmotic stabilizer and, although PVP was far superior, different batches of PVP gave different results. Gooder found the percentage induction frequency to range from 0.001 to 0.3% as compared with the findings of Lawson and Douglas [5], who observed induction frequencies approaching 100% for all strains tested. No consistent pattern was observed on comparing induction frequencies of gonococcal cultures in different growth phases or in different growth media. Similarly, no correlation was found between colony type or number of subcultures since isolation. However, revertant gonococci obtained on transfer of L-forms to medium devoid of penicillin tended to yield L-cultures with a higher induction frequency than the original cultures. By periodic transfer of L-forms to medium free of penicillin, stable L-forms were obtained. These strains were adapted to growth in broth, and two of these strains have been adapted to a defined chemical medium. We have recently obtained one of these strains and have observed luxuriant growth with viable counts above 10^8 CFU/ml in the defined medium described above [7]. In contrast, Lawson and Bacigalupi [10] found that cells from type 4 colonies were induced to the L-form at levels 10- to 100-fold greater than cells from types 1 and 2 colonies. This observation was evident at all concentrations of penicillin tested. In addition revertants from L-forms induced with cells from type 1 colonies usually reinduced to the L-form at the low frequencies typical for type 1 cells. However, revertants from cells obtained from type 1 colonies that have converted to type 4 colonies always induced to the L-form at the high frequencies routinely expected with cells from type 4 colonies. In our laboratory we have adapted gonococcal L-forms isolated on sucrose L-medium to liquid growth without albumin or osmotic stabilizer. In media devoid of penicillin, some reversion will still occur. The revertants were found to have generation times more than four times longer than those of the original parent. These isolates were resistant to antimicrobial agents affecting cell wall biosynthesis but they were much more sensitive to the broad-spectrum antibiotics. Unexpected increases in sensitivities to polymixin B and vancomycin were noted both in the L-forms and the apparently aberrant revertant gonococci.

Ultrastructural studies of the broth adapted L-form revealed the presence of double membrane forms. Both inner and outer membranes appeared as typical "unit" membranes. Peptidoglycan was absent. These findings were in contrast to previous observations that L-forms induced at high frequencies on PVP L-medium appeared to possess only a single membrane whereas L-forms induced at low frequencies on PVP medium or sucrose L-medium were always double-membrane forms. In this context we were never able to adapt L-forms induced at high frequency on PVP L-medium to liquid culture, perhaps indicating a greater tendency for disruption of single membrane forms.

In an attempt to gain insight into regulation of the L-induction process we looked at the role of cyclic adenosine monophosphate (cAMP) on induction frequency. We found that by decreasing the glucose content in the synthetic medium intracellular cAMP levels rose dramatically (11- to 25-fold). This increase however had no effect on L-form induction. Although induction frequencies ranged from 0.12 to 8.97 at the higher intracellular levels of cAMP, and from 0.10 to 1.9 at the lower levels, there were no consistent differences nor was there any consistency in percent induction to the L-form within any range of cAMP levels. The addition of cAMP to the growing cells did not appear to affect induction to the L-forms. However, it was noted that L-forms induced from parent bacteria grown at higher intracellular cAMP levels or in the presence of exogenous cAMP appeared much earlier on the L-media and were somewhat larger than those L-forms induced from parents grown in lower levels of cAMP. Similarly, exogenous cAMP had no effect on the percent reversion to the parental form upon the addition of penicillinase to the induction plate. This lack of a demonstrable effect on cAMP on L-form induction is in contrast to the dramatic effect of cAMP and other regulators of transcription on the morphogenesis of the stable L-form. In unpublished work from our laboratory, we have observed that typical L-form growth occurs when cAMP levels are maintained above 10^{-3}. However, if cAMP levels are depressed by any one of several methods, including stimulation of cAMP phosphodiesterase, the entire L-form culture is converted to a culture of large bodies averaging over 8 μm in diameter. These large bodies are viable and contain within the cytoplasmic membranes dense membranous bodies that are released upon mechanical rupture of the large bodies. These elementary bodies in turn exhibit L-form growth in the presence of high levels of cAMP but convert to large bodies at very low levels.

Ota et al. [11] studied the fine structure of reverting L-forms of the gonococcus. Some reverting colonies consisted of closely packed large cells containing membranous structures of various sizes that were usually double the size of the parent gonococcal cells. The cytoplasm appeared as a thin fibrous network, often including electron-dense spots located near the cytoplasmic membrane. Numerous small vesicular elements of various sizes were noted among the large, reverting L-form cells. The elements usually close to the cell membrane contained electron-dense cores. This same group [12] also looked at the effects of colonial type and strain differences on the induction of L-forms of the gonococcus. Inducibility was found to be constant for each type and strain and to depend only on the amount of penicillin added to the medium. They also found L-form induction more likely and at higher frequencies in cells from T_4 colonies than from T_1 or T_2. These workers also noted that L-forms were induced which lacked any evidence of an outer membrane.

B. Effects of Antibiotics

Roberts [4] in 1966 was the first to compare the antibiotic sensitivities of the gonococcal L-forms with their respective parent strains. The L-forms were found to be resistant to four of eight antibiotics that inhibit bacterial cell wall biosynthesis. The sensitivity to other antibiotics such as novobiocin, tetracycline, and erythromycin was similar to that of the parent strains. Lawson and Bacigalupi

[10] assessed the effects of antibiotics during the induction and/or reversion of the L-forms of *N. gonorrhoeae*. Induction to the L-form was achieved with penicillin G or with the three synthetic derivatives tested. Peak induction frequencies were observed in the presence of 10-20 μg/ml. Surprisingly, L-form induction showed a biphasic response to increasing amounts of penicillin, with a second peak induction occurring at concentrations ranging between 100 and 1000 μg/ml. The induction frequency showed similar fluctuations in the presence of varying amounts of ampicillin and carbenicillin. Cephalothin was found to mediate L-form conversion over a wide concentration range of between 10 and 500 μg/ml. Similarly, in the presence of high concentrations of cycloserine, L-form induction occurred, although the range was more restricted. In the presence of various other antimicrobial agents, in addition to penicillin G, L-form induction did not occur, even though the parental gonococcus was resistant to these drugs at much higher concentrations. Nystatin and colistin had no obervable effect on the induction process in ranges routinely incorporated into medium for the clinical isolation of the gonococcus. Vancomycin at concentrations used in the VCN inhibitor caused a significant decrease in yields of newly induced L-forms, although no effect was noted on the growth of stable L-forms or the parental gonococcus. The difference in sensitivities between parental gonococci and the L-forms may be related to the ease of penetration of the antimicrobial agent as a consequence of the removal of the cell wall barrier. The differences between this data and that of Roberts [4] may be explained by the demonstration that the L-forms induced on sucrose L-medium contained an outer membrane whereas those induced on PVP L-medium at high frequencies appeared to have lost this structure. Others, including Ovchinnikov et al. [13], have also found increased sensitivity of the gonococcal L-form to antibiotics as compared to the parental gonococcus. Mickelsen and Dallon [14] compared the frequencies of spontaneous with antibiotic-induced production of L-forms of *N. gonorrhoeae*. They also found that the ability to grow as L-forms once induced was independent of an antibiotic inducing agent. These findings were similar to those previously reported by Lawson and Douglas [5].

C. In Vivo Isolation

L-forms of *N. gonorrhoeae* have been implicated in certain clinical manifestations of gonorrhea. As early as 1959 Barile et al. [3] reported a case study of a patient who developed recurrent gonorrhea after treatment for gonococcal urethritis with 600,000 units of penicillin. Penicillin tolerance tests were run and during the in vitro studies, L-forms of the particular strain were induced. Ovchinnikov et al. [13] observed L-forms of gonococci by electron microscopy in pus obtained directly from patients. In the United States, Holmes et al. [15] reported the isolation of gonococcal L-forms from sterile synovial fluid by means of an agar overlay containing sucrose and serum. Small nonreverting and reverting colonies were isolated which were identified as *N. gonorrhoeae*. More recently Gnarpe et al. [16,17] isolated L-forms from patients with urethritis who were negative for *N. gonorrhoeae* by standard microbiological methods. A medium supporting the growth of the gonococcal L-form was developed and used in parallel with conventional gonococcal media to detect the presence of L-forms. In about 12% of patients with gonorrhea L-forms were isolated from the urethra or the cervix. Some of the specimens of *N. gonorrhoeae* were isolated only on osmotically stabilized media, and one patient gave only a pure growth of L-forms. They found that by using partly osmotically stabilized media, the number of cases with positive cultures of the parent gonococcus increased by 10%. Olmas [18,19] studied ultrastructural changes during the degeneration of the gonococcus in various media unfavorable to its development. He found a high degree of polymorphism of the intracellular organisms in contrast to the morphological regularity of those localized in the extracellular space. In general cells were of large size and irregular shape; he believed them to be L-forms. He presented little evidence for this conclusion.

In 1980 Hickman and Lawson [20] isolated a stable cell wall-defective form, strain J-14, on medium containing PVP from an exudate of an untreated patient with urethritis. This isolate could not be subcultured on medium stabilized with sucrose or on conventional laboratory media. The isolate on medium devoid of penicillin appeared atypically flat with a dark granular center surrounded by a smooth translucent periphery. The addition of penicillin gave colonies with the typical "fried egg" L-form morphology. The organism was incapable of reverting to a typical gonococcus. It is not certain whether strain J-14 represents a true wall-defective form or the strain possesses an overactive autolytic enzyme system that leads to lysis in the absence of stabilizers. Regardless, the organisms apparently survive in vivo as wall-defective cells that readily grow as L-forms on the addition of an inducer.

II. L-FORMS OF *NEISSERIA MENINGITIDIS*

A. Growth and Development

Initial in vitro studies on the induction of L-forms of *Neisseria meningitidis* have used the penicillin gradient technique originally described by Sharp [21]. Roberts and Wittler [22] adopted this method for the isolation and characterization of meningococcal L-forms. Later, Bohnhoff and Page [23] found that transformation to the L-form occurred readily among all serological groups of *N. meningitidis* in the presence of penicillin, osmotic stabilizer, and high concentrations of horse serum. Transformation to L-growth occurred most readily among strains recently isolated from patients. They found that revertant

L-colonies developed diplococcal colonies on blood agar and L-colonies on sucrose penicillin agar in a ratio of 10% L-colonies. During this same period Koptelova and Mironova [24] found that of 20 strains investigated, eight could be induced to L-forms with penicillin. They used 20% saccharose for osmotic stabilization. Glycine as well as penicillin served as a transforming agent. Koptelova and Mironova [24] further studied the reversion to the parent form of 56 strains of stable and unstable L-forms of the meningococcus. On reversion of the L-forms in subcultures 1-10, the properties of the parent organism were completely restored. In contrast, cultures of L-forms in subcultures 10-23 acquired pigmentation, exhibited polyagglutin ability, and displayed an increased resistance to penicillin. These authors subsequently showed that meningicoccal L-forms after extended subculture underwent changes in serological properties. We have found similar physiological and serological changes in reverting L-forms as have others. Chin and Lawson [25] described cultural conditions that permitted highly efficient conversion of all serogroups of *N. meningitidis* to the L-form. PVP was incorporated into the medium for stabilization. Light and scanning electron microscopy of the L-form inductants showed characteristics distinctive among the strains observed. Bibel and Lawson [26] had previously described similar variations among streptococcal L-form colonies.

Chin and Lawson [25] further investigated the effects of antibiotics other than penicillin on L-form induction of the meningococcus. With cephalothin L-form induction occurred in the presence or absence of penicillin. With novobiocin no L-form induction was observed even at concentrations not found to be inhibitory to the parental meningococcus nor to a stable L-form variant. In contrast to the findings with the gonococcus [10], vancomycin did not inhibit L-form induction or growth in the presence of penicillin. Similarly, colistin, nystatin, and trimethylprim, other components of the VCN inhibitor added to media for the isolation of pathogenic neisseriae, had no effect on L-induction or growth.

B. In Vivo Isolation

Bohnhoff and Page [23] using mucin as a host depressant, compared parent and revertant L-strains for initial pathogenicity and the development of virulence by serial mouse passage. Revertant L-strains appeared to retain the pathogenic characteristics of the parent. However, stable L-strains were completely avirulent, although persistence of L-forms could be demonstrated in peritoneal exudates for 6 days following inoculation. Konstantinova and Koptelova [27] and Koptelova et al. [28-31] isolated L-forms from the cerebrospinal fluid of patients suffering from epidemic cerebrospinal meningitis. In 12 out of 130 patients studied, forms with aberrant growth were observed and in 30 cases actual stable and unstable L-forms were detected. The loss of the capacity to revert prevented species identification of the stable forms; however, subculture of the unstable L-forms on media without penicillin resulted in reversion to the meningococcus of serotype A. Of 19 cultures reverted to the meningococcus, 11 were resistant, and 7 possessed reduced sensitivity to penicillin. Pribnow et al. [32] injected meningococcal L-forms of Group A into the rabbit vitreous. Inflammation occurred that appeared somewhat accelerated as compared with bacterial controls. The L-forms could be cultured from injected eyes for 8 hr postinjection. Heat-killed L-forms also produced ocular inflammation whereas heat-killed meningococcal parental forms did not.

III. CONCLUSIONS

In summary, cell wall-defective (CWD) forms of the neisseriae are readily induced to the L-form in vitro on solid media stabilized with sucrose, NaCl, and especially PVP, with antimicrobial agents interfering with cell wall biosynthesis. Those L-forms induced at high frequency on PVP medium seemed to be devoid of an outer membrane. Induction frequencies were consistently higher with *N. gonorrhoeae* from cells from colonial type 4 than from either types 1 or 2. Little effect on induction frequency was produced by cAMP, but the cyclic nucleotide had a pronounced effect on growth and morphology of the L-form. CWD forms *N. gonorrhoeae* have been isolated from urethral exudates and synovial fluids. Similar forms of *N. meningitidis* have been found in cerebrospinal fluids from patients with meningitis. However, due to the paucity of research in this area, considerable work is still required to determine what role these CWD forms have in clinical disease.

REFERENCES

1. Dienes, L. (1940). L-type growth in gonococcus cultures. *Proc. Soc. Expl. Biol. Med. 44*:470–471.
2. Dienes, L., Bandur, B. M., and Madoff, S. (1964). Development of L-type growth in *Neisseria gonorrhoeae* cultures. *J. Bacteriol. 87*:1471–1476.
3. Barile, M. F., VanZee, C. K., and Yaguchi, R. (1959). The occurrence of failures in penicillin treated gonorrheal urethritis. I. The significance of L-form transformation of *Neisseria gonorrhoeae* to penicillin resistance. *Antibiot. Med. Clin. Ther. 6*:470–479.
4. Roberts, R. B. (1966). L-form of *Neisseria gonorrhoeae*. *J. Bacteriol. 92*: 1609–1614.
5. Lawson, J. W. and Douglas, J. T. (1973). Induction and reversion of the L-form of *Neisseria gonorrhoeae*. *Can. J. Microbiol. 21*:1698–1704.
6. Kellogg, D. S., Jr., Cohen, I., Nores, L., Schroeder, A., and Reising, G. (1968). *Neisseria gonorrhoeae* II Colonial variation and pathogenicity during thirty-five months *in vitro*. *J. Bacteriol. 96*:596–605.

7. Bacigalupi, B. A. and Lawson, J. W. (1973). Defined physiological conditions for the induction of the L-form of *Neisseria gonorrhoeae*. *J. Bacteriol.* 116:778-784.
8. Geary, I. and Watkins, S. (1977). The development of L-phase colonies of *Neisseria gonorrhoeae*. *J. Gen. Microbiol.* 99:233-239.
9. Gooder, H. (1977). Stable L-phase variants of gonococci in *Spheroplasts, Protoplasts and L-Forms of Bacteria*, vol. 64, (J. Roux, ed), INSERM, Paris, p. 57.
10. Lawson, J. W. and Bacigalupi, B. (1977). Induction and reversion of the L-form of *Neisseria gonorrhoeae* in *Spheroplasts, Protoplasts and L-Forms of Bacteria*, vol. 64, (J. Roux, ed.), INSERM, Paris, pp. 91-106.
11. Ota, F., Nukui, K., Ashton, F. E., and Diena, B. B. (1976). The fine structure of reverting L-forms of *Neisseria gonorrhoeae*. *J. Microbiol.* 20:59-62.
12. Ota, F., Ashton, F. E., and Diena, B. B. (1976). Type and strain variation in induction of the L-forms of *Neisseria gonorrhoeae*. *J. Microbiol.* 20:77-82.
13. Ovchinnikov, N. M., Delektorski, V. V., Dmitriev, C. A. and Akyshbaeva, K. S. (1976). Ultrastructure of the L-forms of the gonococcus and its alterations under the influence of kanomycin. *Vestr. Dermatal. Veneral.* 76: 44-48.
14. Mickelsen, P. A. and Dallon, H. P. (1976). Comparison of spontaneous and antibiotic induced L-form production in *Neisseria gonorrhoeae*. *J. Clin. Microbiol.* 4:185-187.
15. Holmes, K. K., Gutman, L. T., Belding, M. E., and Turck, M. (1971). Recovery of *Neisseria gonorrhoeae* from "Sterile" synovial fluid in gonococcal arthritis. *N. Engl. J. Med.* 284:318-320.
16. Gnarpe, H., Wallin, J., and Forsgren, A. (1973). Studies in venereal disease II. Improved diagnosis of gonorrhoeae by the parallel use of conventional L-phase media. *Br. J. Vener. Dis.* 49:505-507.
17. Gnarpe, H., Wallin, J., and Forsgren, A. (1972). Studies in venaral disease I. Isolation of L-phase organisms of *Neisseria gonorrhoeae* from patients with gonorrhoeae. *Br. J. Vener. Dis.* 48:496-499.
18. Olmas, L. (1975). Form L-gonococcus. *Ann. Dermatol. Syphilis (Paris)* 102: 542-546.
19. Olmas, L. (1976). Degeneration of the gonococcus in various media. *Arch. Dermatol. Res.* 256:305-317.
20. Hickman, R. K. and Lawson, J. W. (1980). Isolation of a stable cell wall defective form of *Neisseria gonorrhoeae* from a case of untreated gonococcal urethritis. *J. Clin. Microbiol.* 12:603-605.
21. Sharp, J. T. (1954). L colonies from hemolytic streptococci: New technic in the study of L-forms of bacteria. *Proc. Soc. Exp. Biol. Med.* 87:94-97.
22. Roberts, R. B. and Wittler, R. C. (1966). The L-form of *Neisseria meningitidis*. *J. Gen. Microbiol.* 44:139-148.
23. Bohnhoff, M. and Page, M. I. (1968). Experimental infection with parent and L-phase varients of *Neisseria meningitidis*. *J. Bacteriol.* 95:2027-2077.
24. Koptelova, E. I. and Mironova, T. K. (1968). A method of obtaining L-forms of meningococcus. *Zh. Microbiol. Epidemiol. Immunobiol.* 45:101-104.

25. Chin, W. L. and Lawson, J. W. (1976). Effect of antibiotics on L-form induction of *Neisseria gonorrhoeae. Antimicrob. Agents Chemother. 9*: 1056-1065.
26. Bibel, D. J. and Lawson, J. W. (1972). Scanning electron microscopy of L-phase streptococci on millipore filters. *Can. J. Microbiol. 18*:1179-1184.
27. Konstantinova, N. D. and Koptelova, E. I. (1978). Ultrastructure of the L-forms of Meningococcus. *Zh. Microbiol. Epidemiol. Immunobiol. 55*: 25-27.
28. Koptelova, E. I., Mironova, T. K., Pokrovsky, V. I., and Leschinskaya, E. V. (1973). Isolation of L-forms from the cerebrospinal fluid of patients suffering from epidemic cerebrospinal meningitis. *Zh. Microbiol. Epidemiol. Immunobiol. 50*:107-109.
29. Koptelova, E. I. and Mironova, T. K. (1970). Stabilization and reversion of meningococcus L-forms. *Zh. Microbiol. Epidemiol. Immunobiol. 47*: 16-19.
30. Koptelova, E. I., Mironova, T. K., Pokrovsky, V. I., and Leschinskaya, E. V. (1972). The incidence of L-transformation of *N. meningitidis* isolated from the cerebrospinal fluid of patients suffering from epidemic cerebrospinal meningitis. *Zh. Microbiol. Epidemiol. Immunobiol. 49*:112-115.
31. Kopotelova, E. I., Pakrovsky, V. I., and Mironova, T. K. (1972). Pathogenicity of meningococcal L-forms obtained under the influence of penicillin. *Antibiotiki 17*:1017-1020.
32. Pribnow, J. F., Hall, J. M., Stewart, R. H., and Vedros, N. A. (1973). The occular inflammation produced following intravitreal injections of a stable L-phase varient of *Neisseria meningitidis. Can. J. Ophthalmol. 8*:361-365.

9
L-Forms of *Pseudomonas aeruginosa*

JOHN Z. MONTGOMERIE
Infectious Disease Division, University of Southern California School of Medicine, Los Angeles, California

I.	Introduction	195
II.	In Vitro Production and Propagation of L-Forms of *P. aeruginosa*	195
III.	Morphology	197
IV.	Antibiotic Sensitivities	198
V.	Biochemical Reactions and Immunology	198
VI.	Pathogenicity Studies	199
VII.	Conclusions	201
	References	201

I. INTRODUCTION

There have been few reports of L-forms of *Pseudomonas aeruginosa* (pseudomonas) and there is a general impression that it has been more difficult to produce L-forms of *P. aeruginosa* than L-forms of other gram-negative bacilli. One reason for this is that *P. aeruginosa* was resistant to the penicillin group of antibiotics until the development of carbenicillin. Most of the studies on pseudomonas L-forms have therefore been in the 10–15 years since the introduction of carbenicillin in the 1960s.

II. IN VITRO PRODUCTION AND PROPAGATION OF L-FORMS OF *P. AERUGINOSA*

Watanakunakorn and Hamburger [1] in 1969 induced spheroplasts of *P. aeruginosa* in liquid medium with carbenicillin. Hubert et al. [2] produced and propagated

L-forms of *P. aeruginosa*, using carbenicillin and agar medium. A similar approach was used by White et al. [3] and Bertolani et al. [4] to produce L-forms of a number of strains of pseudomonas. Hubert et al. [2] used gradient plates containing 10 and 30 µg of carbenicillin per ml, 0.5 M sucrose, and 2% bovine serum albumin. Because the L-forms tended to revert on these plates, the concentration of antibiotic needed to prevent reversion was periodically increased until the concentration of carbenicillin was 5000 µg/ml at the 20th transfer. Bertolani et al. [4] also found it necessary to increase the concentration of carbenicillin to prevent reversion after many passages of the L-forms on agar medium. Hubert et al. [2] found that microscopically the colony of pseudomonas L-form was less dense than the bacterial form, it was finely granular, and it did not demonstrate the smooth edge of the bacterial colony. At the 32nd transfer growth was streaked on 0.75% agar plate containing osmotic stabilizer as well as onto the regular 1.5% agar. L-form colonies with the typical fried-egg characteristic and large peripheral vacuoles appeared in the softer agar medium. Several transfers were made on this medium. The L-forms were then again carried on medium containing 1.5% agar with the continuation of classical L-form colony morphology. After 53 transfers, it was possible to subculture the L-form onto medium without carbenicillin without reversion to the bacterial form, and also into broth in the absence of carbenicillin. A wide range of osmotic stabilizers have been used to culture L-forms [5]. L-forms of *P. aeruginosa* grow well on medium containing 0.5 M sucrose or 1.8% NaCl (author's unpublished observations). Others have used polyvinylpyrolidone as an osmotic stabilizer [4].

Spheroplasts of *Pseudomonas* spp. have also been produced using lysozyme [6-8]. Yamamoto and Homma [9] produced L-forms of *P. aeruginosa* when spheroplasts induced by lysozyme EDTA treatment were cultured on a gradient plate containing carbenicillin in an anaerobic environment. The ability of these L-forms to develop related to the ease with which the organisms were converted to spheroplasts following treatment by lysozyme, i.e., those that converted easily to spheroplasts survived more readily. Unstable L-forms were obtained in six out of 11 strains. Stable L-forms were obtained after 10-13 subcultures of unstable L-forms derived from three strains. These organisms were cultured in medium containing bovine serum, but L-forms of two strains could be cultured in media in which the bovine serum was reduced until the medium was serum-free. This method of producing L-forms of pseudomonas with lysozyme seems to have been more successful than the methods using carbenicillin. The significance of the anaerobic environment to the production of L-forms is unclear. These authors considered that the anaerobic environment prevented the reversion of the L-forms to the bacterial form.

L-forms of *P. aeruginosa* can survive lyophilization and freezing at -70°C, although the optimal methods of long-term preservation are unknown (author's unpublished observations).

III. MORPHOLOGY

The gross morphology and light microscopic colony morphology of pseudomonas L-forms have been similar to L-forms of other bacteria. L-form cells have been oval and bounded by a plasma membrane. Cell wall studies of *P. aeruginosa* and its carbenicillin induced L-form have shown major morphological differences at the cellular level [2]. The L-forms had lost the outer triple layer cell wall structure and coarse electron-dense granules seen in the parent bacterial form have been absent (Figure 1). The L-form, but not the bacterial form, of *P. aeruginosa* also contained cores, organelles similar to those that had been previously reported in Group D streptococci [10]. Although the outer triple layer of the cell wall of the bacterial form of *P. aeruginosa* was absent in its stable L-form, the technique used in preserving both forms for electron

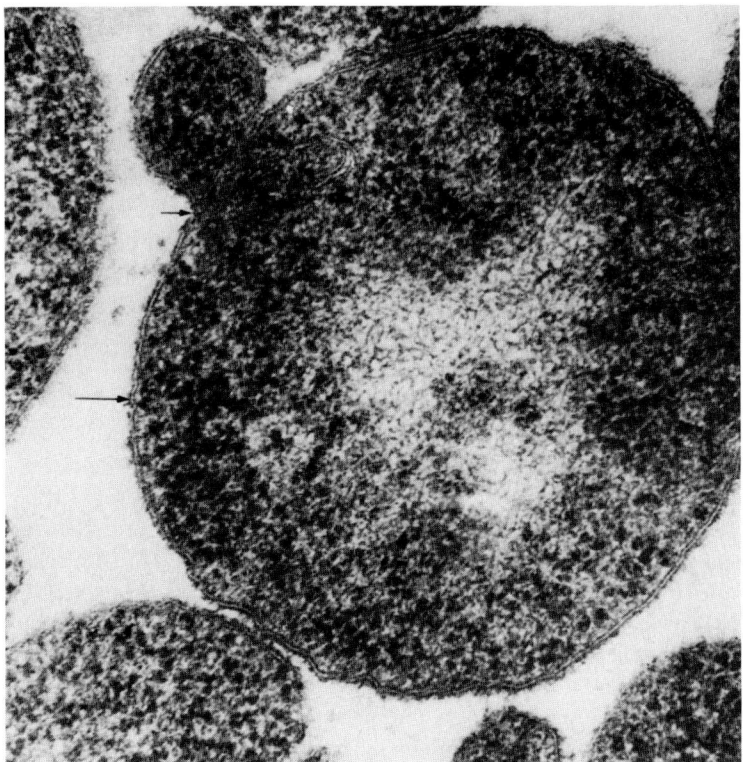

Figure 1 Stable L-form derived from *Pseudomonas aeruginosa*. No cell wall triple layer is evident. (Long arrow) Plasma membrane triple layer; (short arrow) a possible point of emergence of a "daughter" cell from the larger "parent" form. Bar, 0.1 μm.

microscopy did not reveal the presumed lysozyme-sensitive mucopeptide of the bacterial form as a single electron-dense layer between the triple layer of the plasma membrane and the triple layer of the cell wall. Therefore, it was by no means certain that the L-form was incapable of making at least some cell wall substance, since the cell margin was invariably thinly covered with fluffy material [2].

IV. ANTIBIOTIC SENSITIVITIES

The stable L-form of pseudomonas was as sensitive as, or more sensitive than, the bacterial form to most antibiotics, including the tetracyclines and macrolides. However, polymyxin B, colistin sulfate, and gentamicin were more active against the bacterial form than the L-forms [2,11]. These results were confirmed by Yamamoto and Homma [12] who found that L-forms of their strains of pseudomonas were more resistant than parent forms to all the aminoglycoside group. Similar results have been reported with *Proteus* spp. [13]. Yamamoto and Homma found a reduced uptake of an aminoglycoside antibiotic (dibekacin) into L-forms; they suggested that the decreased activity of colistin sulfate, polymyxin B, and the aminoglycosides against the L-forms may result from changes in the biochemistry of the membrane [12]. There are obvious strain differences since others have obtained opposite results with L-forms being more susceptible to aminoglycosides than the parent bacteria [3].

The L-form of pseudomonas was more susceptible to the bactericidal activity of normal human serum [2] and to polymorphonuclear extract [14] than the parent bacterial form.

V. BIOCHEMICAL REACTIONS AND IMMUNOLOGY

Studies of the L-forms of *P. aeruginosa* have shown the colonies to be colorless and to produce insignificant amounts of pyocyanin. Although 0.5 M sucrose in the medium inhibited pigment production by the parent bacterial form, this did not account for the failure of the L-form to produce pyocyanin [2]. This lack of ability to produce the blue-green pigment characteristic of the parent bacteria is similar to that observed in the L-form of *Serratia marcescens* [15]. The L-form of *P. aeruginosa* has been metabolically less active than the parent bacteria and has been unable to give reactions with oxidase, gelatin liquification, and gluconate tests. The L-forms have been nonmotile, but they have still reacted as the parent in nitrate, dextrose, and litmus milk. An L-form of a strain of *P. aeruginosa* that had produced both protease and elastase was found to lack these enzyme activities [9].

To study the cell wall composition of unstable L-forms of *P. aeruginosa*, White et al. [3] extracted lipopolysaccharide from both the parent bacteria and

L-forms. On analysis of this fraction, the overall carbohydrate contents appeared to be similar; however, significantly more phosphorus was found in the lipopolysaccharide fraction isolated from L-form. C11 fatty acids were not found in the parent bacteria whereas the L-form did not contain C20. The significance of these changes in fatty acids is not clear.

Yamamoto and Homma [16] studied serological cross-reactions among stable L-forms of *P. aeruginosa*, *Streptococcus pyogenes*, and Mycoplasma using passive hemagglutination and agar gel diffusion tests. Antiserum to L-forms of *P. aeruginosa* strain IFO-3455 reacted with L-form strain N-10 in passive hemagglutination and agar gel diffusion tests, although it is a serologically different serotype. In addition, the two L-forms of *P. aeruginosa* cross-reacted with an L-form of *Streptococcus pyogenes*. L-forms of *P. aeruginosa* and *S. pyogenes* did not react with five strains of Mycoplasma in PHA and agar gel diffusion tests.

VI. PATHOGENICITY STUDIES

Pseudomonas L-forms have only rarely been isolated from clinical specimens. Table 1 summarizes the reported instances of the isolation of L-forms from clinical specimens, most of them from the urine. The isolation of osmotically fragile *P. aeruginosa* from the urine of a patient was noted by Braude in 1968 [17]. Conner et al. [18] described pseudomonas L-forms in seven patients with

Table 1 Isolation of L-forms from Clinical Specimens

Reference number	Site			Antibiotics[a]	Parent bacteria also isolated	Comments
	Urine	Sputum	Other			
23			1	NK[b]		
17	1			No		Osmotically fragile bacteria
18	7			No	NK	
20	1			Yes		
21	1			Yes		
19	2			Yes		
24		1			NK	
22	1	2	1	Yes		
Total	13	3	2			

[a]Patients receiving antibiotics at the time of culture.
[b]NK, Not known.

urinary tract infection who were not receiving antibiotics at the time of culture. Crowe and Koblasz [19] isolated L-forms that later reverted to *Pseudomonas* spp. from two patients receiving treatment for recurrent urinary tract infections. Swierczewski and Reyes [20] and Domingue and Schlegel [21] each described a single instance of a similar case. Yamamoto and Homma [22] isolated unstable L-forms from clinical specimens of patients with pseudomonas infection during antibiotic therapy. Specimens were inoculated on BHI agar supplemented with 0.5 M sucrose, 10% sucrose, 10% horse serum, and 5000 units of penicillin and incubated in an anaerobic jar. Unstable L-forms were isolated from the sputum of two patients, and the urine and pus of one patient each. In no instance was there any evidence that the L-forms were persistent or causing significant disease. The criteria for L-forms in these papers seems to have been "spheroplast" or "protoplast" bodies seen in broth from the original culture and/or typical L-colonies (fried egg) observed on agar medium without penicillin that later reverted to the parent bacteria. In this study it is important to note that penicillin was included in the medium and the L-forms could have arisen in vitro as a result of this penicillin.

A patient with cervical adenitis yielded a pure growth of *P. aeruginosa* L-forms [23]. Middleton and Chmel [24] found an aberrant form of *P. aeruginosa* in sputum and cerebrospinal fluid that caused infection in a compromised patient. A patient with lymphoma was described who developed meningitis and from whom an aberrant form of *P. aeruginosa* was seen on the gram stain, i.e., a long filamentous gram-negative rod. This organism grew on primary isolation media without the need for hypertonic media. On primary isolation media, it lost its aberrant morphology.

L-forms found in clinical specimens may indicate one or more of the following: (1) the bacteria have been converted to L-forms by the action of antibiotics, lysozyme, or other agents while the true pathogen is the parent bacterium; (2) the L-forms persist while the patient is receiving antibiotics active on cell wall synthesis and revert when antibiotics are withdrawn; or (3) the L-forms persist and are pathogenic. In the cases reviewed there was little evidence that L-forms occurred as persisters and produced further disease on reverting to the parent form. Furthermore, there was no evidence that L-forms of pseudomonas were pathogenic as L-forms in these cases.

There have been few pathogenic studies in animals. Bertolani et al. [4] injected approximately 10^8-10^9 unstable L-forms of pseudomonas into the peritoneum of mice with lethal results in 24–48 hr. The rapid death suggests that this may have been the result of a toxin associated with the L-forms. These authors also raised the possibility that L-form induction and reversion may result in a revertant with different antigenic properties and antibiotic sensitivities. They induced three unstable L-forms from a single strain of *P. aeruginosa*. Cultured in different media they differed in respect to colonial shape on solid medium, growth rate, biochemical properties, antibiotic sensitivities, surface antigen, and virulence for mice. Unfortunately, they did not study the virulence of the revertant in mice. Changes in virulence of revertant bacteria compared with the original bacterial strain has been shown with *Klebsiella pneumoniae* [25].

VII. CONCLUSIONS

In summary, L-forms of *P. aeruginosa* have been produced in vitro and propagated by a number of different methods. The curious resistance of some of these strains to aminoglycosides and polymyxins has not been well studied. L-forms of pseudomonas have been isolated from the urine and other sites of infection in patients. Further work will be necessary to determine the role (if any) for the pseudomonas L-form in the pathogenesis of infectious disease.

REFERENCES

1. Watanakunakorn, C. and Hamburger, M. (1969). Induction of spheroplasts of *Pseudomonas aeruginosa* by carbenicillin. *Appl. Microbiol.* 17:935-937.
2. Hubert, E. G., Potter, C. S., Hensley, T. J., Cohen, M., Kalmanson, G. M., and Guze, L. B. (1971). L-forms of *Pseudomonas aeruginosa*. *Infect. Immun.* 4:60-72.
3. White, C. J. B., Horsman, M. R., Rowe, P. S., and Howells, K. F. (1978). Cell wall characteristics of *Pseudomonas aeruginosa* and its carbenicillin-induced L-form. *Acta Biol. Acad. Sci. Hung.* 29:67-74.
4. Bertolani, R., Edberg, S. S., and Ralston, D. (1975). Variations in properties of L-forms of *Pseudomonas aeruginosa*. *Infect. Immun.* 11:180-192.
5. Montgomerie, J. Z., Kalmanson, G. M., and Guze, L. B. (1967). Effect of osmotic stabilizer on protoplasts and bacterial forms of *Streptococcus faecalis*. *J. Lab. Clin. Med.* 70:539-553.
6. Carson, K. J. and Eagon, R. G. (1966). Lysozyme sensitivity of the cell wall of *Pseudomonas aeruginosa*: Further evidence for the role of the nonpeptidoglycan components in cell wall rigidity. *Can. J. Microbiol.* 12:105-108.
7. Rhodes, M. E. and Payne, W. J. (1967). Influence of cations on spheroplasts of marine bacteria functioning as osmometers. *Appl. Microbiol.* 15:537-542.
8. Klemperer, R. M., Gilbert, P., Meier, A. M., Cozens, R. M., and Brown, M. R. (1979). Influence of suspending media upon the susceptibility of *Pseudomonas aeruginosa* NCTC 6750 and its spheroplasts to polymyxin B. *Antimicrob. Agents Chemother.* 15:147-151.
9. Yamamoto, A. and Homma, J. Y. (1978). L-form of *Pseudomonas aeruginosa*. 1. An effective method for the production of stable L-forms. *Jpn. J. Exp. Med.* 48:219-226.

10. Cohen, M., McCandless, R. G., Kalmanson, G. M., and Guze, L. B. (1968). Core-like structures in transitional and protoplast forms of *Streptococcus faecalis* in *Microbial Protoplasts, Spheroplasts, and L-Forms* (L. B. Guze, ed.), Williams & Wilkins, Baltimore, Maryland, pp. 94–109.
11. Hubert, E. G., Kalmanson, G. M., Montgomerie, J. Z., and Guze, L. B. (1972). Activity of methacycline, related tetracyclines and other antibiotics against various L-forms and their parent bacteria in vitro. *Antimicrob. Agents Chemother.* 2:276–280.
12. Yamamoto, A. and Homma, J. Y. (1978). L-form of *Pseudomonas aeruginosa*. 2. Antibiotic sensitivity of L-forms and their parent forms. *Jpn. J. Exp. Med.* 48:355–362.
13. Daschner, F. D., Hovel, R., and Marget, W. (1973). Action of gentamicin on penicillin G-induced *Proteus* spheroplasts. *Chemotherapy* 18:235–241.
14. Montgomerie, J. Z. (1978). Cell wall-deficient bacteria in the urinary tract in *Infections of the Urinary Tract* (E. H. Kass and W. Brumfitt, eds.), Univ. Chicago Press, pp. 257–260.
15. Hubert, E. G., Potter, C. S., Kalmanson, G. M., and Guze, L. B. (1969). Pigment formation in L-forms of *Serratia marcescens*. *J. Gen. Microbiol.* 55:165–167.
16. Yamamoto, A. and Homma, J. Y. (1978). L-forms of *Pseudomonas aeruginosa*. 3. The serological cross-reactions among stable L-forms of *Pseudomonas aeruginosa*, L-form of *Streptococcus pyogenes* and mycoplasma. *Jpn. J. Exp. Med.* 48:545–551.
17. Braude, A. I., Siemienski, J., and Lee, K. (1968). Spheroplasts in human urine in *Microbial Protoplasts, Spheroplasts and L-Forms* (L. B. Guze, ed.), Williams & Wilkins, Baltimore, Maryland, pp. 396–405.
18. Conner, J. F., Coleman, S. E., Davis, J. L., and McGaughen, F. S. (1968). Bacterial L-forms from urinary-tract infections in a veterans hospital population. *J. Am. Geriatr. Soc.* 16:893–900.
19. Crowe, C. C., and Koblasz, K. K. (1971). Isolation of L-forms in recurrent urinary tract infections. *Am. J. Med. Tech.* 37:367–370.
20. Swierczewski, J. A. and Reyes, R. (1970). Isolation of L-forms in a clinical microbiology laboratory. *Appl. Microbiol.* 20:323–327.
21. Domingue, G. J. and Schlegel, J. U. (1970). The possible role of microbial L-forms in pyelonephritis. *J. Urol.* 104:790–798.
22. Yamamoto, A. and Homma, J. Y. (1979). Isolation of unstable L-forms from clinical specimens with Pseudomonas infection during antibiotic therapy. *Jpn. J. Exp. Med.* 49:362–364.
23. Kagan, B. M. (1968). Role of L-forms in Staphylococcal infections in *Microbial Protoplasts, Spheroplasts, and L-Forms* (L. B. Guze, ed.), Williams & Wilkins, Baltimore, Maryland, pp. 372–378.
24. Middleton, J. and Chmel, H. (1978). Aberrant forms of *Pseudomonas aeruginosa* in sputum and cerebrospinal fluid causing infection in a compromised patient. *J. Clin. Pathol.* 31:351–354.
25. Guze, L. B., Harwick, H. J., and Kalmanson, G. M. (1976). Klebsiella L-forms. Effect of growth as L-form on virulence of reverted *Klebsiella pneumoniae*. *J. Infect. Dis.* 133:245–252.

10
Biology of Cell Wall-Defective Forms of *Nocardia*

BLAINE L. BEAMAN
Department of Medical Microbiology and Immunology, University of California School of Medicine, Davis, California

I.	Introduction	203
II.	The Cell Wall of *Nocardia*	204
	A. Chemical Composition	204
	B. Physical Structure	205
III.	Induction of L-Forms	207
	A. Factors Affecting Cell Morphology and Cell Wall Structure	207
	B. In Vitro and In Vivo Removal of the Cell Wall	209
	C. Isolation, Maintenance, and Growth of L-Forms	213
IV.	Properties of L-Forms	214
	A. Structure	214
	B. Chemical and Physiological Properties	215
V.	L-Form Reversion: Variation of L-Form Revertants	217
VI.	Role of L-Forms in Disease	220
VII.	Conclusions	222
	References	223

I. INTRODUCTION

The major functions of the cell wall are to provide protection of the cell from osmotic lysis, to determine the size and shape of the bacterial cell, and to serve as a physical barrier. Chemical, physical, or structural modifications within the cell walls of most bacteria usually result in alterations of these functional capacities. In some bacteria, these properties are altered during the growth cycle. Thus, within the genus *Nocardia*, cells that are in the stationary phase of growth are usually either short pleomorphic rods, coccobaccilli, or cocci. If these coccoid cells are inoculated into a fresh, nutrient medium they will increase in diameter and elongate. In logarithmic phase of growth, the organisms are normally elongated into slender branching filaments that fragment to shorter cells by transverse septation. As the nutrients become depleted and the organisms enter a stationary phase of growth, the cells fragment further to produce shorter pleomorphic rods and cocci. Studies have determined that there are concomitant changes in the wall during the cellular development of nocardia [1-4].

II. THE CELL WALL OF NOCARDIA

A. Chemical Composition

The nocardiae are gram-positive bacteria that are biologically related to both the corynebacteria and mycobacteria. All of these organisms possess an unusually complex cell envelope composed of a variety of unique substances [5-9]. The cell walls of *Nocardia asteroides* have been studied extensively [1,2,10-12].

In nocardia, the cell walls consist of between 14% to a maximum of 45% peptidoglycan, depending upon the stage of growth and the strain of organism [1,2,11]; and, in actively growing cells of most strains of *N. asteroides* that have been studied, it accounts for approximately 20% of the cell wall weight [1,2,11]. The peptidoglycan of *N. asteroides*, and probably other nocardiae, is composed of β-N-acetylglucosaminyl-1,4-N-glycolyl-muramic acid. The carboxyl group of the N-glycolylmuramic acid is linked to a tetrapeptide composed of L-alanine-Dα-glutamine-meso-diaminopimelic acid-D-alanine which is cross-linked to adjacent tetrapeptides by direct D-alanine to meso-DAP linkages [1,2,8-13].

The cell walls of nocardia contain an arabinogalactan polymer composed of 1-5-linked arabinofuranosyl, 1-4-linked galactopyranosyl, and some 1-2-linked arabinofuranose [10]. This arabinogalactan polymer appears to be covalently bound to the glycolylmuramic acid by way of either a phosphodiester bridge between muramic acid and arabinose or by a direct glycosidic linkage between arabinose and muramic acid. In addition, the arabinogalactan may possess multiple branches consisting of polymers of arabinose, and the nonreducing terminal portion of the arabinogalactan consists of arabinose covalently linked to mycolic acid [9-11]. As a result, the basal structure of the cell wall of nocardia consists of a peptidoglycan-arabinogalactan-mycolate complex.

Mycolic acids are α-branched, β-hydroxylated, long-chain fatty acids with the general formula:

$$R - \underset{R^1}{C} - \overset{OH}{\underset{|}{C}} - COOH$$

[6]. In nocardiae the total number of carbons varies from C40 to C60 and they represent between 10 and 30% of the total cell wall weight, depending upon the stage of growth as well as the specific strain of nocardia [2,10-12]. Some of the mycolic acids are freely associated within the cell envelope; however, most of the mycolates are covalently linked to a moiety such as the arabinose of the arabinogalactan, glucose, or trehalose [2,10-12].

Exterior to the peptidoglycan complex resides a variety of constituents. One of the major outer components is a polypeptide fraction covalently linked to a lipid moiety. In *N. asteroides*, this peptide is composed primarily of alanine, glycine, aspartic acid, leucine, isoleucine, threonine, valine, and phenylalanine linked to a long-chained fatty acid [1,2]. The precise composition of the peptidolipid in the cell wall varies with both culture age and with each strain of nocardia [1,2]. Additional lipoidal components firmly bound to the cell wall are composed of palmitic (C16), oleic (or vaccenic; C18:1), stearic (C18), and tuberculostearic (10 methyl-stearic) acids. The relative amounts of each of these fatty acids also vary with culture age and with each strain of nocardia [1,2]. The cell walls of nocardia contain many additional loosely and firmly associated compounds such as glycolipids (e.g., trehalose dimycolates); long-chain ketones (nocardones); pigments; lipid-soluble, iron-binding compounds (nocobactins); and probably additional, yet undefined substances [1,2,10-12]. Thus, the chemical makeup of the cell envelope of nocardia is complex and dynamic.

B. Physical Structure

Electron microscopy has shown that cell walls of the nocardiae are structurally complex. Further, the ultrastructural appearance changes during the normal growth and development of the cells and significant modifications are induced by both environmental and nutritional factors [1,3,4]. Thin sections of cells demonstrate that the cell wall is multilayered. During early stages of growth (lag phase), the outermost layer is greatly enlarged and as the filaments elongate during log phase of growth, the outer region, which appears to be bound by a nonunit membrane, becomes very thin giving the cell wall a trilayered appearance [1,3]. During fragmentation into rods and coccoid cells, the outer region of the wall becomes thickened and more diffuse with a less distinct border, while the innermost layer increases in both thickness and osmiophilic density [1,3,4].

Freeze-fracture replicas reveal significant ultrastructural detail of the cell envelope (Fig. 1). The basal peptidoglycan layer, which lies adjacent to the cytoplasmic membrane, is a relatively smooth structure that is overlain by a thin granular substance. Interspersed along the surface of the basal layer and embedded within the cell wall matrix are rope-like strands of mycolic acids (Fig. 1B). Surrounding the mycolic acid-arabinogalactan-peptidoglycan complex is

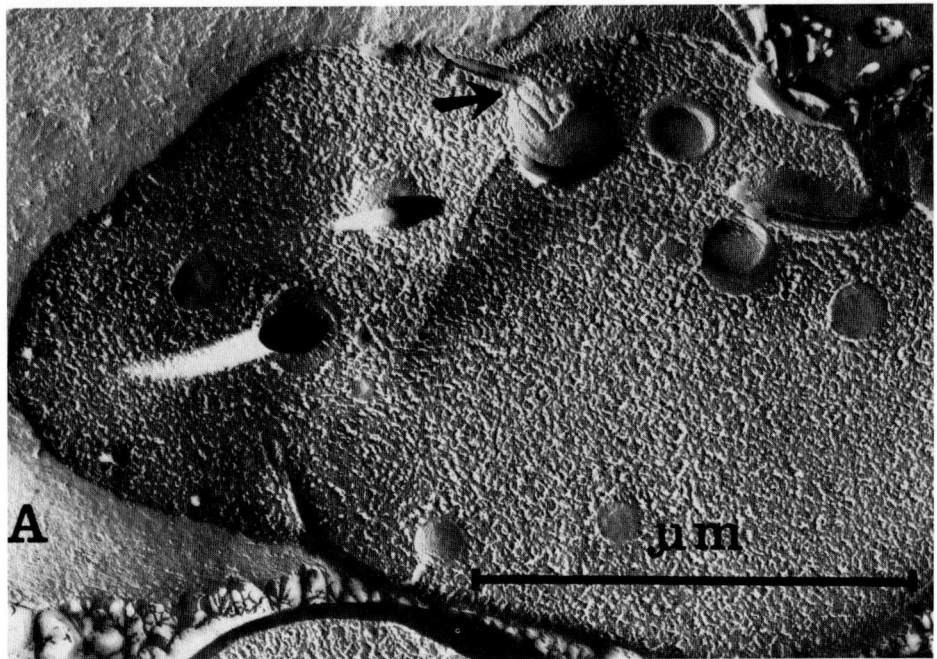

Figure 1 Freeze-fracture replicas of nocardia. The cells were not chemically fixed; colonies were scraped from the agar surface, placed on gold specimen stubs, quickly frozen in liquid Freon 22 in a liquid nitrogen bath, and the samples cleaved and etched in a Balzers as described by Beaman and Shankel [4]. (A) Nocardia grown on BHI agar for 16 hr. Note the tubulovesicular mesosome associated with septum formation originating from the cytoplasmic membrane (arrow). (B) N. asteroides grown on BHI agar for 16 hr showing the surface structure of the cell. Note the presence of fibers across the cell surface (arrow). (C) Nocardia grown on BHI agar for 24 hr showing the cell surface and cytoplasm with a membrane extending into the cytoplasm (arrow). Note the surface structure of the cytoplasmic membrane and the outer layer of the cell wall. (D) N. asteroides clearly showing the multilayer nature of the cell wall (arrows). (E) Nocardia grown on BHI agar for 24 hr. Note the thickened outer, wrinkled nature of the cell wall (bent arrow) and the granular nature of the cell membrane.

the outer layer that has the appearance of a wrinkled or folded membrane (Fig. 1C,D,E). This outermost layer is composed of peptidolipid, mycolic acid, glycolipid as well as other lipoidal material [1,2]. The total architecture of the cell envelope is dynamic, and modifications that occur in this structure result in changes in cellular morphology, surface permeability, cellular rigidity, and resistance to environmental factors (i.e., drying) [1-3,14].

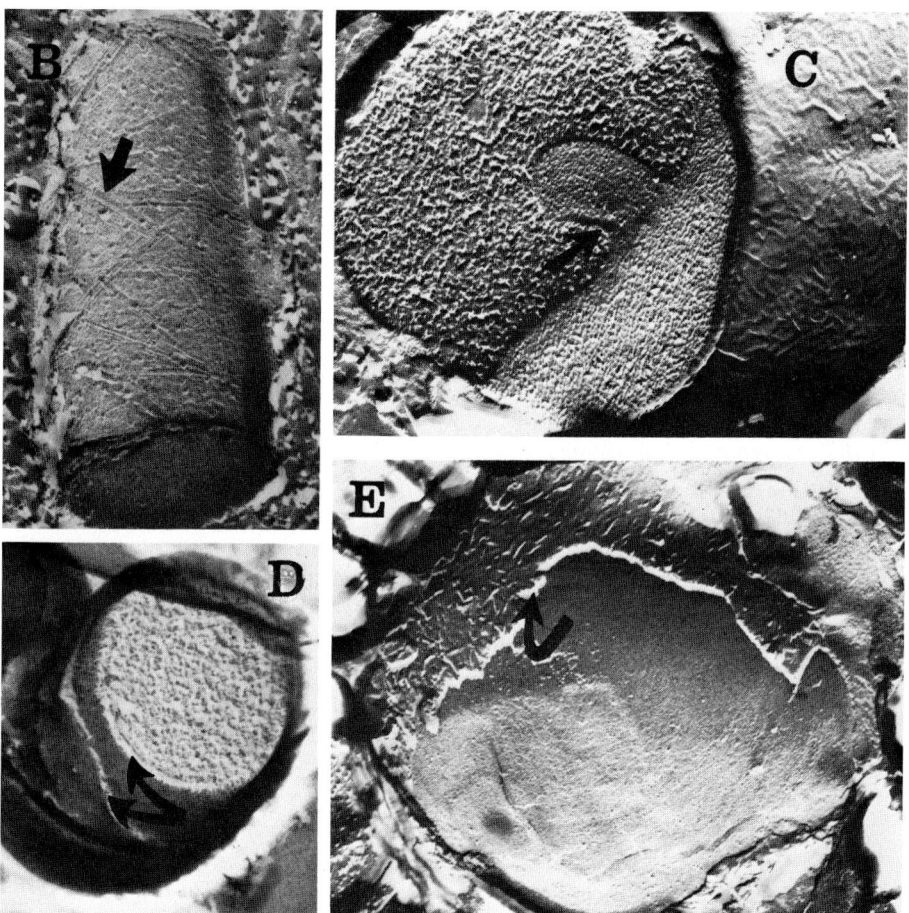

III. INDUCTION OF L-FORMS

A. Factors Affecting Cellular Morphology and Cell Wall Structure

Environmentally induced alterations in cellular morphology of certain strains of nocardia have been reported [4,15-17]. When grown in brain-heart infusion (BHI), some isolates of *N. rubra* (*Rhodococcus* spp.) form large, involuted, and bulbous to spherical-shaped cells that do not demonstrate a regular pattern of septation [4]. These greatly enlarged cells produce multiple and random septae that divide them into irregular shaped bodies of varying sizes [4]. Further, the enlarged, bulbous cells are significantly more susceptible to lysis in distilled water, and they are less resistant to dehydration than the smaller, more regularly shaped organisms from the same culture (B. L. Beaman, unpublished data). In contrast, these same isolates of nocardia grown on either nutrient agar or a chemically defined mineral salts medium do not undergo this pattern of altered morphology; instead, they form cells that have a more typical and uniform structure [4]. Similar modification of cellular morphology observed in BHI can be induced when these organisms are grown in a chemically defined mineral salts medium supplemented with large amounts of either D,L-alanine (0.5%), arabinose (5%), galactose (5%), or glycine (4%) (B. L. Beaman, Ph.D. thesis, University of Kansas, Lawrence, 1968).

Webly [17] reported that *N. opaca* produced bulbous and involuted cells when grown in a chemically defined medium that was deficient in either iron, manganese, or zinc. However, the morphology of these cells was not altered when grown in a medium deficient in either copper, molybdenum, or boron [17]. Webb et al. [15] reported that *N. corallina* formed large, involution forms which became multicellular when grown at temperatures above 35°C. In addition it has been shown that increased CO_2 during growth, as well as growth on certain hydrocarbons, vegetable oils, and fatty acids, significantly affects the morphological development of strains of nocardia [16]. Since the cellular alterations induced by the various conditions described above are similar, it appears that the control mechanisms of cell wall biosynthesis and cell division of nocardia may be affected significantly by a variety of exogenous environmental stimuli and nutrients.

Numerous strains of nocardia have been injected into a variety of experimental animals, and ultrastructural and histological analysis of the events leading to experimental infections have been studied [3,18-26]. Most of the nocardiae used as the inoculum are not acid-fast when grown in a medium such as BHI; however, these strains become strongly acid-alcohol-fast when grown in animals. Further, unlike the stable acid-fastness reported in mycobacteria [5], the acid-fastness of in vivo-grown nocardiae is removed by pyridine extraction [27]. In addition, all strains of nocardia are uniformyl gram-positive when grown in BHI, but they become somewhat gram-variable and highly beaded in appearance when grown in vivo. With some strains such as *N. asteroides* 10905, large numbers of gram-negative, club-shaped, and involuted cells are localized to form bacterial granules within the lesions [18]. The more virulent strains such as *N. asteroides* GUH-2 undergo the least cellular modification within the host whereas the less virulent organisms are affected the most. Histochemical studies reveal addition alterations in both the host response and the nocardial cell structure. Thus, in tissues of infected mice, the periodic acid Schiff reaction is positive for the less virulent strains (*N. asteroides* 10905 and *N. farcinica*-C) and negative for the more virulent organisms (*N. asteroides* GUH-2, and *N. asteroides*-Mahvi). Acid haematein staining is positive for *N. asteroides*-Mahvi and *N. farcinica*-C, which share several similarities in cell wall mycolic acid structure, while it is negative for *N. asteroides* GUH-2 and *N. asteroides* 10905, which have different cell wall mycolates (B. L. Beaman, unpublished data). All of these staining reactions are negative for all of the strains when grown in BHI broth. The prominent beads within the in vivo-grown cells of *N. asteroides* are acid-fast, gram-positive, Sudan Black-B positive (for lipid inclusions), acid haematein positive (for phospholipids), and metachromatic with Toluidine Blue (for phosphate inclusions) after pyridine extraction. Within lesions in the mouse 2 weeks after infection by the less virulent strains of *Nocardia* (*N. asteroides* 10905), the organisms become strongly positive for calcium. In contrast, the more virulent organisms (*N. asteroides* GUH-2) give little or no staining reaction for calcium even after several months within the tissues (B. L. Beaman, unpublished data). These observations indicate that all strains of nocardia undergo both chemical and biological modification when grown within the host's tissues. Further, the changes that are observed appear to be closely associated with the type of infection induced within the host (i.e., chronic mycetomatous response vs. acute or chronic invasive nocardiosis), and with the varying degree of pathogenicity observed for each strain of nocardia. Ultrastructural analysis confirms that significant structural alterations occur in the cell envelope of many strains of nocardia as they adapt to grow within the host [18].

B. In Vitro and In Vivo Removal of the Cell Wall

Most strains of nocardia are resistant to the lytic action of lysozyme, penicillin, or D-cycloserine when grown in a chemically defined mineral salts medium [28]. However, by supplementing the medium with 2% glycine in combination with these substances, dramatic alterations in cellular morphology occur, and the cells lyse during growth. By the addition of osmotic stabilizers such as 0.35 M sucrose or 5% NaCl, the cells are prevented from lysis and they are converted to either protoplasts or spheroplasts (Fig. 2A) [28].

Glycine potentiates enhanced susceptibility of *Nocardia* to cell wall inhibitors such as penicillin and D-cycloserine, and it facilitates the action of lysozyme directly on the nocardial peptidoglycan backbone because glycine is incorporated into the peptidoglycan and the cell wall peptidolipid in place of D- and L-alanine [28,29]. As a consequence of this substitution by glycine, the peptide cross-linkages within the peptidoglycan cannot occur, and the cell wall is weakened significantly. Additionally, peptidoglycan precursors that contain glycine in place of alanine are poor substrates in the transpeptidation reaction during cell wall biosynthesis [29]. Thus, as the nocardial cells grow in a glycine-rich medium, the newly synthesized cell wall is either weakened or inhibited. The cytoplasm, constrained only by the cell membrane, is then extruded through the breaks in the newly synthesized cell wall, and the protoplast is released from the terminal end of the bacterial cell [28].

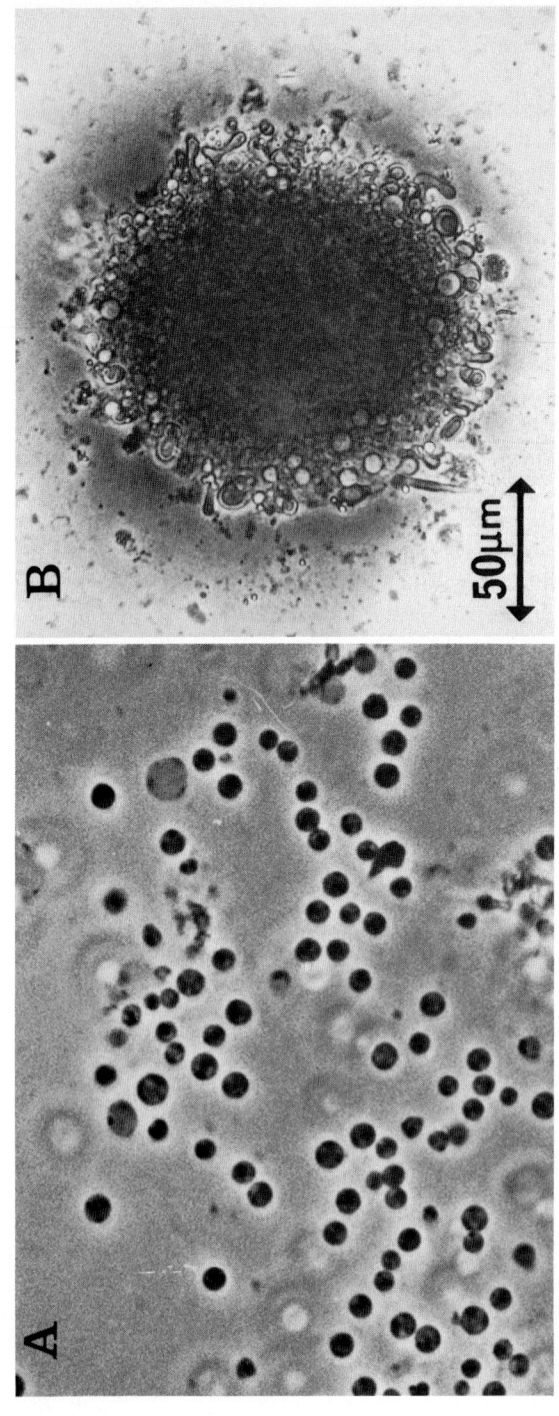

Figure 2 In vitro induction of L-forms of nocardia. (*A*) Phase-contrast micrograph of spheroplasts of *N. asteroides* after 8 days of incubation in a liquid induction medium containing glycine and lysozyme. (*B*) Phase-contrast micrograph of an L-form colony of *N. caviae* grown for 1 week on BYE-L agar. Note that the colony is composed entirely of refractile spheres, granules, and membranous extrusions (L-form colonies of *N. asteroides* usually have a similar appearance). (*C*) Electron micrograph of a thin section of L-forms of *N. asteroides* GUH-2 after 3 weekly transfers in BYE-L broth. Note the absence of the cell wall and the accumulation of intracytoplasmic structures. Smaller, membrane-bound bodies are prominent. Arrow notes the presence of large amounts of extracellular membranous and granular material that may be cell wall substances secreted into the medium by the L-forms during growth. (*D*) Electron micrograph of a thin section of Type A L-forms of *N. caviae* 112 after 3 weekly transfers in BYE-L broth. Arrow notes the absence of the cell wall.

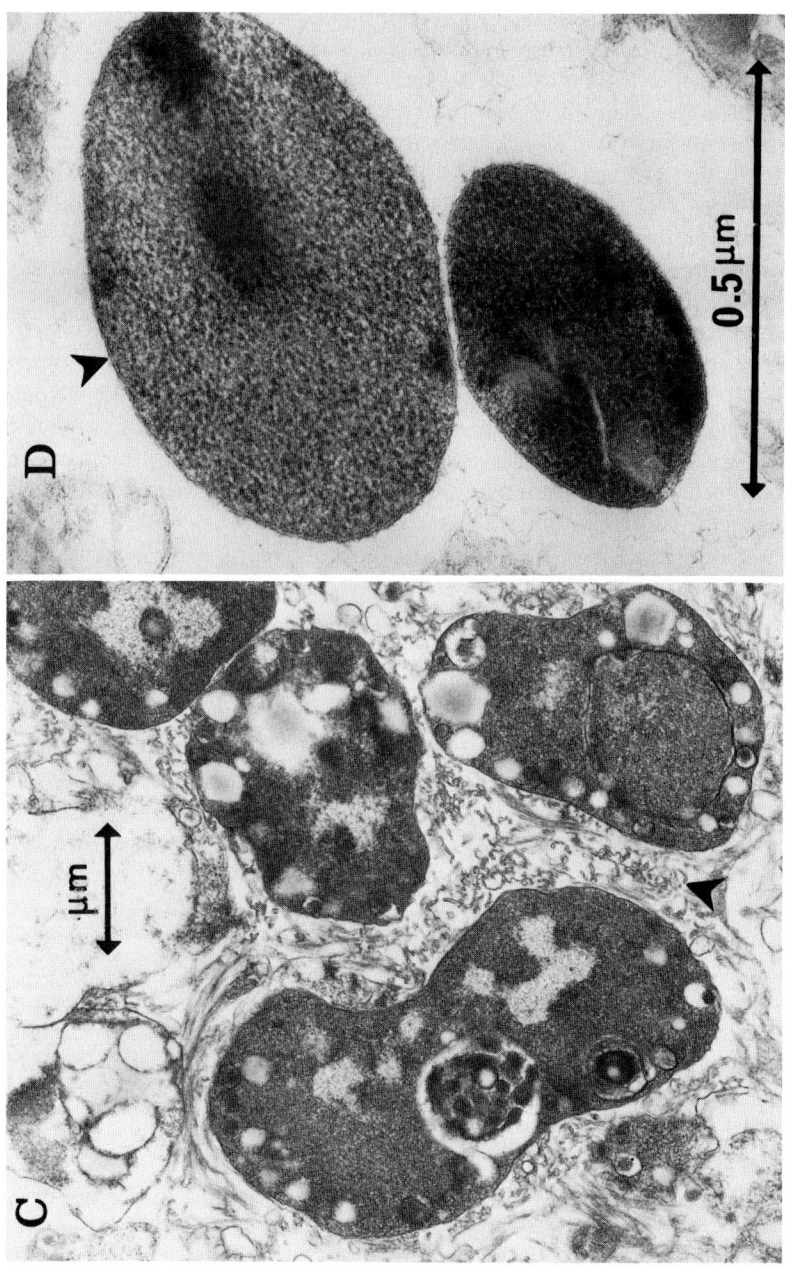

Generally, other methods used to remove the cell wall from bacteria in order to induce protoplasts and spheroplasts (i.e., EDTA + lysozyme) are not effective when applied to the nocardiae. However, Prasad and Bradley recovered a cell wall-defective variant of *N. rubra* after mutagenesis with quinacrine [30]. Serrano (Abstract, Proc. Electron Microscopy Soc. of Amer. 1972, pp. 330-331) reported the selection of mutants of nocardia with disorganized septation followed by transformation to L-forms resulting from serial transfer of the organisms in media containing penicillin or D-cycloserine; however, using the same strains of nocardia (i.e., *N. asteroides* 14759), Bourgeous was not able to reproduce these results using penicillin or D-cycloserine alone [28].

There have been many reports documenting the removal of the cell wall from a variety of bacteria both within the host and by host cells such as macrophages [31-34]. It was shown that spheroplasts or protoplasts of cells of *N. asteroides* 10905 are induced within in vitro maintained peritoneal macrophages obtained from mice [32], and protoplasts of *N. caviae* 112 are induced within tissues of mice infected either intranasally, intraperitoneally, or intravenously [35-37]. The specific mechanisms by which the host removes the cell walls from nocardia are not known; however, the phagocytic cells (polymorphonuclear neutrophils and macrophages) possess lysosomal bodies that contain a variety of degradative enzymes including lysozyme. It is probable that several components within the lysosome can replace glycine and thus potentiate the action of lysozyme on the bacterial cell wall. Thacore and Willet reported that lysosomal extracts obtained from macrophages facilitated the action of lysozyme on the induction of spheroplasts of *Mycobacterium tuberculosis* [38]. The lysosomal components believed to be responsible for this induction of the spheroplasts from *M. tuberculosis* are lysozyme, acid-phosphatase, and phospholipase C [38]. In addition, nonenzymatic factors such as the unavailability of free iron or other essential trace metals (i.e., zinc or manganese) within the macrophage phagolysosome may play an important role in altering the cell structure of nocardia [17]. As described above, Webley demonstrated that reduced availability of either iron, manganese, or zinc results in bulbous, pleomorphic cells of *N. opaca* [17]. It was observed that restricting iron availability to *N. asteroides* 10905 in whole serum induces bulbous, pleomorphic, and greatly swollen cells (B. L. Beaman, unpublished data), and similar morphological changes are observed when *N. asteroides* 10905 is grown in medium containing 2% (w/v) glycine [28]. The iron within macrophages is bound, and thus the available free iron that the nocardiae can use for growth is severely restricted. Therefore, it is likely that restricted iron availability, as well as the presence of enzymes such as acid phosphatase and phospholypase C within the phagolysosome enhance the affects of lysozyme on the cells of nocardia resulting in the formation of either protoplasts or spheroplasts during cellular growth within the macrophage. These wall-less cells would be protected from osmotic lysis within the macrophage by a combination of increased osmolarity within the phagolysosomes and by the integrity of the macrophage membrane surrounding the phagolysosome [32,35].

C. Isolation, Maintenance, and Growth of L-Forms

Both in vitro- and in vivo-induced protoplasts or spheroplasts of *N. asteroides* and *N. caviae* will grow as L-forms when inoculated into an appropriate culture medium [3,28,32,35-37]. A variety of incubational procedures combined with different media have been studied extensively to determine the optimal conditions for the induction, maintenance, and growth of L-forms of *N. asteroides, Nocardia brasiliensis*, and *Nocardia caviae* (B. L. Beaman, unpublished data). It was found that most L-forms of nocardia could grow to some extent (some strains more poorly than others) on Barile, Yaguchi, and Eveland agar (BYE) [39]. The induction of L-forms of nocardia is both strain specific and dependent upon the specific stage of growth during the induction process. The type of medium used to induce L-forms is critical; thus, even though several hundred varieties of induction media have been explored, several strains of *N. asteroides* and *N. brasiliensis* could not be successfully induced into L-forms. Nevertheless, L-forms of *N. asteroides* strains GUH-2, (Beaman), GUH-5 (Beaman), 10905 (Rozanis), 287 (Causey), N-852 (Kurup), and 14759 (ATCC) have been produced. All strains of *N. caviae* that have been studied thus far [*N. caviae* 112 (Causey), 260 (Causey), and 14629 (ATCC)] have been induced to grow as L-forms. In contrast, even though spheroplasts or protoplasts of several strains of *N. brasiliensis* could be produced, L-forms of these strains have not yet been grown (B. L. Beaman, unpublished data). The L-forms derived from *N. asteroides* GUH-2, GUH-5, 10905, and 287 and *N. caviae* 112 have been studied most extensively (B. L. Beaman, unpublished data). The optimal conditions for obtaining L-forms from the most difficult to induce of these strains (*N. asteroides* GUH-2) are described below.

Single cell suspensions of the log-phase (16 hr) of *N. asteroides* GUH-2 [40] grown in BHI broth were obtained by passing the growth suspension through a sterile glass wool column followed by differential centrifugation. The cell pellet was resuspended in fresh induction medium that consisted of 4% BHI (powder, w/v), 0.4% yeast extract (w/v), 15% sucrose (w/v), 3% NaCl (w/v), 4% glycine (w/v), 10% horse serum (v/v), and 2 mg/ml lysozyme added to double glass-distilled water. The medium was sterilized by filtration. The cell concentration within the induction medium was adjusted to an absorbance of 0.1 ($\lambda = 580$ nm), and 200 ml of this suspension was placed in sterile 2800-ml Fernback flasks. The flasks were incubated at $37°C$ with rotational agitation (150 rpm) for 6 hr followed by stationary incubation at $37°C$ in a CO_2 incubator (5% CO_2 in air) for 1 week. The refractile spheres and granules were collected and transferred to fresh induction medium [Transfer 2 (T_2)] as described above, except that

D-cycloserine (0.2 mg/ml) was added in place of lysozyme. After 1 week of incubation at 37°C in CO_2, the L-forms were transferred to fresh induction medium (T_3) without either inducing agent (lysozyme or D-cycloserine). The L-forms were then transferred at weekly intervals in the above medium (BYE broth) prepared without glycine. L-forms of *N. asteroides* GUH-2 grew well in BYE broth, but they grew poorly on the surface of agar plates prepared from BYE supplemented with 0.8% Noble agar. Even slight variations in these procedures resulted in the inability either to induce or maintain the L-forms of *N. asteroides* GUH-2. In contrast, different media and experimental procedures were most successful for the induction and growth of L-forms of *N. asteroides* GUH-5, *N. asteroides* 10905, and *N. asteroides* 287 [28].

Nocardia caviae 112 could be induced and maintained as L-forms more readily than *N. asteroides*, and a wide variety of manipulations resulted in L-form growth. Further, L-form colonies obtained from *N. caviae* 112 could be readily recovered on BYE agar (0.8% Noble agar). The methods that yielded the best recovery of L-forms of *N. caviae* 112 failed to induce either spheroplasts or protoplasts of *N. asteroides* GUH-2 [28].

In addition to strain specificity and stage of growth, many factors influence greatly the ability to grow L-forms of nocardia. For example, it was discovered that different preparations of BHI broth, yeast extract, and serum affect significantly the recovery of L-forms from either animal lesions or in vitro-induced broth cultures. Further, some L-form isolates will not grow beyond the second or third transfer in fresh BYE, and it appears as though some essential metabolite is absent in the culture medium. Also the temperature of incubation as well as the level of CO_2 greatly influence L-form growth and development (B. L. Beaman, unpublished data).

IV. PROPERTIES OF L-FORMS

A. Structure

When protoplasts or spheroplasts of nocardia (Fig. 2A) are incubated in BYE, the phase dense spheres enlarge in size and they become highly refractile when observed by phase-contrast microscopy. The large refractile spheres develop numerous intracellular granules, and small refractile spheres and granules extend from and proliferate near the surface of these larger bodies. Within 1 week in BYE broth incubated at 37°C, numerous clumps of large refractile spheres become surrounded by masses of smaller, irregular granules and refractile spheres. On BYE agar, the development of L-form colonies is similar to that observed in broth except the colonies usually develop a central core of larger spheres that grow into the agar. This core is surrounded by granules, spheres, and membranous extensions that give the colony its characteristic "fried-egg" appearance (Fig. 2B). The cell wall-deficient organisms that produce this type of colony are defined as L-forms; however, not all of the wall-less cells of nocardia produce this type of colony, and many colonial variations have been recognized [41,42]. The organisms that produce colonies with an altered morphology (i.e., not having the "fried-egg" appearance) are defined as L-form variants (Fig. 4D) of nocardia [37].

Electron microscopy reveals considerable variation within the structure of L-forms and L-form variants when grown either in BYE broth or on BYE agar (B. L. Beaman, unpublished data) [3,28,35–37]. L-forms that are actively growing are filled with internal membranous structures, and numerous membrane bound bodies are formed at the periphery of the cell (Fig. 2C). Large quantities of membranous and granular material are produced within the culture supernatant (Fig. 2C); however individual protoplasts, with no visible evidence of cell wall, predominate (Fig. 2D, 4A). Many of the larger L-form bodies of *N. asteroides* GUH-2 possess core structures (Fig. 3) that have an overall morphology of microtubules. Similar core structures have been observed in the L-forms of *Pseudomonas aeruginosa* [43], *Streptococcus faecalis* [44], *Staphylococcus aureus* [45], and *Escherichia coli* [46]. The L-forms that have no cell wall material are defined as Type A (Fig. 2D, 4A) [42]. In contrast, some of the induced L-forms produce colonial variants that, when observed by electron microscopy, consist of cells of extremely variable size and shape (Fig. 4B). These cells possess the outer portion of the cell wall; usually as a thick granular structure enclosed by a single membranous layer. The peptidoglycan or basal layer of the walls of these cells is missing, and the organisms have lost their shape and rigidity (Fig. 4B). The cells with an altered wall are defined as Type B L-form variants [42]. One of the major characteristics of Type B L-forms of *N. asteroides* is that the cells possess very large lipid inclusion granules within their cytoplasm which result in a beaded appearance when observed by light microscopy (Fig. 4B). These granules, but not the cells, tend to stain positive with the gram stain, they are acid-fast, and they stain positively with Sudan Black-B (for lipids). In contrast, the cells are gram-negative, nonacid-fast, and osmotically fragile.

B. Chemical and Physiological Properties

Because the L-forms of nocardia grow only in complex BYE medium supplemented with serum, it is not possible to compare many of their physiological properties (i.e., sole carbon source and carbohydrate utilization) with those of the parental strains from which they were derived. However, since the nocardial envelope contains several unique constituents, it is important to determine whether these substances are produced by the wall-deficient organisms. Chemical analysis of both Type A and Type B L-forms of *N. asteroides* 10905, GUH-2,

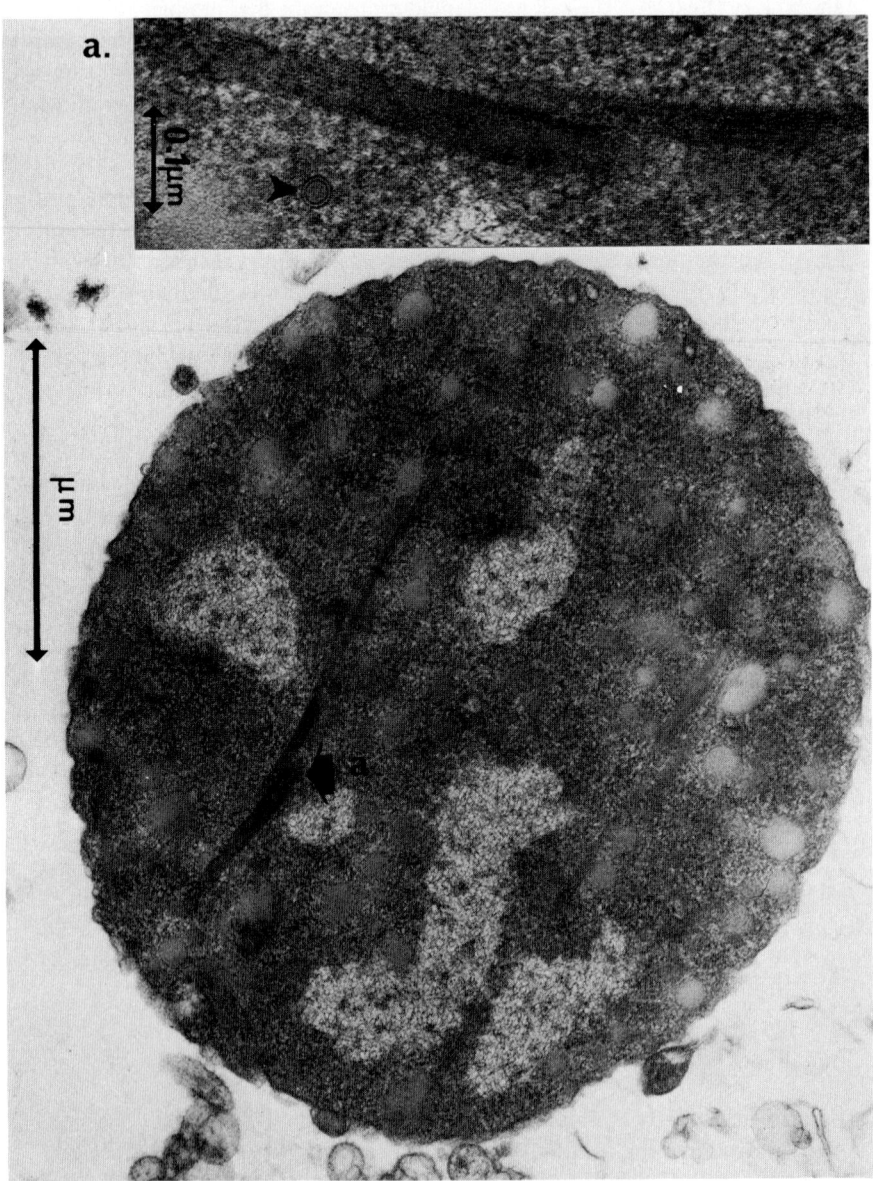

Figure 3 Electron micrograph of a thin section of an L-form cell of *N. asteroides* GUH-2 transferred four times in BYE-L broth (at weekly intervals). Many of the large cells contain microtubule-like cores. (*a*) High-magnification insert showing core structure; arrow points to the cross-section of a core filament revealing its tubular nature.

GUH-5 and 287, as well as *N. caviae* 112, have been performed using thin-layer chromatography, gas chromatography, and amino acid analysis (B. L. Beaman, unpublished data). None of the L-forms that were studied had detectable levels of muramic acid, and all strains contained significantly decreased levels of meso-diaminopimelic acid (DAP) and glucosamine as compared with the normal organisms. Type B L-forms had more meso-DAP, arabinose, and galactose than Type A L-forms. Even though arabinose and galactose were present in Type A L-forms, the amounts represented only approximately 10% of the levels detected in the normal cells, and glucose always represented the major sugar detected in whole-cell hydrolysates of both Type A and Type B L-forms. The fatty acid and lipid composition of the L-forms of nocardia was qualitatively similar to the parental strains; however, major quantitative shifts were observed. Tuberculostearic acid (10-methyl-stearic acid) is a unique cell membrane and cell wall marker among mycobacteria and nocardia [1,2,5,10]. This fatty acid was detectable in significant amounts in all forms of nocardia; however, it was the major fatty acid found in Type B L-forms. In addition, mycolic acids were present in varying amounts in both Type A and Type B L-forms, but Type A L-forms had significantly less mycolic acid than either Type B L-forms or the parental bacteria. The data suggest that the large amounts of membranous and granular material secreted into the medium (Fig. 2C) during growth of the L-forms is composed of mycolic acid, arabinogalactan, peptidolipid, and other components usually found in the outer portion of the cell wall of nocardia [1,2,6,7].

L-forms of nocardia grow in BYE broth more slowly than the normal organisms, and the L-form growth is enhanced significantly by incubation in 5% CO_2 in air. L-form colonies grown on BYE agar are catalase negative, whereas the colonies of the normal organisms produce large amounts of catalase. Further, the addition of specific antiserum against nocardia to BYE agar inoculated with L-forms inhibit the growth of the L-forms but not of the normal bacteria.

V. L-FORM REVERSION: VARIATION OF L-FORM REVERTANTS

The induction and growth of bacteria in the cell wall-less state presents a unique opportunity for protoplast fusion, indiscriminate uptake of exogenous DNA, and loss of endogenous chromosomal material through randomized and uncontrolled cellular division, and they may potentiate mutation because of membrane-DNA perturbations during chromosomal replication. In addition, nonmutationally induced alterations may occur in the reassembly of the cell envelope during the reversion process.

There have been many reports indicating that L-form revertants of various bacterial species differ substantially from the parental strain [47-50]. While screening L-form revertants of several strains of *N. asteroides*, it was observed

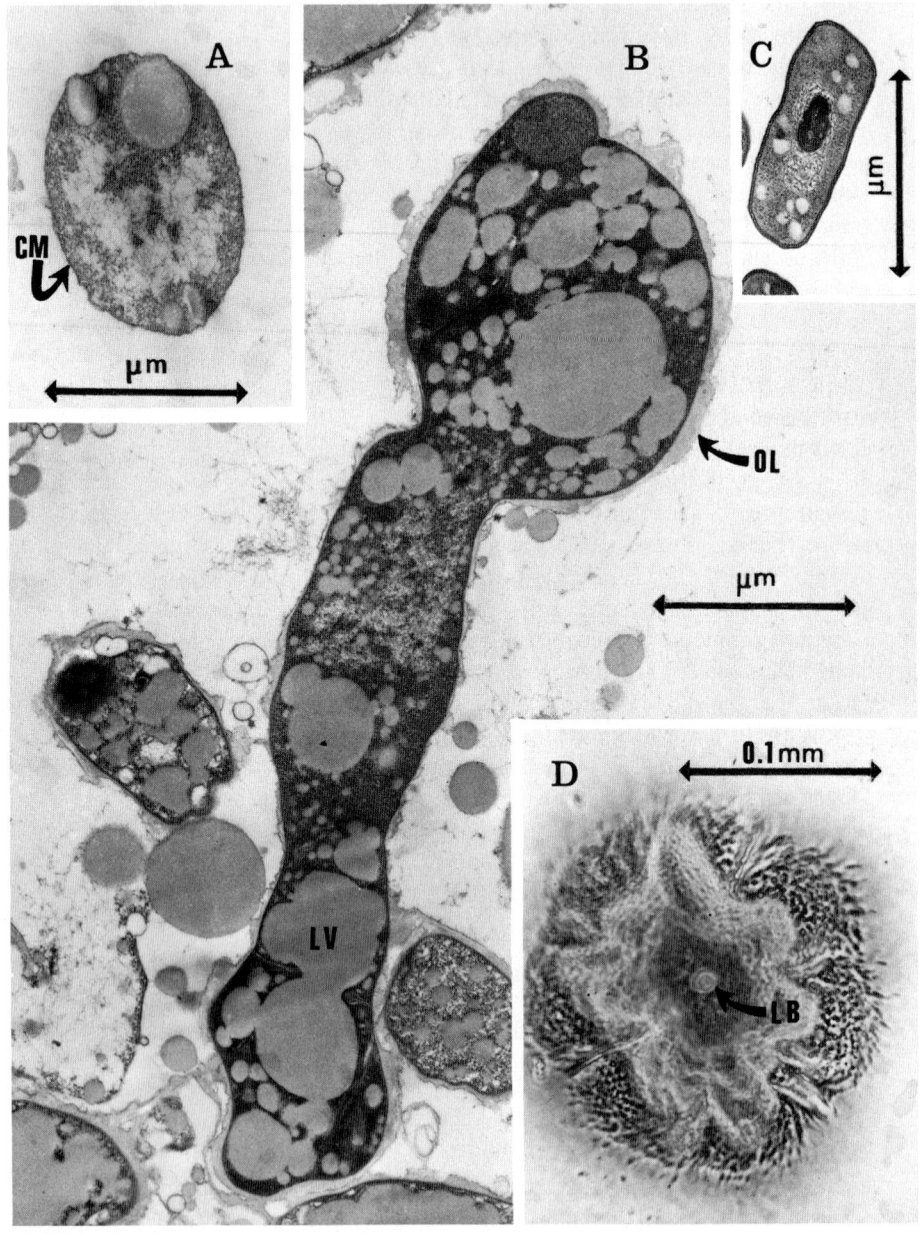

that every isolate that was studied (of more than 100) had at least one property different from the parental strain of *N. asteroides* and some revertants exhibited numerous alterations in colonial, cellular, and physiological properties [2,14].

Revertants were recovered from either macrophage or in vitro-induced L-forms of *N. asteroides* 10905. Their cell walls, colonial and cellular morphology, metabolic capacities, mycolic acid composition, and virulence for animals were studied [2,14]. It was shown that the cell walls of each revertant differed from the parental strain. Thus, in some of the revertants the mycolic acids and peptidolipid of the outer portion of the cell envelope were altered whereas in other revertants the sugar, fatty acids, and mycolic acids were changed. There were major shifts in both relative amounts and relative sizes of mycolic acids [2]. It appeared that the method of inducing the L-forms and the length of time the L-forms were maintained before reversion affected the degree of alteration in the composition of the cell envelope. Changes in the chemical makeup of the outer portion of the cell wall, particularly in mycolic acid composition, would be expected to affect the hydrophobic nature of the surface of the cells. As a consequence of this alteration in the surface lipids, there should be concomitant changes in cell-to-cell interactions during growth within the culture. This should result in modifications in colonial morphology when grown on solid media [14]. Further, modification of the envelope would affect uptake of nutrients, rate of growth, and probably host-parasite interactions. All of these types of changes were observed, to varying degrees, within the L-form revertants of *N. asteroides* 10905 [2,14]. The physiological and biochemical changes observed within the revertants were stable and probably reflected mutational events. Thus, the induction of L-forms of nocardia, followed by reversion, appears to potentiate or select for either multiple mutational events or polyfunctional mutations that result in changes in gene expression. These observations concerning biological alterations as the result of passage of nocardial cells through the L-form of growth may provide a possible explanation for the taxonomic heterogeneity of species of nocardia [51-54].

Figure 4 Electron microscopy of an L-form variant colony of *N. asteroides* 10905. (*A*) A thin section of a Type A L-form grown on BYE-L agar for 1 week. Arrow notes the absence of the cell wall. (*B*) A thin section of a Type B L-form grown on BYE-L agar for 1 week. Compare the size, shape, and structure of the Type B L-form with its normal parent (*C*). Note the altered outer portions of the cell wall (OL) and the abundant lipid inclusions (LV). (*C*) A thin section of a normal cell of *N. asteroides* 10905 grown on BHI agar for 1 week. Compare with *A* and *B*. *A*, *B*, and *C* are enlarged approximately the same amount. (*D*) Phase-contrast micrograph of an L-form variant colony of *N. asteroides* 10905 (BYE-L agar for 1 month). LB, Large body. Compare with the L-form colony shown in Fig. 2*B*. (Reproduced with permission from Beaman, Ref. 19.)

VI. ROLE OF L-FORMS IN DISEASE

It has been demonstrated that host defense mechanisms can induce L-forms of nocardia and nocardial L-forms have been recovered from both experimentally infected mice and humans [28,31,32,35-37]. It was shown that L-forms of *N. caviae* 112 could persist within the murine host for more than 1 year, and the growth of these L-forms appeared to be intimately involved in the induction and formation of mycetomatous lesions [37]. In addition, the intranasal administration of normal cells of *N. caviae* into the lungs of mice resulted in acute pneumonia. When the lungs of these dying mice were cultured for both conventional bacteria and L-forms, it was found that only L-forms could be recovered from many of the animals [35]. It appeared that the L-forms induced within the lungs of these mice played an active role in the disease process, because when greater amounts of either formalin or heat-killed cells of *N. caviae* were aspirated into the lungs of control mice, no animals developed pulmonary symptoms [35].

The role of L-forms of nocardia in infections of humans has not been studied adequately; however there is considerable evidence suggesting that nocardial L-forms are induced within humans (B. L. Beaman, unpublished data) [3,19, 55-59]. Further, L-forms may play an important role in persistence, latency, and pathogenesis of disease [37]. Although a systematic search for L-forms in patients suspected of having nocardial infections has not been done, there is considerable indirect evidence suggesting that nocardial cells may frequently be present in an altered cellular state within infected tissues [55-59]. There are several reports of an inability to visualize cells of nocardia in tissues from which organisms can be readily isolated, and numerous investigators stress that often nocardial cells cannot be isolated from tissues even though the organisms can be visualized microscopically [55-59]. In one case, a patient presented with pulmonary nocardiosis secondary to polymyositis. The patient received appropriate antinocardial drugs for several weeks prior to developing clinical symptoms of brain infection. Cerebrospinal fluid (CSF) of this patient had a high leukocyte count, but bacteria could neither be visualized in nor isolated from repeated samples of the CSF. Several months following the initial onset of disease, the CSF of this patient was inoculated onto BYE-L agar and evaluated for the presence of L-forms. After 1 week of incubation at 37°C in 5% CO_2, approximately 10^4 L-form colonies per milliliter of CSF were isolated. Refrigeration of the CSF at 4°C for 24 hr abrogated the ability to isolate L-forms from this CSF. The CSF was obtained from this patient three more times at 1- to 2-week intervals, and approximately 10^4 L-forms per milliliter of CSF was recovered each time. The L-forms were suspected as being derived from *N. asteroides* because they had the following properties: immunofluorescent when treated with antibody against *N. asteroides*; fatty acid profiles obtained by gas

Table 1 Comparative Antibiotic Sensitivities of *N. asteroides* GUH-5 (lung isolate) and its L-form Revertant (CSF isolate)[a]

Strain	Ampicillin	Bacitracin	Carbenicillin	Gentamycin	Penicillin	Tetracycline	Sulfachloropyridazine	Vancomycin[b]
Parent (lung isolate)	31	21	26	34	32	No zone	46	32
L-form revertant (CSF isolate)	25	No zone	No zone	29	No zone	No zone	38	No zone

[a]Values represent diameter (in mm) of zone of inhibition surrounding antibiotic disks at 24 hr incubation by the standard Kirby-Bauer method of determining antibiotic sensitivities for bacteria.
[b]Both strains of *N. asteroides* were resistant to all other antibiotics tested.

chromatography demonstrated tuberculostearic acid; and partially acid-fast by the auramine-rhodamine fluorescent stain. During agar block transfers of the L-forms obtained from the patient's CSF, the L-forms reverted to normal cells of *N. asteroides* (approximately 1 month after the initial isolation of the L-forms). Metabolically and culturally, the L-form revertant strains obtained from the CSF appeared to be identical to the normal organism isolated directly from the lungs of this patient. Antibiotic sensitivities of both strains were performed, and it was found that the L-form revertant had very different antibiotic sensitivities as compared with the parent (Table 1). The patient died from disseminated disease, and it was believed that the L-form contributed to the inability to successfully treat the brain infection in this patient (B. L. Beaman, unpublished data).

Whether or not L-forms of bacteria per se are pathogenic has been a subject of controversy for several years. "Koch's postulates" have not been satisfactorily fulfilled because L-forms, when injected into laboratory animals, either fail to induce a host response, or they revert to the classical bacterial form before disease is recognized. In a series of experiments designed to ascertain the pathogenicity of L-forms of *N. caviae* 112, mice were injected with stable L-forms induced in vitro. It was observed that 100% of the mice injected with L-forms developed chronic mycetomatous lesions approximately 6 months to 1 year after injection. Both L-forms and normal cells of *N. caviae* were isolated from the lesions present in most of the mice (9/10) infected for 1 year; however, in one mouse that had a massive lesion (approximately 50 gm weight) only L-forms could be isolated from the lesion. Light and electron microscopy demonstrated only spheroplast-like bacterial cells within this lesion. L-forms isolated from this mouse were grown in BYE-L broth and injected into several additional mice. Approximately 1 year after infection these mice (4/5) had mycetomatous lesions, and only L-forms could be recovered from two of these mice. Thus, "Koch's postulates" appear to have been fulfilled showing that in vitro-induced L-forms of *N. caviae* 112 are pathogenic for mice. Further, these L-forms induce a mycetomatous disease almost indistinguishable from the disease caused by the normal organisms (B. L. Beaman, unpublished data).

VII. CONCLUSIONS

Several strains of nocardia can be induced to grow as L-forms when inoculated into a hypertonic medium supplemented with high concentrations of glycine combined with a variety of cell wall inhibitors such as D-cycloserine. The precise conditions required for induction and growth of nocardial L-forms appear to be strain specific. In general, those isolates that are induced readily into L-forms in vitro are also induced into the cell wall-deficient state when grown in the host. Considerable evidence suggests that L-forms may be important in host-parasite interactions, and L-forms may be involved in bacterial persistence, latency, and recrudescence of disease caused by certain strains of nocardia. The in vitro-induced L-forms of *N. caviae* 112 and *N. asteroides* GUH-2 have been shown to be pathogenic for mice. In addition, L-forms of *N. asteroides* GUH-5 were isolated from the cerebrospinal fluid of a human prior to the terminal onset of disseminated disease.

The nocardiae are normally saprophytic bacteria growing within the soil. No experimental evidence has been presented to indicate either the presence or survival of L-forms of nocardia within the environment. Therefore, their role, if any, in nature has not been investigated. It is known, however, that there is a large amount of taxonomic heterogeneity in isolates of nocardia recovered from both environmental and clinical sources [51-54]. Beaman and Bourgeois [14] demonstrated that passage of *N. asteroides* 10905 through the L-form resulted in considerable alteration in the physiological morphological, ultrastructural, and biochemical properties of this organism. Further, the longer the organism remained as an L-form prior to reversion, the greater the changes in these properties. Additional L-form revertants of *N. asteroides* have been studied, and it could be demonstrated that every L-form revertant possessed at least one metabolic or physiological property distinct from the parental strain (B. L. Beaman, unpublished data). Most of these alterations appear to be stable and they apparently represent mutational changes. Thus, passage of cells of *N. asteroides* through a cell wall-deficient form either potentiates mutations or selects for multifunctional mutational events. These observations could explain the mechanisms of the diversity and heterogeneity that are characteristic of the genus *Nocardia*. Therefore, the induction and growth of L-forms of nocardia may have considerable significance in understanding the basic biology of these organisms both within the environment and the host.

ACKNOWLEDGMENTS

Much of the work discussed in this review was supported by Public Health Service Research Grants from the National Institutes of Health, NIAID, AI-13167 and AI-15114.

REFERENCES

1. Beaman, B. L. (1975). Structural and biochemical alterations of *Nocardia asteroides* cell walls during its growth cycle. *J. Bacteriol.* 123:1235-1253.
2. Beaman, B. L., Bourgeois, A. L., and Moring, S. E. (1981). Cell wall modification resulting from *in vitro* induction of L-phase variants of *Nocardia asteroides*. *J. Bacteriol.* 148:600-609.

3. Beaman, B. L., Serrano, J. A., and Serrano, A. A. (1978). Comparative ultrastructure within the Nocardia. *Zentralblatt fur Bakteriologie, Supple.* 6, pp. 201-220.
4. Beaman, B. L. and Shankel, D. M. (1969). Ultrastructure of *Nocardia* cell growth and development on defined and complex agar media. *J. Bacteriol.* 99:876-884.
5. Barksdale, L. and Kim, K. S. (1977). *Mycobacterium. Bacteriol. Rev.* 41: 217-372.
6. Beaman, B. L., Kim, K. S., Laneelle, M. A., and Barksdale, L. (1974). Chemical characterization of organisms isolated from leprosy patients. *J. Bacteriol.* 117:1320-1329.
7. Beaman, B. L., Kim, K. S., Salton, M. R. J., and Barksdale, L. (1971). Amino acids of the cell wall of *Nocardia rubra. J. Bacteriol.* 108:941-943.
8. Cummins, C. S. (1965). Chemical and antigenic studies on cell walls of Mycobacterium, Corynebacterium and Nocardia. *Am. Rev. Resp. Dis.* 92: 63-72.
9. Goren, M. B. and Brennan, P. J. (1979). Mycobacterial lipids: Chemistry and biology activities in *Tuberculosis* (G. P. Youmans, ed.), W. B. Saunders, Philadelphia, pp. 63-193.
10. Azuma, I., Kanetsura, F., Tanaka, Y., Mera, M., Yanagihara, Y., Mifuchi, I., and Yamamura, Y. (1973). Partial chemical characterization of the cell wall of *Nocardia asteroides* strain 131. *Jpn. J. Microbiol.* 17:154-159.
11. Michel, G. and Bordet, C. (1976). Cell walls of Nocardiae, in *The Biology of the Nocardiae* (M. Goodfellow, G. H. Brownell, and J. A. Serrano, eds.), Academic, London, pp. 141-159.
12. Vacheron, M-J., Guinard, M., Michel, G., and Ghuysen, J-M. (1972). Structural investigations on cell walls of Nocardia sp.: The wall lipid and peptidoglycan moieties of *Nocardia kirovani. Eur. J. Biochem.* 29:156-166.
13. Azuma, I., Thomas, D. W., Adam, A., Ghuysen, J. M., Bonaly, R., Petit, J. F., and Lederer, E. (1970). Occurrence of N-glycolylmuramic acid in bacterial cell walls. A preliminary survey. *Biochim. Biophys. Acta* 208: 444-451.
14. Beaman, B. L. and Bougeois, A. L. (1981). Variations in properties of *Nocardia asteroides* resulting from growth in the cell wall-deficient state. *J. Clin. Microbiol.* 15:574-578.
15. Webb, R. B., Clark, J. B., and Chance, H. L. (1954). A cytological study of *Nocardia corallina* and other actinomycetes. *J. Bacteriol.* 67:498-502.
16. Webley, D. M. (1954). The morphology of *Nocardia opaca* Waksman Henrici (*proactinomyces opacus* Jensen) when grown on hydrocarbons, vegetable oils, fatty acids and related substances. *J. Gen. Microbiol.* 11: 420-425.
17. Webley, D. M. (1960). The effect of deficiency in iron, zinc, and manganese on the growth and morphology of *Nocardia opaca. J. Gen. Microbiol.* 23: 87-92.
18. Beaman, B. L. (1973). An ultrastructural analysis of *Nocardia* during experimental infections in mice. *Infect. Immun.* 8:828-840.

19. Beaman, B. L. (1976). Possible mechanism of nocardial pathogenesis in *Biology of the Nocardiae* (M. Goodfellow, G. H. Brownell, and J. A. Serrano, eds.), Academic, London, pp. 386–417.
20. Beaman, B. L. and Maslan, S. (1977). The effect or cyclophosphamide on experimental *Nocardia asteroides* infection in mice. *Infect. Immun. 16*: 995–1004.
21. Beaman, B. L., Goldstein, E., Gershwin, M. E., Maslan, S., and Lippert, W. (1978). Lung response of congenitally athymic (nude), heterozygous, and Swiss Webster mice to aerogenic and intranasal infection by *Nocardia asteroides*. *Infect. Immun. 22*:867–877.
22. Folb, P. I., Jaffe, R., and Altman, G. (1976). *Nocardia asteroides* and *Nocardia brasiliensis* infections in mice. *Infect. Immun. 13*:1490–1496.
23. Folb, P. I., Timme, A., and Horowitz, A. (1977). Nocardia infections in congenitally athymic (nude) mice and other inbred mouse strains. *Infect. Immun. 18*:459–466.
24. Kurup, P. V., Randhawa, H. S., Sands, R. S., and Abraham, S. (1970). Pathogenicity of *Nocardia caviae, N. asteroides* and *N. brasiliensis*. *Mycopathol. Mycol. Appl. 40*:113–130.
25. Macotella-Ruiz, E. and Mariat, F. (1963). Sur la production de mycetoma experimentaux par *Nocardia brasiliensis* et *Nocardia asteroides*. *Bull. Soc. Pathol. Exot. 89*:426–431.
26. Uesaka, I., Oiwa, K., Yasuhira, K., Kobara, Y., and McClung, N. M. (1971). Studies on the pathogenicity of *Nocardia* isolates for mice. *Jpn. J. Exp. Med. 41*:443–457.
27. Beaman, B. L. and Burnside, J. (1973). Pyridine extraction of nocardial acid fastness. *Appl. Microbiol. 26*:426–428.
28. Bourgeois, L. and Beaman, B. L. (1976). In vitro spheroplast and L-form induction within the pathogenic nocardiae. *J. Bacteriol. 127*:584–594.
29. Hammes, W., Schleifer, K. W., and Kandler, O. (1973). Mode of action of glycine on the biosynthesis of peptidoglycan. *J. Bacteriol. 116*:1029–1053.
30. Prasad, I. and Bradley, S. G. (1972). Cell wall-defective variants of *Nocardia rubra*. *J. Gen. Microbiol. 70*:571–572.
31. Beaman, B. L. and Smathers, M. (1976). Interaction of *Nocardia asteroides* with cultured rabbit alveolar macrophages. *Infect. Immun. 13*:1126–1131.
32. Bourgeois, L. and Beaman, B. L. (1974). Probable L-forms of *Nocardia asteroides* induced in cultured mouse peritoneal macrophages. *Infect. Immun. 9*:576–590.
33. Hatten, B. A. and Sulkin, S. E. (1966). Intracellular production of Brucella L-forms. I. Recovery of L-forms from tissue culture cells infected with *Brucella abortus*. *J. Bacteriol. 91*:285–296.
34. O'Beirne, A. J. and Eveland, W. C. (1974). Induction of the L-phase of *Listeria monocytogenes* by rabbit alveolar macrophages in vitro. *Can. J. Microbiol. 20*:963–966.
35. Beaman, B. L. (1980). The induction of L-phase variants of *Nocardia caviae* within the intact murine lung. *Infect. Immun. 29*:244–251.

36. Beaman, B. L. (1981). The possible role of L-phase variants of *Nocardia* in chronic infections. *Zentralblatt fur Bakteriologie* Suppl. 11, pp. 221–227.
37. Beaman, B. L. and Scates, S. M. (1981). Role of L-forms of *Nocardia caviae* in the development of chronic mycetomas in normal and immunodeficient murine models. *Infect. Immun. 33*:893–907.
38. Thacore, H. and Willet, H. P. (1963). Formation of spheroplasts of *Mycobacterium tuberculosis* by lysozyme treatment. *Proc. Soc. Exp. Biol. Med. 114*:43–47.
39. Barile, M. J., Yaguchi, R., and Eveland, W. C. (1958). A simplified medium for the cultivation of Pleuropneumonia-like organisms and the L-forms of bacteria. *Am. J. Clin. Pathol. 30*:171–176.
40. Beaman, B. L. and Maslan, S. (1978). Virulence of *Nocardia asteroides* during its growth cycle. *Infect. Immun. 20*:290–295.
41. Madoff, S. and Pachas, W. N. (1970). Mycoplasma and the L-forms of bacteria in *Rapid Diagnostic Methods in Medical Microbiology* (C. D. Graber, ed.), Williams & Wilkins, Baltimore, pp. 195–217.
42. Madoff, S. and Pachas, W. N. (1977). Clinical significance of mycoplasma and bacterial L-forms in *Significance of Medical Microbiology in the Care of Patients* (V. Lorian, ed.), Williams & Wilkins, Baltimore, pp. 149–158.
43. Hubert, E. G., Potter, C. S., Hensley, T. J., Cohen, M., Kalmanson, G. M., and Guze, L. B. (1971). L-forms of *Pseudomonas aeruginosa. Infect. Immun. 4*:60–72.
44. Cohen, M., McCandless, R. G., Kalmanson, G. M., and Guze, L. B. (1968). Core-like structures in transitional and protoplast forms of *Streptococcus faecalis* in *Microbial Protoplasts, Spheroplasts and L-Forms* (L. B. Guze, ed.), Williams & Wilkins, Baltimore, pp. 94–109.
45. Eda, T., Kanda, Y., Mori, C., and Kimura, S. (1977). Microtubular structures in a stable staphylococcal L-form. *J. Bacteriol. 132*:1024–1026.
46. Eda, T., Kanda, Y., Mori, C., and Kimura, S. (1979). Core-like and microtubular structures in a stable L-form of *Escherichia coli. Microbiol. Immunol. 23*:915–920.
47. Mattman, L. (1974). *Cell Wall Deficient Forms*, CRC Press, Cleveland, Ohio, pp. 293–301.
48. Simon, H. J. and Yin, E. J. (1970). Penicillinase studies on L-phase variants, G-phase variants, and reverted strains of *Staphylococcus aureus. Infect. Immun. 2*:644–654.
49. Watanakunakorn, C. and Glotzbecker, C. (1975). In vivo behavior of revertants from *Staphylococcus aureus* L-phase variants compared with the parent strain. *Infect. Immun. 11*:1182–1186.
50. Wieckiewicz, J. (1979). Loss of virulence of revertants from *Staphylococcus aureus* L-phase variants in comparison with the parent strain. *J. Hyg. Epidemiol. Microbiol. Immunol. 23*:328–331.
51. Kurup, P. V. and Schmitt, J. A. (1973). Numerial taxonomy of *Nocardia. Can. J. Microbiol. 19*:1035–1048.
52. Mishra, S. K., Gordon, R. E., and Barnett, D. A. (1980). Identification of Nocardiae and Streptomycetes of medical importance. *J. Clin. Microbiol. 11*:728–736.

53. Orchard, V.A. and Goodfellow, M. (1980). Numerical classification of some named strains of *Nocardia asteroides* and related isolates from soil. *J. Gen. Microbiol.* 118:295–312.
54. Schaal, K. P. and Reutersberg, H. (1978). Numerical taxonomy of *Nocardia asteroides*. *Zentrabl. fur Bakt, Parasitenk, Infektionskrank, and Hyg. Suppl.* 6:53–62.
55. Causey, W. (1974). *Nocardia caviae*: A report of 13 new isolations with clinical correlation. *Appl. Microbiol.* 28:192–198.
56. Causey, W. A., Arnell, P., and Brinken, J. (1974). Systemic *Nocardia* cavial infection. *Chest* 65:360–362.
57. Greer, K. (1974). Nocardial mycetoma. *Virginia Medical Monthly 101*: 193–195.
58. Neu, H. C., Silva, M., Hazen, E., and Rosenheim, S. H. (1967). Necrotizing nocardial pneumonitis. *Ann. Int. Med.* 66:274–284.
59. Stropes, L., Bartlett, M., and White, A. (1980). Multiple recurrences of nocardial pneumonia. *Am. J. Med. Sci.* 280:119–122.

11

L-Forms as Models for the Study of Antibiotic Activities

JANINE SCHMITT-SLOMSKA
U.65 INSERM: National Institute of Health and Medical Research, Department of Microbiology, Faculty of Medicine, Nimes, France

I.	Introduction	229
II.	Studies on the Susceptibility of L-Forms to Antibiotics	230
III.	L-Forms as Models for the Study of Antibiotic Activity	233
	A. The Response of L-Forms to Penicillins and Other Inhibitors of Wall Synthesis	233
	B. The Response of L-Forms to Antibiotics Affecting Function of the Cytoplasmic Membrane	235
	C. The Response of L-Forms to Inhibitors of Nucleic Acid Synthesis	244
	D. The Response of L-Forms to Antibiotics Inhibiting Protein Synthesis	244
IV.	Chromosomal and Plasmid-Mediated Antibiotic Resistance in L-Forms	248
V.	Concluding Remarks	252
	References	255

I. INTRODUCTION

A study of the mode of action of an antibiotic should attempt to elucidate its biochemical effect on susceptible organisms and their organelles. One such region of the cell is the envelope, a complex of the cell wall and the cell membrane, which controls the permeation of antibiotics into bacterial cells. Furthermore, to inhibit the enzyme systems, antibiotic molecules must penetrate layers of the cell envelope unrelated to the specific inhibitory activity of the antibiotic. Although cell walls vary widely, ranging from the chemically simple walls of some gram-positive species to the very complex multilayered walls of smooth strains of gram-negative bacteria, the cytoplasmic membrane has a relatively consistent chemical composition and molecular structure [1-4].

The mechanisms by which many antibiotics gain access to their site of action within the target cell are not well known. The biological mechanisms involved in antibiotic resistance of bacterial cells could be changes in the permeability of the cell envelope, in the accessibility of specific targets, or in the metabolic activity [5]. The resistance to many important antibiotics appears to be due to a failure to build up an adequate concentration of the antibiotic within the bacterial cell [6].

The use of cell wall-defective or cell wall-deficient bacterial cells showed that changes in susceptibility to an antibiotic were not always due to removal of the cell wall or other barriers to transport. In stable L-forms there may be other modifications besides the loss of the cell wall. The relationship of such modifications to changes in the patterns of susceptibility to antibiotics present a very useful tool for studies of mechanisms of antibiotic resistance [7]. Antibiotic-resistant L-form strains provide a particularly interesting model for such a study.

II. STUDIES ON THE SUSCEPTIBILITY OF L-FORMS TO ANTIBIOTICS

In the past 30 years, numerous studies of antibiotic susceptibility of L-forms and other wall-defective bacterial cells have been reported. In 1952 Tulasne and Minck [8] showed the resistance of *Proteus* L-forms to penicillin and increased susceptibility to streptomycin, chloramphenicol, and tetracyclines. In 1958, Ward et al. [9] compared the antibiotic susceptibility of L-form and *Mycoplasma* strains. Since then, many workers have reported that L-forms are not susceptible to β-lactams and other drugs acting on cell wall synthesis; they have also reported increased susceptibility of the L-forms to antibiotics acting on metabolic processes of cells [10-15]. On the other hand the loss of L-form susceptibility to antibiotics acting on the cytoplasmic membrane has been reported [7,16,17]. Although much work has been performed on the action of antibiotics against wall-less cells [18,19], it is difficult to compare the data obtained with different types of wall-defective or wall-deficient cells variously called spheroplasts, protoplasts, L-variants, and unstable and stable L-forms. These growth forms were, moreover, obtained from many different bacterial strains by the action of several antibacterial agents. Many of the investigators did not describe the criteria used to identify a growth form as the L-state. Also, methodology for testing of antimicrobial activity was not always appropriate. Spheroplasts and protoplasts obtained by lysozyme-EDTA treatment have often been used in such studies [20]. It is known, however, that the inducer also changes the cell metabolism and thus the response of the protoplasmic body or membrane to antimicrobial drugs [21].

Finally, the results of studies of L-form susceptibilities may also have been contradictory because most of these organisms are fragile and may require a long period of adaptation before they are completely stabilized and adapted to growth. The addition of antibiotics during this period may affect the growth of the cells and lead to lysis, even though the same drugs have no effect on adapted wall-deficient cells. Given this background, a short, accurate, and critical summary of antibiotic susceptibilities and their biochemical bases is difficult, but may be supported by our data from the study of stable penicillin-induced L-forms [7]. The antimicrobial products tested in our studies are listed in Table 1 and the microorganisms in Table 2.

In our preliminary assays, the most reproducible results were obtained with trypticase soy broth (TSB) and trypticase soy agar (TSA) supplemented with 10% heat-inactivated horse serum and either 0.3 M sucrose or 1.5% NaCl. Supplemented media were called TSB-L and TSA-L. Bacteria were grown for 18 hr and L-forms for 48 hr. Inocula were standardized to 10^5-10^6 colony-forming units (CFU). Antibiotic susceptibility was measured by the agar dilution and agar diffusion (using bioDiscs, BioMerieux) methods on TSA and TSA-L plates. The agar dilution method could be used when L-form growth was poor and when antibiotics were inactivated enzymatically or by the incubation

Table 1 Antibiotics Used in the Study of the Susceptibility of L-Forms

Inhibitors of cell wall synthesis	β-Lactams: penicillin G, ampicillin, oxacillin, cephalosporins Others: D-cycloserine, ristocetin, bacitracin (Ba), vancomycin (Vm), novobiocin (Nv)
Affecting the function of the cytoplasmic membrane	Polymyxin B (Px), colistin
Inhibitors of nucleic acid synthesis	Actinomycin D, rifampicin (Rf), nalidixic acid (Na)
Inhibitors of protein synthesis (ribosome function)	Tetracyclines: tetracycline (Tc), vibramycin minocycline (Min) Chloramphenicol (Cm) Macrolides and related drugs: erythromycin (Em), oleandomycin (Ol), spiramycin (Spi), lincomycin (Lm), streptogramins (Sg), synergistins, fusidic acid (Fa) Aminoglycosides: streptomycin (Sm), kanamycin (Km), tobramycin (Tm), gentamycin (Gm)

Table 2 Bacterial and L-Form Strains Used in the Studies of Antibiotic Susceptibilities

Bacterial strain			
Species	Resistance markers[a]	Collection L-form strains were derived from	Forms studied[b]
Staphylococcus aureus 209 P(6538 P)	—	Our laboratory, U65 INSERM, Nîmes	B, L, R, Ls
S. aureus BM 3002	Tm Km Sg Cd Fa Nv Rf		B, L, R, Ls
Streptococcus pneumoniae K 23	—	G. Ya. Kagan, Gamaleya Institute (Moscow)	B, Ls
Group A *Streptococcus* G1-8	—	Our laboratory, U65 INSERM, Nîmes	B, L, R, Ls
Group A *Streptococcus* type 49	Tc		B, L, R, Ls
Group B *Streptococcus* BM 6101	Tc Cm Em Lm Sg		B, L, R, Ls
Listeria monocytogenes type 4b	—	S. Madoff, Mass. Gen. Hosp. (Boston)	B, L, R, Ls
Brucella suis 1330 type I	—	Our laboratory, U65 INSERM, Nîmes	B, R, Ls
Neisseria gonorrhoeae	—		B, R, Ls
Salmonella typhimurium LT2	—		B, L, R
Salmonella typhimurium LT2 sm^r	Sm		B, L, R
Proteus vulgaris P 18	—		B, L, Ls
Proteus mirabilis VI	—	E. Schuhmann and J. Gumpert, Inst. of Microbiol. Jena	B, Ls
Escherichia coli B	—		B, Ls

We defined the stabilized L-forms or stable L-forms as those that can be propagated for a long time in the L-form state after withdrawal of the inducing agent.
[a]See Table 1 for symbols.
[b]B, parent bacterium; L, L-form reversible; R, revertant; Ls, stabilized L-form.

conditions. Resistant cells could be selected from a large L-form population. Nevertheless, inoculum size and incubation times greatly affected the results of testing L-form susceptibility.

Resistance to an antibiotic was, therefore, often a qualitative rather than a quantitative judgment and had to be compared every time with the susceptibility of the parent strain and of the control osmotically insensitive L-form strain tested under the same conditions.

In our study, L-forms were universally resistant to β-lactam antibiotics (three penicillins and three cephalosporins). Similar results were obtained with other drugs known to inhibit cell wall synthesis. The values obtained with L-form strains growing in osmotically protective TSA-L media did not differ from those obtained with control strains adapted to growth without osmotic support and in the absence of serum. Thus the possibility of nonspecific inhibition of antibiotic effects by components of the medium was eliminated [22].

The responses of L-forms to antibiotics of other groups indicate the utility of these growth forms in investigating the mechanism of antibiotic action, and the ways in which membranes may be altered. For this reason, the results obtained in our laboratory will be discussed further in the following section.

III. L-FORMS AS MODELS FOR THE STUDY OF ANTIBIOTIC ACTIVITY

A. The Response of L-Forms to Penicillins and Other Inhibitors of Wall Synthesis

1. Penicillins

The interaction of β-lactams with live bacteria remains the focal point of extensive investigations. Until quite recently it seemed to be clear that the synthesis of bacterial cell wall murein was the general target of penicillin action. Since the early 1950s the major focus of biochemical work with penicillin has been the effort to identify a penicillin-sensitive enzyme in the synthesis of bacterial murein. For a long time the morphological effects of penicillin were considered to be consequences of a structural damage to the cell wall, but the biochemical mechanism of penicillin action was more difficult to explain. The insensitivity of L-forms and the changed susceptibility of their revertants to penicillins observed by several authors [7,23,24], was attributed to reduction in the physiological importance of the cell wall target, to some decreased importance of the target enzymatic system, or to metabolic properties that were thought to be impaired in revertants. In 1967 Panos et al. [25] suggested that penicillin-binding sites in streptococcal L-forms are probably distinct from those concerned with cell-wall formation.

2. Penicillin-Binding Proteins

In recent years, studies on the interaction of β-lactams with live bacterial cells showed the existence of multiple, functionally different penicillin targets: penicillin-binding proteins (PBPs), penicillin-sensitive enzymes, and murein hydrolases, were described [26,27]. β-Lactam antibiotics bind to PBPs, integral constituents of bacterial cytoplasmic membranes. In different bacterial species, the PBPs differ in number and molecular size [28]. Suginaka [29] showed with ampicillin-induced stable *Staphylococcus aureus* L-forms that these organisms bound radioactively labeled penicillin. This observation suggests that these stable wall-less cells may possess transpeptidase or lack other enzymes of cell wall synthesis. Martin et al. [30] showed the presence of membrane proteins with the specific ability to bind penicillin in two strains of stable L-forms of *Proteus mirabilis*. On the basis of the PBP pattern of the normal bacteria and that of the corresponding stable L-forms, the authors have suggested that the permanent inability of the L-forms to synthesize a normal peptidoglycan might be related to the hereditary and selective loss of PBP 4 (D-alanyl-D-alanine-cleaving peptidase).

Recently, Rousset et al. [31] confirmed the results obtained by Martin et al. [30] and expanded them by showing that the stable L-form derived from *Proteus vulgaris* P18 has kept the ability of the parent strain to synthesize all of the enzymes known to be involved in peptidoglycan cross-linking and its further maturation during the bacterial life cycle. However, during growth the stable L-forms secrete the highly penicillin-sensitive, D'D-carboxypeptidase-transpeptidase penicillin-binding protein PBP 4 (which in normal bacteria is located in the periplasmic region (see Chapter 6).

3. Other Inhibitors of Wall Synthesis

The biochemical modes of action of other inhibitors of peptidoglycan synthesis (e.g., D-cycloserine, ristocetin, bacitracin, and vancomycin) are poorly understood [1,2]. Neither D-cycloserine nor ristocetin had any effect on the growth of L-forms [7]. Bacitracin combines with the carrier molecules in the cell membrane and induces L-forms [32]. Further studies on protoplasts and L-forms with bacitracin have not elucidated the extent of damage by this antibiotic to the cytoplasmic membrane [7,10,32]. Storm and Strominger [33] found that bacitracin may induce changes in the membrane permeability. Controversial data have also been obtained with ristocetin and vancomycin [34,35].

Perkins and Nieto [36] showed that particular membrane systems that synthesize peptidoglycan were inhibited by vancomycin. Watanakunakorn [37] induced *S. aureus* L-forms using vancomycin and attributed the low-growth yield of L-forms to the additional effects of this antibiotic on the cytoplasmic membrane. Similar results were obtained with vancomycin-induced L-forms of

Neisseria gonorrhoeae [38]. In our recent study with a penicillinase-producing *S. aureus* strain, vancomycin was used with success as an L-form inducer. However, the L-form colonies obtained with vancomycin could not be propagated in the presence of this antibiotic for more than eight to ten transfers. This suggests that high concentrations of vancomycin affect the fragile L-form growth during the stabilization period; vancomycin had no effect against stabilized L-forms of the same *S. aureus* strain that was cultured in parallel on oxacillin-containing medium (J. Schmitt-Slomska, unpublished data).

Novobiocin also has an action on cell wall synthesis that has not been elucidated [39]. In our studies, the drug was active against all stable L-forms, no matter whether they were derived from susceptible gram-positive cocci or from novobiocin-resistant gram-negative bacilli, confirming that it acts specifically on a cellular compartment other than the cell wall [7]. Increase of membrane permeability and effects on RNA synthesis have been proposed as biochemical mechanisms [40]. Slabyj and Panos [41] reported that the stable L-forms of *Streptococcus pyogenes* growing in the presence of novobiocin contained only 17% of teichoic acid found in control cells. Concentrations of novobiocin greater than 1000 μg/ml were used by Cherepova et al. [42] to induce L-forms of *Erysipelothrix rhusiopathiae*. When lower concentrations of the antibiotic were employed structural alterations of bacterial envelope were observed.

Therefore, the targets of some antibiotics thus lie within the cell envelope, as in the case of β-lactams and novobiocin, which interfere with peptidoglycan synthesis and membrane metabolism. Envelope damage may also be produced by other antibiotics, such as polymyxins, that attack both envelope membranes and often render wall-defective or wall-deficient cells more susceptible to penetration by additional molecules.

B. The Response of L-Forms to Antibiotics Affecting Function of the Cytoplasmic Membrane

1. Polymyxins

According to most of the previous studies on polymyxin activity, the susceptibility of biological membranes may depend on whether this antibiotic penetrates its target within the cytoplasmic membrane [1,2]. Gram-positive bacteria and their L-forms are unaffected by polymyxin, whereas minimum inhibitory concentrations (MICs) for gram-negative bacteria range from 0.05 μg/ml to 1000 μg/ml (Table 3). It has been reported that the cell wall as a barrier could be responsible for the resistance of some gram-negative bacilli [5,6] to polymyxins. The mechanism of polymyxin activity has been intensively studied in the past 25 years [43–45]. It acts on the bacterial membrane and interacts with membrane phospholipids. The morphological changes that it induced in the cytoplasm and outer membrane of bacterial cells were also described [46].

The use of spheroplasts and stable L-forms has helped to clarify the mechanism of polymyxin resistance. A direct demonstration of polymyxin action at the cell surface, both in bacterial and spheroplast-type cells of *Escherichia coli*, was shown by Koike et al. [47].

In 1969 Teuber [48] found increased susceptibility to polymyxin in L-forms derived from a resistant *P. mirabilis* strain and suggested that the cell wall barrier could be responsible for polymyxin resistance in *Proteus* species. This observation was confirmed in our study [7]. Nevertheless, the polymyxin-resistant L-form variants could be selected from polymyxin-susceptible L-form populations of *P. mirabilis* and *E. coli* strains (Fig. 1).

Several authors reported that some wall-less bacterial cells derived from gram-negative bacteria may retain or acquire resistance to polymyxin [7,16,17,49,50].

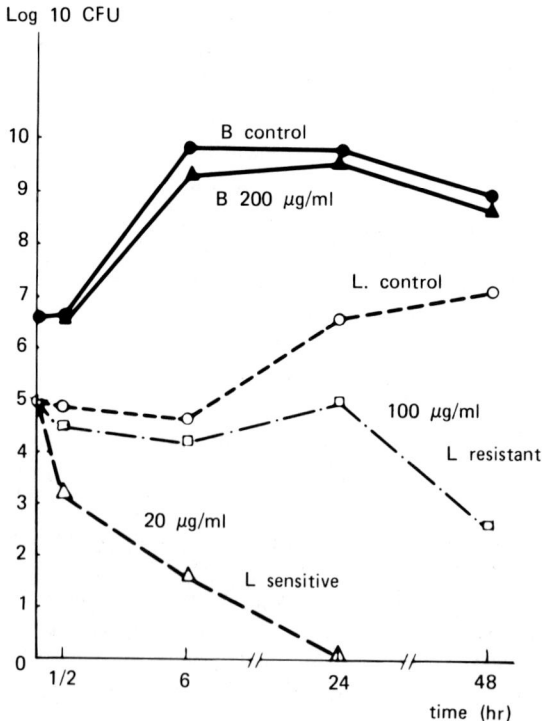

Figure 1 Growth of *P. mirabilis* VI and its L-forms in the presence of different concentrations of polymyxin B. B, Bacteria; L, L-forms; control, growth in the absence of polymyxin in culture broth; 20, 100, and 200 μg/ml concentration of polymyxin/ml of broth; L-sensitive, L-form population susceptible to polymyxin; L-resistant, selected L-form polymyxin-resistant mutants.

Table 3 Resistance of Bacteria and L-Forms to Polymyxins

Strains	Minimum inhibitory concentration (µg/ml)			
	Polymyxin B		Colistin	
	Bacteria	L-forms	Bacteria	L-forms
S. aureus 209 P	100[a]	100	100	100
Group A Streptococcus	100	100	100	100
L. monocytogenes	100	100	100	100
N. gonorrhoeae	100	6.25	100	6.25
S. typhimurium	0.4	0.1	0.8	0.2
E. coli B	0.4	0.1 (6.25[b])	0.2	0.1 (6.25[b])
P. vulgaris P 18	100	3.12	100	6.25
P. mirabilis VI	100	3.12 (50[b])	100	3.12 (25[b])

[a]The highest concentration used in the study.
[b]Selected L-form-resistant variants.

These findings suggested that the resistance to polymyxin is not due merely to the cell wall barrier of gram-negative bacteria. In our laboratory, comparative structural and biochemical studies on the polymyxin resistance in stable L-forms selected from the usual and predominant susceptible L-forms of *P. mirabilis* VI and *E. coli* B strains were undertaken. The electron microscopy study of Louis and Schmitt-Slomska [51] showed marked changes of the cytoplasmic membrane in polymyxin-resistant L-forms growing in the presence of a high concentration of drug (Fig. 2). Freeze-etching analysis confirmed the membrane modifications showing an unusual distribution of the membrane-associated particles on the cytoplasmic face of the membrane (Fig. 3). These findings confirmed that a purely mechanical explanation of resistance to polymyxin, invoking just the barrier effect of the cell wall is not sufficient. Kozdroj et al. [52] further studied this phenomenon. The activity and substructural localization of polymyxin B in *P. mirabilis* VI and *E. coli* B bacteria and L-forms were investigated using polymyxin coupled to dansyl chloride-D (PXD), which is fluorescent in UV light as described by Newton [53]. Fractionation of the cells and subsequent gradient centrifugations confirmed that the fluorescence was bound exclusively to the membrane fractions of the bacteria and the L-forms. The concentration of PXD was higher in polymyxin-susceptible *E. coli* bacterial and L-form cells than in *P. mirabilis* cells resistant to polymyxin. The acrylamide-gel electrophoresis of L-forms labeled with PXD confirmed that the fluorescence was protein bound. The comparative study of the phospholipid

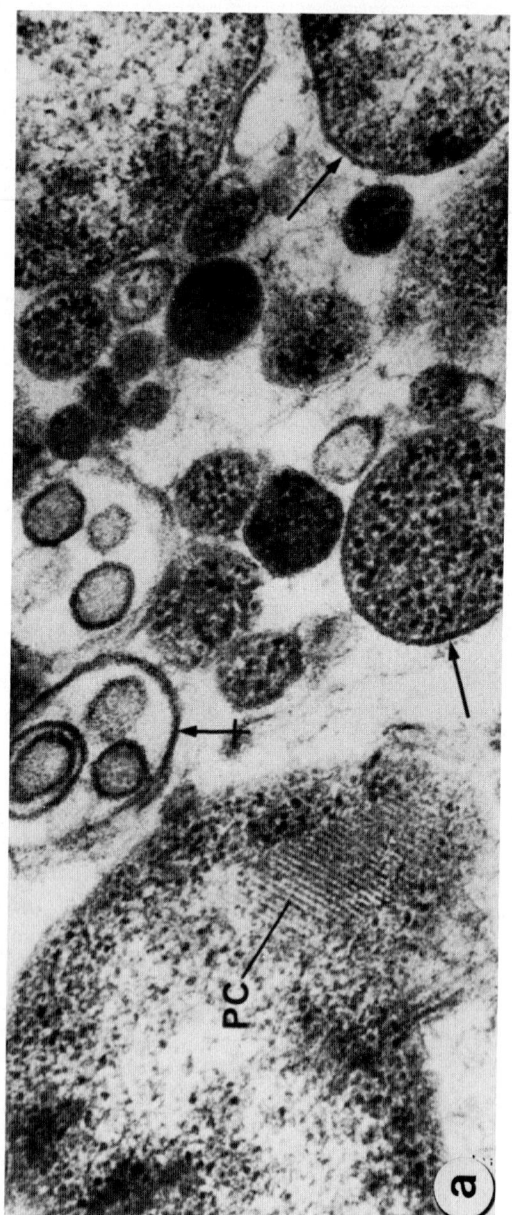

Figure 2 Electron microscopy study of *P. mirabilis* VI stable L-forms (C. Louis and J. Schmitt-Slomska (1977). Effect of polymyxin B on the ultrastructure of the stable *Proteus mirabilis* L-forms, in *Spheroplasts, Protoplasts and L-forms of Bacteria* (J. Roux, ed.), Ed. INSERM, vol. 64, Paris, pp. 197–210, with permission.

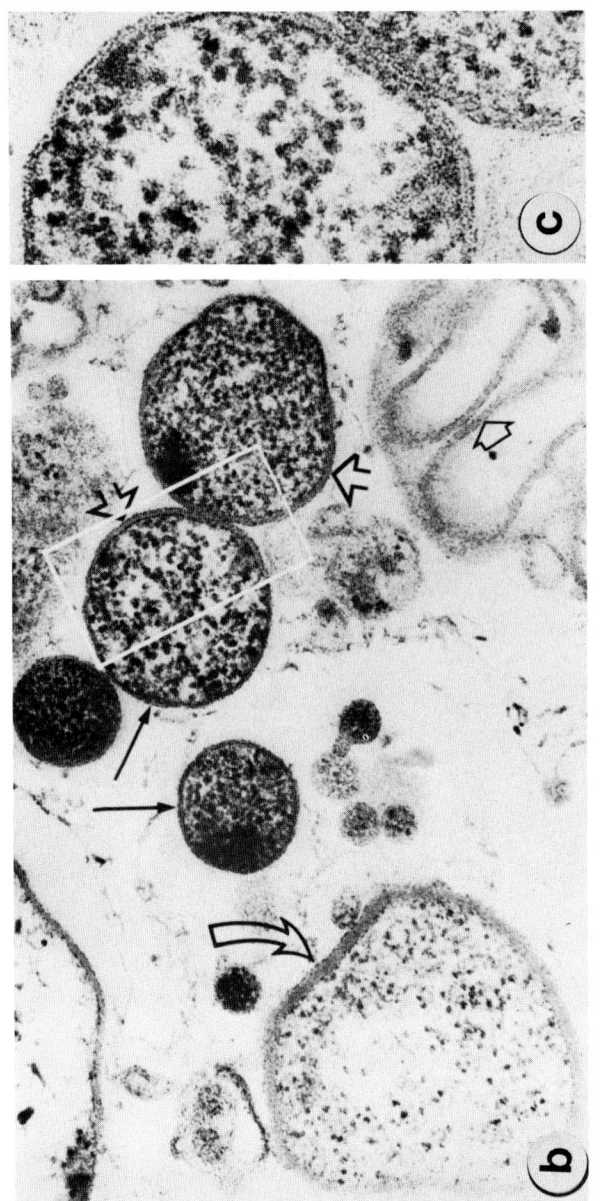

(a) Polymyxin-susceptible L-forms. Ultrathin section of L-form colony growth on medium without antibiotics. The L-forms are bounded only by one unit membrane (→). They show an apparently normal ultrastructure; (→) tubules; (*) dense bodies. Magnification ×80,000. (b–c) Polymyxin-resistant L-forms growing in the presence of high doses of polymyxin (100 μg/ml). L-form bodies present a partially transformed membrane, showing swelling. (⇦) Moderate thickening; (⇨) important thickening; (⇦) extracellular thickened membranes. (d and e, ×120,000.)

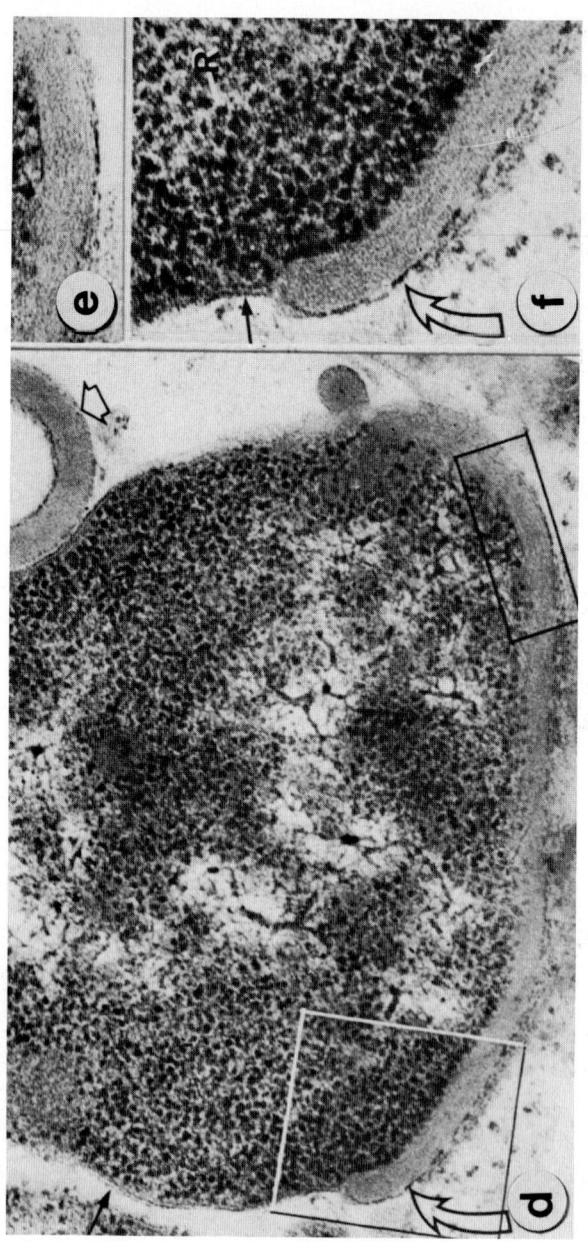

Figure 2 (Continued)

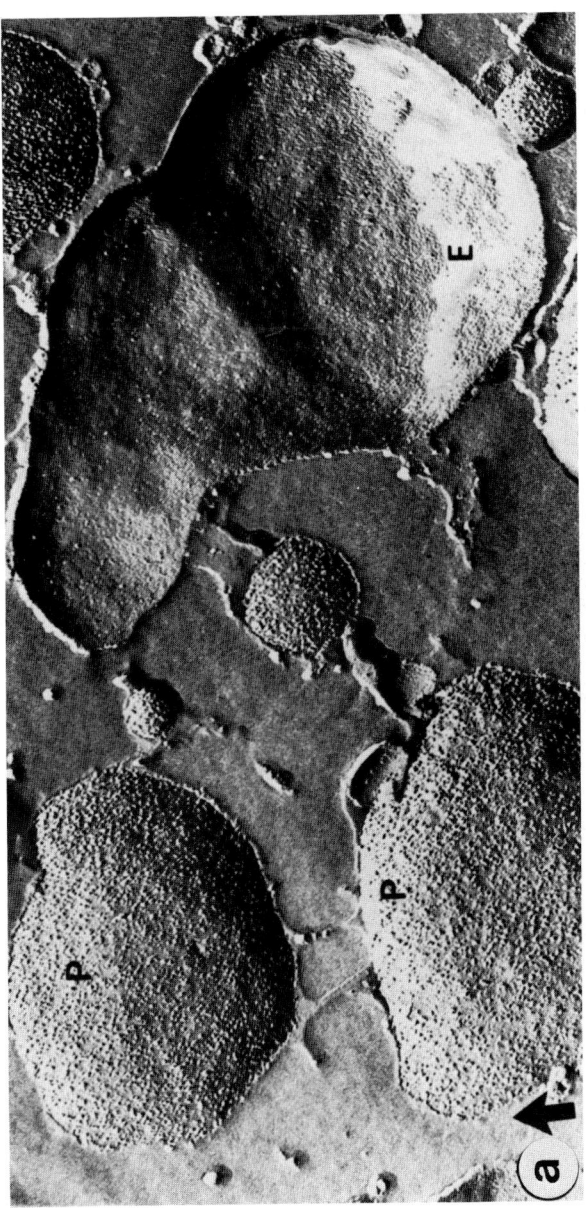

Figure 3 Freeze-etching of L-colonies of *P. mirabilis* VI on solid medium. (P) "Plasmic" face of cleavage of the cytoplasmic membrane; (E) "external" face of cleavage of the plasma membrane. (∗) Patch (particle-less area); (➔) direction of the shadowing. (*a*) Polymyxin-resistant L-forms growing without antibiotics (control). Magnification ×64,000. (*b*) As (*a*) but in presence of 100 μg/ml of polymyxin. Particleless zone (patch ∗), and depressions (⇌) corresponding to the thickened part of the membranes on the sections. Magnification ×90,000. (*c*) As (*b*), particle-less zone showing remnants of the intermediate substance. (⇧) Depressions are seen on the P- and E-faces. Magnification ×50,000. (From Ref. 51 with permission.)

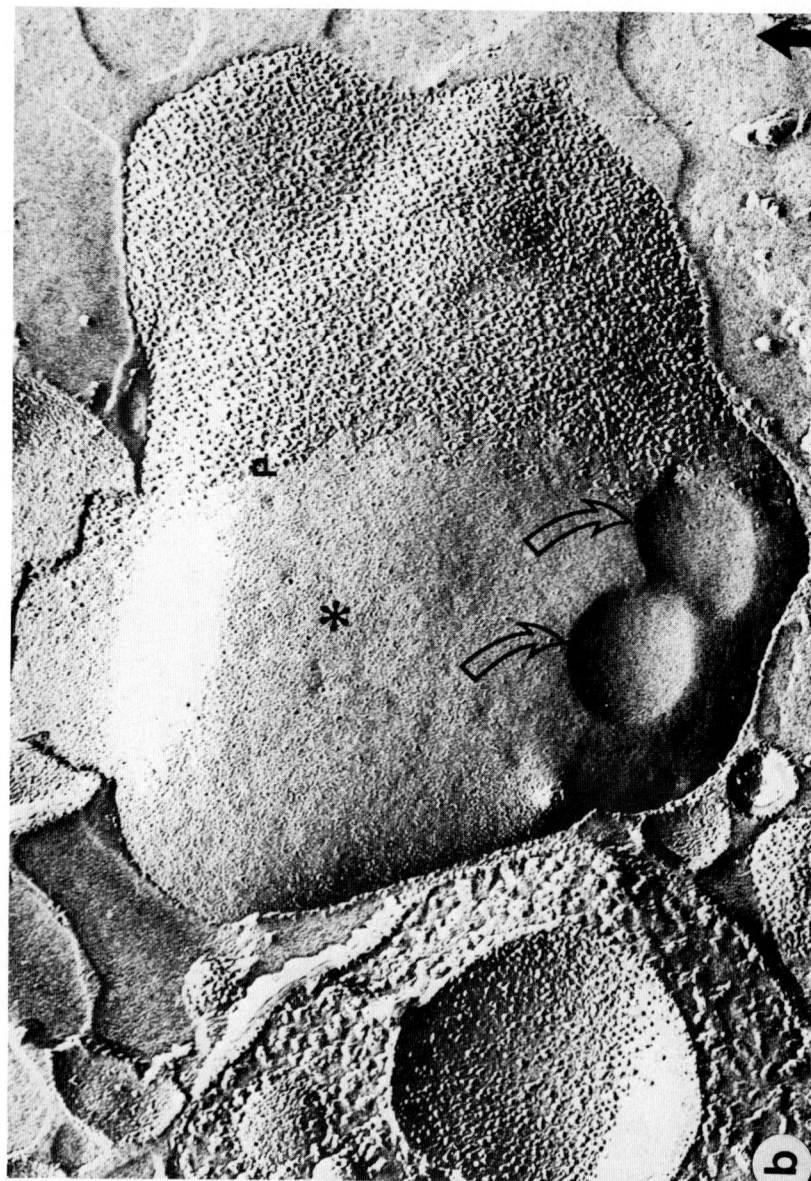

Figure 3 (Continued)

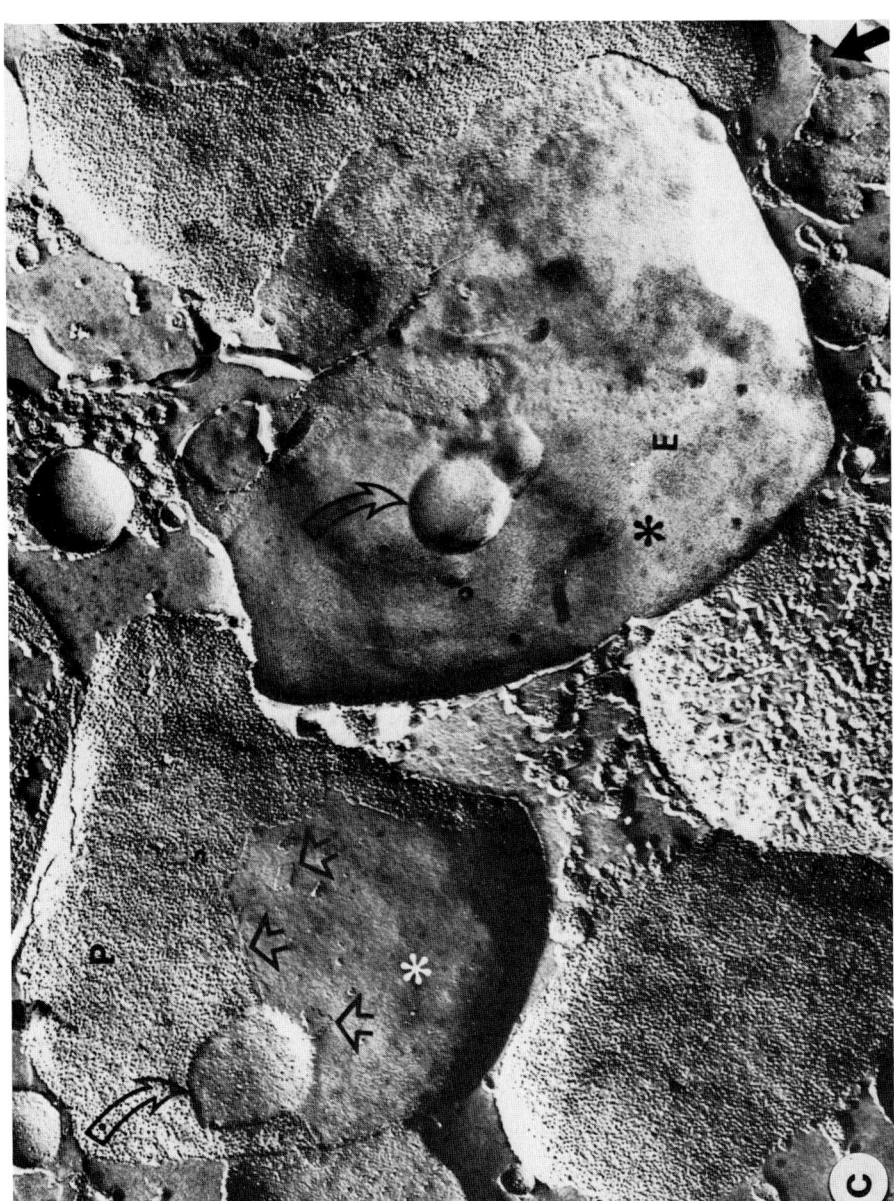

Figure 3 (Continued)

composition of polymyxin-resistant *P. mirabilis* VI bacteria and derived polymyxin-suscepitibile L-forms showed marked changes in the ratios of membrane phospholipids, but did not account for the mechanism of resistance to polymyxin [54].

These results indicate that membrane proteins play a role in the activity of polymyxin on the metabolism of the bacterial cell. More detailed chemical investigations are necessary to determine the precise targets of polymyxin activity within the cytoplasmic membrane and the mechanism of bacterial resistance to this group of antibiotics. The use of polymyxin-resistant wall-less cells may be helpful in such studies. Finally, L-forms were also used by Montgomerie et al. [55] to study the mechanism of synergism of polymyxin and sulfonamides.

2. Polyene Macrolide Antibiotics

Polyenes, such as nystatin, filipin, amphotericin, and others, produce lethal alterations in the permeability of sterol-containing cytoplasmic membranes. These antibiotics are active against yeasts, fungi, and other eukaryotic cells, but are usually inactive against bacteria [56]. The resistance of bacteria to polyene antibiotics is generally attributed to the absence of sterols in their membrane. Studies of Haupt et al. [57] on the action of these antibiotics on normal cells and wall-less stable L-forms of *E. coli* showed that although no inhibition of the normal bacteria was detected, the growth of L-forms was inhibited by all of the polyenes tested (12 drugs). Moreover, it has been shown that differences in sterol content do not account for differences in susceptibility of normal and L-form cells. From these results it was concluded that the cell wall of the normal cells functions as a barrier to polyene antibiotics.

The use of L-forms thus has increased knowledge of the mechanism of resistance of some microorganisms to antibiotics that act on the cytoplasmic membrane. Moreover, the study of response of microbial cells to polyene antibiotics may be helpful for elucidating the structure and the function of cell membranes.

C. The Response of L-Forms to Inhibitors of Nucleic Acid Synthesis

Among inhibitors of DNA synthesis, actinomycin D is the best-known and most widely used antibiotic [1]. The differences in susceptibility to actinomycin D between different types of cells probably arise mainly through differences in permeability. Ehrenfeld and Koch [58] showed that the increased permeability of *E. coli* spheroplasts rendered them susceptible to actinomycin D, which did not enter the intact bacteria. Similar observations have been reported by others [59,60] and confirmed in our study with L-forms of gram-negative bacteria.

Rifampicin, a semisynthetic derivative of rifamycin B, at low concentrations, inhibits the growth of gram-positive bacteria and *Mycobacterium tuberculosis*.

In intact bacteria it selectively inhibits RNA synthesis [1,2]. We found that the stable L-forms derived either from rifampicin-susceptible coccal strains or from rifampicin-resistant gram-negative bacilli were susceptible to this antibiotic.

Nalidixic acid, another inhibitor of nucleic acid synthesis, was effective against gram-negative bacterial and L-form cells while L-forms of gram-positive cocci remained resistant (J. Schmitt-Slomska and G. Negre, unpublished data).

D. The Response of L-Forms to Antibiotics Inhibiting Protein Synthesis

Previous studies have shown that L-forms are at least as susceptible to tetracyclines, macrolides, and aminoglycosides as are bacterial cells [11-14,35,61,62]. Kagan [12] related this phenomenon to the ease of antibiotic penetration into the L-form body as a consequence of the removal of the cell wall barrier. There were, however, certain exceptions, where the bacterial form was more susceptible than the L-forms [14]. Recently, Yamamoto and Homma [17] have shown that L-forms of *Pseudomonas aeruginosa* are more resistant than their parent forms to gentamicin, streptomycin, and dibekacin, and more susceptible to tetracycline, chloramphenicol, and macrolides.

In our study, the tetracyclines, the macrolides and related antibiotic molecules showed at least as strong activity against L-forms as against parent bacterial antibiotic-susceptible or antibiotic-resistant strains (Fig. 4). The L-forms derived from the tetracycline-resistant Group A *Streptococcus* type 49 were found to be susceptible to the drug. Similarly, increased antibiotic-susceptibility was observed with the L-forms derived from gram-negative bacteria resistant to fusidic acid. In contrast, streptomycin was more effective against the streptococci than against their L-forms (Fig. 4). The mechanism by which L-forms become more resistant than their parent forms to aminoglycoside-group antibiotics was studied by Yamamoto and Homma [17] by investigation of the uptake of tritiated dibekacin by L-forms of *P. aeruginosa*. The uptake of antibiotic into the L-form was approximately 40% of the total uptake into its parent strain.

1. Resistance to Tetracycline in the L-State

A tetracycline-susceptible strain of *Listeria monocytogenes* type 4^b was converted to the stable L-state by penicillin (S. Madoff). The tetracycline-resistant (Tc-r) L-form variants were then selected from a predominantly tetracycline-susceptible (Tc-s) L-form population on media containing penicillin and increasing concentrations of tetracycline. The relationship of Tc-r L-forms to the parent listeria strain was confirmed biochemically by immunofluorescence and by polyacrylamide gel electrophoresis. Scanning and transmission electron microscopy showed the typical L-form structure and the complete lack of wall

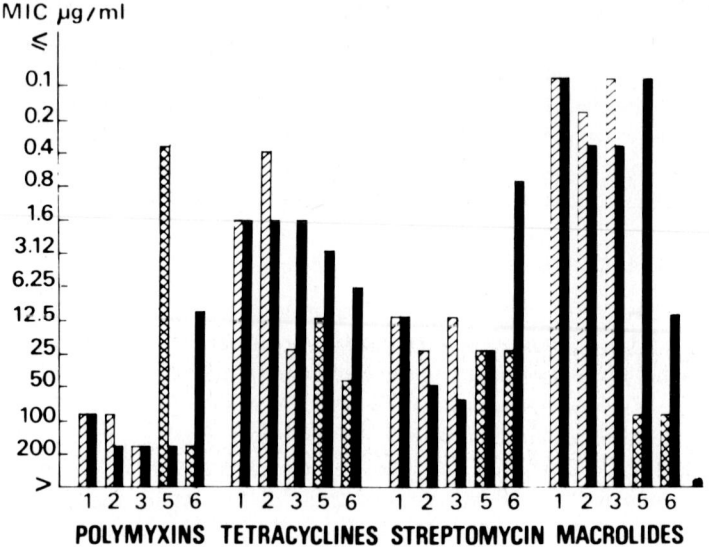

Figure 4 Susceptibility of parent bacteria and their stable L-forms to polymyxins and antibiotics inhibiting protein synthesis. (MIC μg/ml) Minimal inhibitory concentration of antibiotic in agar medium. 1. *S. aureus* 209P; 2. *Str.* A G1-8; 3. *Str.* A 49; 5. *E. coli* B; 6. *P. mir.* VI. Bacteria G−, ▨▨▨ ; L-forms, ▬ ; Bacteria G+, ▧▧▧ .

in both L-form strains. The level of tritiated tetracycline uptake was lower in tetracycline resistant than in susceptible cells. These studies demonstrated that tetracycline resistance can develop in the absence of bacterial cell wall. The preliminary studies did not show the presence of plasmid DNA in Tc-r L-forms. It is probable that the resistance of these variants is the result of multistep chromosomal mutations [63].

Although the molecular basis of tetracycline resistance has been actively explored, relatively little is known about the mechanism of tetracycline accumulation in bacterial cells [64]. Franklin [65] reported that acquisition of tetracycline resistance in *E. coli* was accompanied by an alteration of tetracycline uptake. Penicillin-induced *E. coli* spheroplasts accumulated about 30% less tetracycline than intact bacteria. The development of tetracycline resistance in gram-positive bacteria may depend, at least in part, upon a modification of cell envelope permeability [64,66]. In L-forms of gram-positive bacteria, the changes in the structure of membrane might be responsible for resistance to tetracyclines. Panos et al. [67,68] demonstrated quantitative protein differences in the membrane of *Streptococcus pyogenes* and its stabilized L-form. Gilpin et al.

[69] showed that conversion of *Bacillus subtilis* to an L-form also resulted in the redistribution of membrane proteins. Chopra and Howe [64] concluded "the principal difficulty in establishing the function of any of the proteins associated with mechanism of tetracycline resistance stems from lack of detailed knowledge of the mechanisms of tetracycline accumulation by sensitive bacteria." The study of differences in tetracycline susceptibility of L-forms may possibly serve as a model for understanding some phases of metabolism in whole bacterial cells.

2. Resistance to Streptomycin

The effect of the aminoglycoside group of antibiotics on L-forms is more difficult to interpret. Although L-forms derived from gentamicin- or kanamycin-susceptible parent strains were always susceptible to these antibiotics, this relationship was not always true for streptomycin. In 1958, Lederberg and St. Clair [70] reported the loss of streptomycin-resistance in penicillin-induced spheroplasts of *E. coli*. In contrast, Hewitt et al. [71] found that spheroplasting had no effect on the resistance to streptomycin (MIC greater than 100 µg/ml) in enterococcal mutant strains. In our study, the L-form resistance to streptomycin and related aminoglycosides was found to be dependent on the level of resistance of the parental bacterium. The L-forms of the streptomycin-resistant (MIC greater than or equal to 1000 µg/ml) *Salmonella typhimurium* LT2 mutant strain remained resistant. Moreover, similar MIC values obtained on penicillin-containing and penicillin-free agar confirmed the previous data of Hewitt et al. [72] that the synergistic effect of penicillin and streptomycin may apply only to the parent strain.

It has been shown that the spheroplasts of streptomycin-dependent parent strains were genetically stable [73]. In contrast, antibiotic resistance of a bacterium may be lost upon conversion to the L-state. In 1959 Schoenfeld [23] demonstrated that L-form revertants often differed from the original bacterium. Loss of resistance to several antibiotics (chloramphenicol, tetracycline, erythromycin) was found in *S. aureus* after two to 12 passages as L-forms before reversion; however, the resistance to streptomycin and tyrothrycin was still present up to 19 passages. When resistance was lost, the trait remained in subsequent transfers.

It is known that the high level of resistance to antibiotics acting on protein synthesis generally results from chromosomal mutation, while moderate resistance is mediated by R plasmids. All of these observations on changes of susceptibility patterns in the L-form state have led us to study the genetic basis of this phenomenon in L-forms derived from antibiotic-resistant strains.

IV. CHROMOSOMAL AND PLASMID-MEDIATED ANTIBIOTIC RESISTANCE IN L-FORMS

The marked loss of resistance to antibiotics in the L-state of bacteria has been reported, but the genetic nature of the phenomenon is poorly understood. All the essential genetic information in bacteria is located on the chromosome, which is able to replicate. The bacteria may also contain other autonomous replicons called plasmids [74]. Antibiotic resistance may be encoded by chromosomal and plasmid genes (R plasmids). In 1963 Jacob et al [75] suggested that the cell wall is involved in plasmid maintenance. They postulated that all autonomous replicons are permanently attached to the inner surface of the cell membrane and that this attachment is essential for replication and partition. In 1965, Kawakami and Landman [76] reported that coordinated distribution of episomes (plasmids) with the chromosome persisted in the L-state.

Our approach to the genetic problem of the loss of resistance in the L-state was to study the antibiotype and plasmid DNA content in L-forms obtained from multiresistant bacterial strains carrying chromosomal and plasmid genes coding for resistance characters. A series of findings involving penicillin induced L-forms of Group B *Streptococcus* and *Staphylococcus aureus* strains showed that the loss of plasmid-mediated antibiotic resistance was associated with the simultaneous loss of extrachromosomal DNA in the stabilized L-forms [77,78]. Penicillin-induced L-forms were derived from Group B *Streptococcus* strain BM 6101, serotype II (kindly supplied by T. Horodniceanu). The parent strain is resistant to tetracycline (Tc), chloramphenicol (Cm), erythromycin and other macrolides, lincosamins, and streptogramins (MLS). Genetic and physical studies of this strain (previously referred to as strain B96) allowed the isolation and characterization of two 20-Mdal plasmids (RIP 500 and RIP 501) coding for Tc and Cm-MLS resistance, respectively [77].

Agar dilution MICs of the parent strain and its derived L-forms are shown in Table 4. Both the unstable and the stable L-forms were resistant to penicillin and other inhibitors of cell wall synthesis. Variations in their antibiotic susceptibility were observed according to the stability of the L-forms. While the unstable L-forms and their revertants showed the same phenotypic pattern of resistance to non-β-lactam antibiotics as their parent bacteria, the stable L-forms had lost the resistance characters carried by the plasmid genes. The concurrent change from an unstable to a stable L-form state with the loss of antibiotic resistance, reproduced in three successive independent attempts, suggested a change in plasmid content. A band of extrachromosomal DNA demonstrable in the parent strain DNA by equilibrium centrifugation was not present in the stable L-forms (Fig. 5). Thus, the penicillin induction of a Group B *Streptococcus* strain into cell wall-deficient forms was associated with the loss of the resistance characters carried by the "large" plasmids (greater than or equal to 20 kb) and with the loss of plasmid DNA [78,79].

Table 4 Antibiotic Susceptibility Patterns of Group B *Streptococcus* BM 6101 Strain[a] and its L-Forms

Strains		Pen (U/ml)	Tc (µg/ml)	Cm (µg/ml)	Em (µg/ml)	Lm (µg/ml)
			\multicolumn{4}{c}{MIC (agar dilution method)}			
Parent bacterium BM 6101		0.8	50	25	1000	250
Unstable L-forms BM 6101		1000	25	25	50	125
Revertants BM 6101		1.6	25	25	500	125
Stable L-forms BM 6101		1000	0.4	0.4	0.2	0.4
Control:	Bacteria	0.006	0.4	0.2	0.2	0.2
Group A *Streptococcus* G1-8	L-forms	1000	0.2	0.2	0.1	0.2

[a] BM 6101, parental strain harboring R plasmids RIP 500 (Tc, tetracycline), and RIP 501 (Cm, chloramphenicol; Em, erythromycin; Lm, lincomycin); Pen, penicillin G used as control of L-form growth.

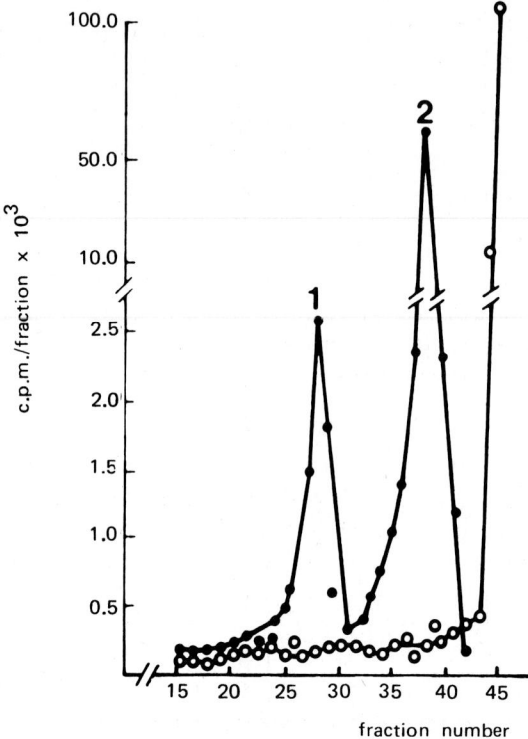

Pic 1: RIP 500 + RIP 501

Figure 5 Disappearance of extrachromosomal DNA in the stable L-forms derived from the Group B *Streptococcus* BM 6101 carrying R plasmids strain. Parent strains (●) and its stable L-forms (○) were labeled with 5 and 8 µg Ci/ml of [^{3}H]methyl thymidine (42 mCi/mM), respectively, and lysed. (J. Schmitt-Slomska, R. Caravano, and N. El-Solh, 1979. Loss of plasmid-mediated resistance after conversion of a Group B *Streptococcus* strain to a stable cell wall deficient variant. *Ann. Microbiol. (Inst. Pasteur)* 130 A:23-27, with permission.)

Novick et al. [80] reported the plasmid curing effect observed during the regeneration of protoplasts produced by the action of lysostaphin on *S. aureus* strains carrying R plasmids. Protoplast formation and regeneration result in the curing of small plasmids (less than or equal to 5 kb) but not of larger ones (greater than or equal to 20 kb). According to these authors, the plasmid elimination could have occurred during the several protoplast divisions before cell wall regeneration was completed, and was due to a disruption of the plasmid partition system as a consequence of removal of the cell wall.

We approached the problem by studying the antibiotypes and plasmid DNA content of L-forms induced by β-lactams from multiresistant *S. aureus* strains carrying both large and small plasmids and chromosomal resistance genes [81]. The parent strains and their derived L-forms were characterized by biological methods and by analysis of DNA [78,82].

The unstable and stable L-forms had classical morphology (Fig. 6). Comparative biological studies of revertants and stable L-forms showed their reduced enzymatic activities and loss of phage susceptibility. Plasmid-encoded drug resistance was also different. The conversion into stable L-forms was always associated with the loss of all extrachromosomal DNA species harbored by the parent strains. In contrast, the resistance characters that were known to be encoded by chromosomal genes were kept both in revertants and in the stable L-form strains.

The clones of stable L-forms in which the plasmid resistance genes had translocated to the chromosome were selected on tobramycin (Fig. 7). Thus, the conversion with β-lactam antibiotics into stable L-forms allowed us to isolate L2-BM3002 carrying Tm-resistance genes on the chromosome [79,82]. The maintenance of resistance characters can provide indirect evidence of their location on the chromosome, even those arising from translocation of plasmid DNA in the stable L-forms.

These data (confirmed by N. El Solh and J. Schmitt-Slomska with another *S. aureus* multiresistant strain [82], suggest that defects in plasmid maintenance in stable L-forms may also be attributed to fundamental changes in the attachment of extrachromosomal DNA to cell membrane. Such attachment, which seems to be involved in the replication/equipartition process of new DNA molecules in daughter cells, might be located on mesosomes. They have never been found in stable L-forms [83-85]. This hypothesis needs further study.

The persistence of chromosomal antibiotic resistance markers in the stable L-forms of *S. aureus* confirms that a chromosome-membrane association like that of the parent strain is retained. The DNA-sequences, DNA-membrane complex, and the involvement of the "rigid" cell wall in DNA replication events have been intensively studied in the past 2 decades. Protoplasts and stable L-forms were often used as models for such studies [86-94].

In conclusion, the wall-defective and -deficient forms derived from bacteria with genetic markers are a useful tool not only in the molecular study of antibiotic resistance but also for further studies on membrane-DNA association and DNA distribution. In 1969 Luria [95] pointed out that the interactions of plasmids with bacterial mutants deficient in cell envelope components have provided much needed experimental evidence of this more widely accepted view.

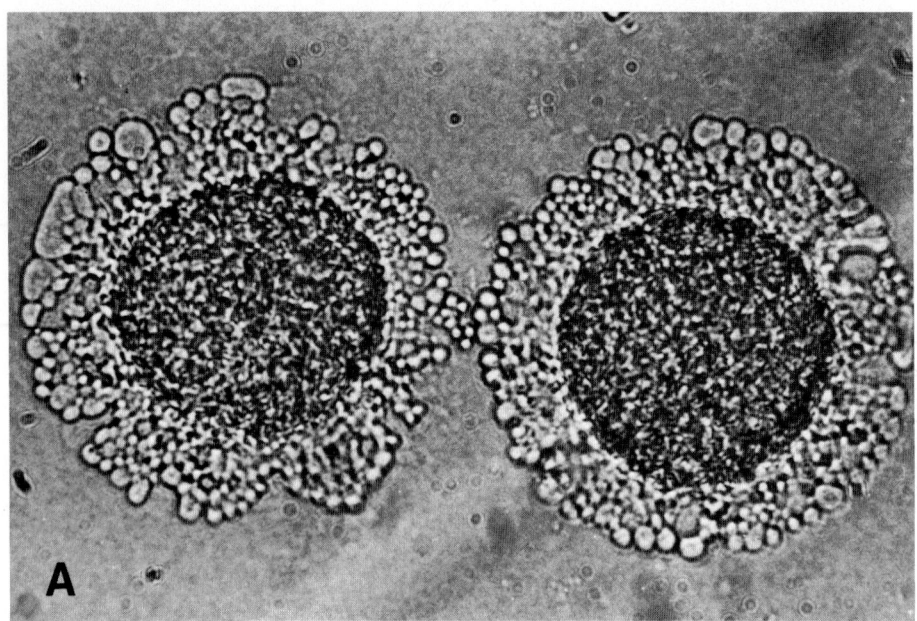

Figure 6 L-forms of *S. aureus* obtained from 10th transfer on penicillin-agar (unstable L-forms). (*A*) Typical aspect of L-form colonies (×400). (*B*) Electron micrograph (×69,000) shows variability in size and shape typical of L-type organisms [102], absence of cell wall. The stable L-forms show the same morphology. [Electron micrograph (*B*) courtesy of Roger M. Cole, NIH, Bethesda, Maryland.]

The curing of antibiotic resistance with penicillin was observed by Lacey and Chopra [96] and is confirmed in our studies [78,79,82].

V. CONCLUDING REMARKS

The wall-deficient bacteria may serve as models for the study of some attributes of the parental bacteria. Studies of responses of L-forms to antibiotics indicate the increasing usefulness of these forms in investigating the mechanisms of antibiotic activity. Moreover, such studies may provide a better understanding of: (1) bacterial cell wall biosynthesis; (2) ways in which membranes may be altered, with associated changes in function; (3) loss (or gain) of DNA-encoded information; (4) genetic location of genes specifying resistance to antibiotics; and (5) membrane-DNA association. Regeneration of protoplasts obtained with β-lactam antibiotics or selection of L-forms may be proposed as a way to cure bacterial cells of plasmids of different sizes.

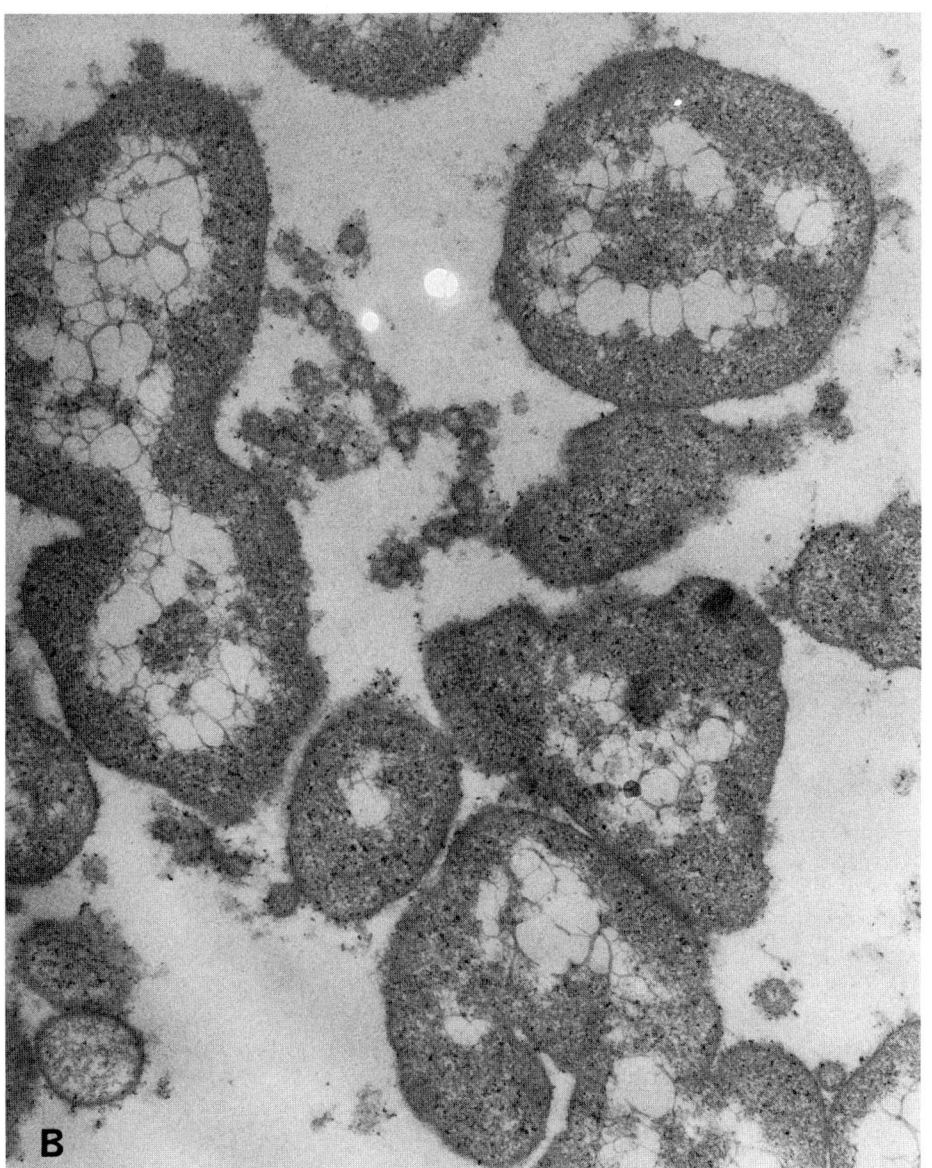

However, findings derived from different wall-deficient cell models must be interpreted cautiously. There is increasing evidence that wall-less cells obtained with penicillin differ completely from those obtained with lysozyme alone or by lysozyme-EDTA treatment [97]. Lysozyme hydrolyzes a specific structural linkage within the cell wall's rigid layer, which consequently is solubilized.

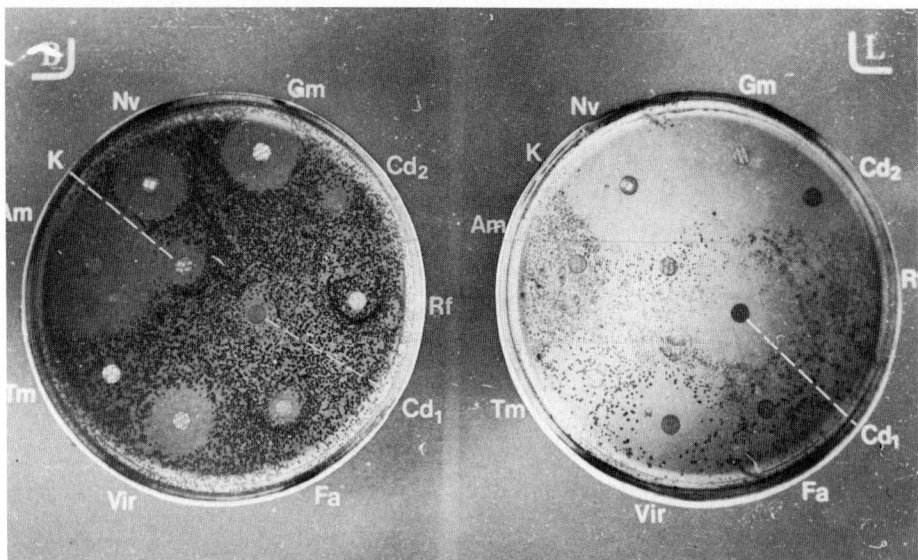

Figure 7 Selection of Tm resistant L-form mutants (L2) from L-form (L1) population of *S. aureus* BM 3002 strain. (*B*) Parent bacterium resistant to (a) virginiamycin (Vir), tobramycin (Tm), kanamycin (K), and cadmium salts (two concentrations: Cd1 and Cd2), all plasmid-encoded resistance characters; (b) rifampicin (Rf), novobiocin (Nv), and fusidic acid (Fa)–chromosomal resistance. Susceptible to ampicillin (Am) strain. (*L*) L-forms are resistant to Am, Rf, and Fa; they show increased susceptibility to Nv, Gm, Vir, Cd, Tm, and K, but Tm- and K-resistant mutants (L2) appeared as satellite colonies around tobramycin and kanamycin disks.

Unlike lysozyme, penicillin has no lytic action on resting cells; to induce the loss of cellular integrity, it must act on actively growing bacteria. Lysozyme-EDTA treatment produces cytoplasmic membrane alteration. It has been shown that the so-called "pericytoplasmic enzymes" are released during this treatment, while the penicillin-obtained spheroplasts of gram-negative bacteria retain these enzymes [98]. The lysozyme-induced changes are reversible in regeneration process; thus no "information" is lost during wall removal and growth as protoplasts. It has also been found that membranes prepared without EDTA contain approximately 25% of the RNA of the whole cells whereas membranes prepared in the presence of EDTA contain less than 2% of the RNA of the whole cells [98]. Short exposure to EDTA alone released about one-half of the lipopolysaccharide from the outer membrane and made *Salmonella* cells and *E. coli* susceptible to antibiotics [99]. It has been demonstrated that EDTA alone, without lysozyme, permits entry of various antibiotic molecules normally excluded from intact cells [100,101]. All findings show that susceptibility to antibiotics judged by experiments in which EDTA was used to treat whole cells may be different from that obtained with penicillin-induced L-forms.

We must recall, however, that other changes besides loss of the cell wall occur in stable L-forms that have been long passaged in the laboratory and from which a selection for certain properties has often been made. Moreover, a homogeneous culture population, which is very important in the use of wall-less bacteria as models, can rarely be obtained; L-colony selection and cloning is very complex. It is also well known that L-forms divide abnormally, giving rise to cells of all sizes, many without nucleoids [88,102].

All these remarks should be taken into consideration for the interpretation of studies of susceptibility to antibiotics of wall-less bacteria. We must also be cautious in the clinical use of findings derived from L-form models; L-forms induced and propagated in vitro may be different from cell-wall-less bacteria that appear in vivo.

ACKNOWLEDGMENTS

I am grateful to N. El Solh, R. Caravano, and H. Kozdroj for the critical reading of the manuscript. The excellent technical assistance of M. C. Marmouset and M. Anoal and the expert secretarial help of M. O. Blervaque are gratefully acknowledged. I wish to thank J. R. King for reviewing and editing this chapter.

I am indebted to the following pharmaceutical laboratories for supplying documentation and antibiotic standard samples: Abott (erythromycin); Beecham-Sévigné (carbenicillin); Bristol (oxacillin); Eli Lilly (vancomycin); Léo (fusidic acid); Le Petit (rifampicin); Pfizer (polymyxin B and tetracyclines); Roger Bellon S.A. (colistin); Roussel Uclaf (bacitracin); Smith Kline & French (virginiamycin); Specia-Rhone Poulenc (penicillin G, streptomycin, and pristinamycin); Theraplix (novobiocin); Unilabo (gentamycin).

Research in my laboratory has been supported by contract No. 75-21 of Fondation de l'Industrie Pharmaceutique pour la Recherche, Paris.

REFERENCES

1. Gale, E. F., Cundliffe, E., Reynolds, P. E., Richmond, M. H., and Waring, M. J. (1972). *The Molecular Basis of Antibiotic Action*, Wiley, London.
2. Corcoran, J. W. and Hahn, F. E. (1975). *Antibiotics III, Mechanism of Action of Antimicrobial and Antitumor Agents*, Springer-Verlag, New York,
3. Singer, S. J. (1974). The molecular organisation of membranes. *Ann. Rev. Biochem. 43*:805-833.

4. Salton, M. R. J. and Owen, P. (1976). Bacterial membrane structure. *Ann. Rev. Microbiol.* 30:451-482.
5. Costerton, J. W. and Cheng, K. J. (1975). The role of the bacterial envelope in antibiotic resistance. *J. Antimicrob. Chemother.* 1:367-377.
6. Franklin, T. J. and Snow, G. A. (1975). *Biochemistry of Antimicrobial Action*, 2nd ed., Chapman and Hall, London.
7. Schmitt-Slomska, J. and Roux, J. (1977). Cell wall defective organisms as a model for the study of antibiotic activity in *Spheroplasts, Protoplasts and L-forms of Bacteria* (J. Roux, ed.), Editions INSERM, vol. 64, Paris, pp. 185-196.
8. Tulasne, R. and Minck, R. (1952). Sensibilité comparée des formes normales et des formes L de deux souches de *Proteus* vis-à-vis de quelques antibiotiques. *C. R. Soc. Biol. (Paris)* 146:778-780.
9. Ward, J. R., Madoff, S., and Dienes, L. (1958). In vitro sensitivity of some bacteria, their L-forms and pleuropneumonia-like organisms to antibiotics. *Proc. Soc. Exp. Biol. Med.* 97:132-135.
10. Shockman, G. D. and Lampen, J. O. (1962). Inhibition by antibiotics of the growth of bacterial and yeast protoplasts. *J. Bacteriol.* 84:508-512.
11. Kagan, B. M., Zolla, S., Busser, R., and Liepnieks, S. (1964). Sensitivity of coccal and L-forms of *Staphylococcus aureus* to five antibiotics. *J. Bacteriol.* 88:630-632.
12. Kagan, B. M. (1968). Antibiotic sensitivities of staphylococcal L-forms, in *Microbial Protoplasts, Spheroplasts and L-forms* (L. B. Guze, ed.), Williams & Wilkins, Baltimore, pp. 314-318.
13. Montgomerie, J. Z., Kalmanson, G. M., and Guze, L. B. (1968). The susceptibility of protoplast and bacterial forms of *Streptococcus faecalis* to antibiotics in *Microbial Protoplasts, Spheroplasts and L-forms* in (L. B. Guze, ed.), Williams & Wilkins, Baltimore, pp. 306-310.
14. Hubert, E. G., Kalmanson, G. M., Montgomerie, J. Z., and Guze, L. B. (1972). Activity of methacycline, related tetracyclines, and other antibiotics against various L-forms and their parent bacteria in vitro. *Antimicrob. Agents Chemother.* 2:276-280.
15. Kalvodova, D. (1974). L-forms of *Listeria monocytogenes*. Induction in vitro and sensitivity to antibiotics. *Cs. Epidem. Mikrobiol. Immunol.* 23:276-281.
16. Shakhovsky, K. P. (1964). Resistance of bacterial L-forms to the effect of antibiotics. *Antibiotiki (Moskva)* 3:220-225.
17. Yamamoto, A. and Homma, J. Y. (1978). L-form of *Pseudomonas aeruginosa*. II. Antibiotic sensitivity of L-forms and their parent forms. *Jpn. J. Exp. Med.* 48:355-362.
18. Hijmans, W., Van Boven, C. P. A., and Clasener, H. A. L. (1970). Fundamental biology of the L-phase of bacteria in *The Mycoplasmatales and the L-phase of Bacteria* (L. Hayflick, ed.), Appleton-Century-Crofts, New York, pp. 67-143.
19. Mattman, L. (1974). *Cell Wall Deficient Forms*, CRC Press, Cleveland.

20. Spicer, A. B. and Spooner, D. F. (1974). The inhibition of growth of *Escherichia coli* spheroplasts by antibacterial agents. *J. Gen. Microbiol.* 80:37-50.
21. Cheng, K. J., Costerton, J. W., Singh, A. P., and Ingram, J. M. (1973). Susceptibility of whole cells and spheroplasts of *Pseudomonas aeruginosa* to actinomycin D. *Antimicrob. Agents Chemother.* 3:399-406.
22. Godzeski, C. W., Brier, G., and Pavey, D. E. (1962). L-phase growth induction as a general characteristic of antibiotic bacterial interaction in the presence of serum. *Antimicrob. Agents Chemother.* 2:843-853.
23. Schönfeld, J. K. (1959). L-forms of Staphylococci; their reversibility: changes in the sensitivity pattern after several intermediary passages in the L phase. *Antonie van Leeuwenhoek* 25:325-331.
24. Watanakunakorn, C., Phair, J. P., and Hamburger, M. (1970). Increased resistance of *Pseudomonas aeruginosa* to carbenicillin after reversion from spheroplast to rod form. *Infect. Immun.* 1:427-430.
25. Panos, C., Cohen, M., and Eagan, G. (1967). Antibiotic inhibition and binding studies with a group A streptococcal L-form. *J. Gen. Microbiol.* 46:299-304.
26. Strominger, J. L., Willoughby, E., Kamiryo, T., Blumberg, P. M., and Yocum, R. R. (1974). Penicillin-sensitive enzymes and penicillin-binding components in bacterial cells in *Mode of action of antibiotics on microbial walls and membranes* (M. R. J. Salton and A. Tomasz, eds.), *Ann. N. Y. Acad. Sci.* 235:210-224.
27. Tomasz, A. (1979). The mechanisms of the irreversible antimicrobial effects of penicillins: How the beta-lactam antibiotics kill and lyse bacteria. *Ann. Rev. Microbiol.* 33:113-137.
28. Spratt, B. G. (1978). The mechanism of action of penicillin. *Sci. Progr. Oxford* 65:101-128.
29. Suginaka, H. (1976). Comparison of the binding of penicillin G to staphylococcal L-form and its parent strain membranes. *Antimicrob. Agents Chemother.* 9:544-545.
30. Martin, H. H., Schilf, W., and Schiefer, H. G. (1980). Differentiation of Mycoplasmatales from bacterial protoplast L-forms by assay for penicillin binding proteins. *Arch. Microbiol.* 127:297-299.
31. Rousset, A., Nguyen-Distèche, M., Minck, R., and Ghuysen, J. M. (1982). Penicillin-binding proteins and carboxypeptidase/transpeptidase activities in *Proteus vulgaris* P18 and its penicillin-induced stable L-forms. *J. Bacteriol.* 152:1042-1048.
32. Rotta, J., Karakawa, W. W., and Krause, R. M. (1965). Isolation of L-forms from group A Streptococci exposed to bacitracin. *J. Bacteriol.* 89:1581-1585.
33. Storm, D. D. and Strominger, J. L. (1974). Binding of bacitracin to cells and protoplasts of *Micrococcus lysodeikticus*. *J. Biol. Chem.* 249/6:1823-1827.
34. Jordan, D. C. and Reynolds, P. E. (1975). Vancomycin, in *Antibiotics III, Mechanism of Action Antimicrobial and Antitumor Agents* (J. W. Corcoran and F. E. Hahn, eds.), Springer-Verlag, Berlin, pp. 704-718.
35. Montgomerie, J. Z., Kalmanson, G. M., and Guze, L. B. (1966). The effects of antibiotics on the protoplast and bacterial forms of *Streptococcus faecalis*. *J. Lab. Clin. Med.* 68:547-551.

36. Perkins, H. R. and Nieto, M. (1974). The chemical basis for the action of the vancomycin group of antibiotics in *Mode of action of antibiotics on microbial walls and membranes* (M. R. J. Salton and A. Tomasz, eds.), *Ann. N.Y. Acad. Sci. 235*:348-363.
37. Watanakunakorn, C. (1971). Vancomycin induction of L-colonies of *Staphylococcus aureus. Infect. Immun. 3*:709-710.
38. Lawson, J. W. and Bacigalupi, B. (1977). Induction and reversion of the L-forms of *Neisseria gonorrhoeae* in *Spheroplasts, Protoplasts and L-forms of bacteria* (J. Roux, ed.), Ed. INSERM, vol. 64, Paris, pp. 91-106.
39. Todorov, T. (1976). Induction of L-forms of *Erysipelothrix insidiosa* using antibiotics and lysozyme. *Acta Microbiol. Virol. Immunol., Bulg. Ac. Sci. 4*:39-45.
40. Yudkin, M. D. (1963). The effect of penicillin, novobiocin, streptomycin and vancomycin on membrane synthesis by protoplasts of *Bacillus megaterium. Biochem. J. 89*:290-296.
41. Slabyj, B. M. and Panos, C. (1976). Membrane lipoteichoic acid of *Streptococcus pyogenes* and its stabilized L-form and the effect of two antibiotics upon its cellular content. *J. Bacteriol. 127*:855-862.
42. Cherepova, N., Mihailova, L., and Golubor, S. (1975). Electron microscopic studies on altered forms of *Erysipelothrix rhusiopathiae* obtained under the effect of novobiocin. *Zentralbl. Bakteriol. I. Abt. Orig. A 233*: 245-252.
43. Few, A. V. (1955). The interaction of polymyxin E with bacterial and other lipids. *Biochim. Biophys. Acta 16*:137-145.
44. Newton, B. A. (1956). The properties and mode of action of the polymyxins. *Bacteriol. Rev. 20*:14-27.
45. Feingold, D. S., Hsu, C. C., and Sud, I. J. (1974). Basis for the selectivity of action of the polymyxin antibiotics on cell membranes in *Mode of action of antibiotics on microbial walls and membranes* (M. R. J. Salton and A. Tomasz, eds.), *Ann. N. Y. Acad. Sci. 235*:480-492.
46. Schindler, P. R. G. and Teuber, M. (1975). Action of polymyxin B on bacterial membranes: morphological changes in the cytoplasm and in the outer membrane of *Salmonella typhimurium* and *Escherichia coli* B. *Antimicrob. Agents Chemother. 8*:95-104.
47. Koike, M., Iida, K., and Matsuo, T. (1969). Electron microscopic studies on mode of action of polymyxin. *J. Bacteriol. 97*:448-452.
48. Teuber, M. (1969). Susceptibility to polymyxin B of penicillin G-induced *Proteus mirabilis* L-forms and spheroplasts. *J. Bacteriol. 98*:347-350.
49. Gumpert, J. (1970). Vergleichende untersuchungen zur wirkung von antibiotika auf bakterielle zellwände und cytoplasmatische membranen in *Mechanisms of Action of Fungicides, Antibiotics and Cytostatics*, Int. Symp., Akademic-Verlag, Berlin, pp. 231-232.
50. Adair, F. W., Manniello, J., and Heymann, H. (1976). Effect of polymyxin B and benzalkonium chloride on spheroplasts of *Pseudomonas cepacia. Abstr. Annu. Meet. Am. Soc. Microbiol* (A 25), p. 5.

51. Louis, C. and Schmitt-Slomska, J. (1977). Effect of polymyxin B on the ultrastructure of the stable *Proteus mirabilis* L-forms in *Spheroplasts, Protoplasts and L-forms of Bacteria* (J. Roux, ed.), Ed. INSERM, vol. 64, Paris, pp. 197-210.
52. Kozdroj, H., Caravano, R., and Schmitt-Slomska, J. (1977). Interest of diethylamino-1-naphthalene sulfonyl-5-chloride (dansyl)-complexed polymyxin for the study of membrane-associated proteins of bacteria and L-forms in *Spheroplasts, Protoplasts and L-forms of Bacteria* (J. Roux, ed.), Ed. INSERM, vol. 64, Paris, pp. 221-231.
53. Newton, B. A. (1955). A fluorescent derivate of polymyxin: Its preparation and use in studying the site of action of the antibiotic. *J. Gen. Microbiol.* 12:226-236.
54. Cavard, D. and Schmitt-Slomska, J. (1977). Phospholipid composition of L-forms and bacteria of *Proteus mirabilis* and modifications observed under the action of polymyxin B in *Spheroplasts, Protoplasts and L-forms of Bacteria* (J. Roux, ed.), Ed. INSERM, vol 64, Paris, pp. 211-219.
55. Montgomerie, J. Z., Kalmanson, G. M., and Guze, L. B. (1973). Synergism of polymyxin and sulfonamides in L-forms of *Staphylococcus aureus* and *Proteus mirabilis. Antimicrob. Agents Chemother.* 3:523-525.
56. Hamilton-Miller, J. M. T. (1973). Chemistry and biology of the polyene macrolide antibiotics. *Bacteriol. Rev.* 37:166-196.
57. Haupt, I., Schuhmann, E., Geuther, R., and Thrum, H. (1976). Effects of polyene macrolide antibiotics on normal and protoplast type L-form cells of *E. coli* W. 1655 F. *J. Antibiot. Jpn.* 29:44-49.
58. Ehrenfeld, E. R. and Koch, A. L. (1968). RNA synthesis in penicillin spheroplasts of *Escherichia coli. Biochim. Biophys. Acta* 169:44-57.
59. Haywood, A. M. and Sinsheimer, R. L. (1963). Inhibition of protein synthesis in *Escherichia coli* protoplasts by actinomycin D. *J. Mol. Biol.* 6: 247-249.
60. Mach, B. and Tatum, E. L. (1963). Ribonucleic acid synthesis in protoplasts of *Escherichia coli*. Inhibition by actinomycin D. *Science* 139:1051-1052.
61. Taubeneck, U. (1962). Susceptibility of *Proteus mirabilis* and its stable L-forms to erythromycin and other macrolides. *Nature* 196:195-196.
62. Watanakunakorn, O., Goldberg, L. M., Carleton, J., and Hamburger, M. (1969). Staphylococcal spheroplasts and L-colonies. IV. Antimicrobial susceptibility of stable methicillin-induced and lysostaphin-induced spheroplasts. *Antimicrob. Agents Chemother.* 8:382-387.
63. Schmitt-Slomska, J., Marmouset, M. C., Louis, C., Bally, R., Starka, G., and Madoff, S. (1982). Tetracycline-resistant L-forms isolated from an antibiotic susceptible strain of *Listeria monocytogenes. Antimicrob. Ag. Chemother.* 22:678-685.
64. Chopra, I. and Howe, T. G. B. (1978). Bacterial resistance to the tetracyclines. *Microbiol. Rev.* 42:707-724.
65. Franklin, T. J. (1967). Resistance of *Escherichia coli* to tetracyclines. Changes in permeability to tetracyclines bearing transferable resistance factors. *Biochem. J.* 105:371-378.

66. Franklin, T. J. (1973). Antibiotic transport in bacteria. *Br. Rev. Microbiol.* 2:253-272.
67. Panos, C. (1969). Chemical and physiological aspects of the bacterial L-phase variants in *The Mycoplasmatales and the L-phase of Bacteria* (L. Hayflick, ed.), Appleton-Century-Crofts, New York, pp. 503-524.
68. Panos, C., Fagan, G., and Zarkadas, C. G. (1972). Comparative electrophoretic and amino acid analyses of isolated membranes from *Streptococcus pyogenes* and stabilized L-form. *J. Bacteriol.* 112:285-290.
69. Gilpin, R. W., Young, F. E., and Chatterjee, A. N. (1973). Characterization of a stable L-form of *Bacillus subtilis* 168. *J. Bacteriol.* 127:1018-1021.
70. Lederberg, J. and St. Clair, J. (1958). Protoplasts and L-type growth of *Escherichia coli. J. Bacteriol.* 75:143-158.
71. Hewitt, W. L., Seligman, S. J., and Deigh, R. A. (1968). Relationship of the antibiotic sensitivity of enterococci to acquired resistance in their L-forms in *Microbial Protoplasts, Spheroplasts and L-forms* (L. B. Guze, ed.), Williams & Wilkins, Baltimore, pp. 311-313.
72. Hewitt, W. L., Seligman, S. J., and Deigh, R. A. (1966). Kinetics of the synergism of penicillin-streptomycin and penicillin-kanamycin for enterococci and its relationship to L-phase variants. *J. Lab. Clin. Med.* 67:792-807.
73. Szybalski, W. and Pitzurra, M. (1959). Mechanism of chemical mutagenesis III. Induced mutations in spheroplasts of *Escherichia coli. J. Bacteriol.* 77:621-622.
74. Novick, R. P. (1969). Extrachromosomal inheritance in bacteria. *Bacteriol. Rev.* 33:210-235.
75. Jacob, F., Brenner, J. F. S., and Cuzin, F. (1963). On the regulation of DNA replication in bacteria. *Cold Spring Harbor Symp. Quant. Biol.* 28:329-348.
76. Kawakami, M. and Landman, O. E. (1966). Retention of episomes during protoplasting and during propagation in the L-state. *J. Bacteriol.* 92:398-404.
77. Horodniceanu, T., Bouanchaud, D. H., Bieth, G., and Chabbert, Y. A. (1976). R plasmid in *Streptococcus agalactiae* (Group B). *Antimicrob. Ag. Chemotherap.* 10:795-801.
78. Schmitt-Slomska, J., Caravano, R., and El Solh, N. (1979). Loss of plasmid mediated resistance after conversion of a group B Streptococcus strain to a stable cell wall deficient variant. *Ann. Microbiol. (Inst. Pasteur) 130A*: 23-27.
79. Schmitt-Slomska, J., and El Solh, N. (1979). Etude de la résistance aux antibiotiques des variants bactériens à paroi défectueuse ou déficiente. S.F.M. Symp. Agents antibactériens, Inst. Pasteur, Paris, Abstr. C23.
80. Novick, R., Sanchez-Rivas, C., Gruss, A., and Edelman, I. (1980). Involvement of the cell envelope in plasmid maintenance: plasmid curing during the regeneration of protoplasts. *Plasmid 3*:348-358.
81. El Solh, N., Fouace, J. M., Shalita, Z., Bouanchaud, D. H., Novick, R. P., and Chabbert, Y. A. (1980). Epidemiological and structural studies of *Staphylococcus aureus* R plasmids mediating resistance to tobramycin and streptogramin. *Plasmid* 4:117-120.

82. El Solh, N., and Schmitt-Slomska, J. (1985). Plasmid loss in *Staphyloccocus aureus* wall deficient cell. *Chemioterapia 4*:686-688.
83. Fitz-James, P. H. (1964). Fate of the mesosomes of *Bacillus megaterium* during protoplasting. *J. Bacteriol. 87*:1483-1491.
84. Ryter, A., and Landman, O. E. (1964). Electron microscope study of the relationship between mesosome loss and the stable L-state (or protoplast state) in *Bacillus subtilis. J. Bacteriol. 88*:457-467.
85. Greenawalt, J. W. and Whiteside, L. T. (1975). Mesosomes: membranous bacterial organelles. *Bacteriol. Rev. 39*:405-463.
86. Levashev, V. S. (1965). Genetic mechanisms of the L-form bacteria formation and prospects for further research. *Vestn. Akad. Med. Nauk. SSSR 20*: 32-37.
87. Ryter, A. (1968). Association of the nucleus and the membrane of bacteria: A morphological study. *Bacteriol. Rev. 32*:39-54.
88. Ryter, A. and Landman, O. E. (1968). Morphological study of the attachment of nucleoid to membrane in bacilli; protoplasts and reverting protoplasts of *Bacillus subtilis*, in *Microbial Protoplasts, Spheroplasts and L-forms* (L. B. Guze, ed.), Williams & Wilkins, Baltimore, pp. 110-123.
89. Hoyer, B. H. and King, J. R. (1969). Deoxyribonucleic acid sequence losses in a stable streptococcal L-form. *J. Bacteriol. 97*:1516-1517.
90. Wyrick, P. B. and Rogers, H. J. (1973). Isolation and characterization of cell wall defective variants of *Bacillus subtilis* and *Bacillus licheniformis. J. Bacteriol. 116*:456-465.
91. Wyrick, P. B., McConnell, M., and Rogers, H. J. (1973). Genetic transfer of the stable L-form state to intact bacterial cells. *Nature 244*:505-507.
92. Horowitz, S., Doyle, R. J., Young, F. E., and Streips, U. N. (1979). Selective association of the chromosome with membrane in a stable L-form of *Bacillus subtilis. J. Bacteriol. 138*:915-922.
93. Doyle, R. J., Streips, U. N., Imada, S., Fan, V. S. C., and Brown, W. C. (1980). Genetic transformation with cell wall-associated deoxyribonucleic acid in *Bacillus subtilis. J. Bacteriol. 144*:957-966.
94. Götz, F., Ahrné, S., and Lindberg, M. (1981). Plasmid transfer and genetic recombination by protoplast fusion in staphylococci. *J. Bacteriol. 145*:74-81.
95. Luria, S. E. (1969). Opening remarks in *Bacterial Episomes and Plasmids* (G. E. W. Wolstenholme and M. O'Connor, eds.), Ciba Found. Symp., I. & A. Churchill, London, pp. 1-3.
96. Lacey, R. W. and Chopra, I. (1974). Genetic studies of a multi-resistant strain of *Staphylococcus aureus. J. Med. Microbiol. 7*:285-297.
97. Ghuysen, J. M. (1968). Use of bacteriolytic enzymes in determination of wall structure and their role in cell metabolism. *Bacteriol. Rev. 32*:425-464.
98. Kaback, H. R. (1971). Bacterial membranes. *Methods Enzymol. 22*:99-120.
99. Nakae, T. and Nikaido, H. (1975). Outer membrane as a diffusion barrier in *Salmonella typhimurium* penetration of oligo- and polysaccharides into isolated outer membrane vesicles and cells with degraded peptidoglycan layer. *J. Biol. Chem. 250*:7359-7365.

100. Hamilton-Miller, J. M. T. (1966). Damaging effects of EDTA and penicillins in permeability barriers in gram negative bacteria. *Biochem. J. 100*: 675–682.
101. Leive, L. (1974). The barrier function of the gram-negative envelope, in *Mode of action of antibiotics on microbial walls and membranes* (M. R. J. Salton and A. Tomasz, eds.), *Ann. N.Y. Acad. Sci. 235*:109–129.
102. Cole, R. M. (1971). Some implications of the comparative ultrastructure of bacterial L-forms in *Mycoplasma and the L-forms of Bacteria* (S. Madoff, ed.), Gordon & Breach, New York, pp. 49–83.

12

Immunology of Bacterial L-Forms

RAYMOND J. LYNN
Department of Microbiology, University of South Dakota, School of Medicine, Vermillion, South Dakota

I.	Introduction	263
II.	Antigenic Characteristics	264
	A. Components in Common with Cell Walls	264
	B. Components Unique to the Membrane	265
	C. Components Elaborated by the L-Form	267
III.	Immunity: Humoral Response	267
	A. Serum Antibody	267
	B. Secretory Antibody	268
IV.	Immunity: Cellular Response	268
	A. Delayed Hypersensitivity	268
	B. Granulomatous Reactions	268
V.	L-Forms as Agents of Immune Modulation	269
	A. Mitogens	269
	B. Suppressors	269
VI.	Conclusions	270
	References	270

I. INTRODUCTION

The L-forms of bacteria offer a unique tool to investigate further the area of membrane antigenicity and immunoregulation. Early reports indicated that the L-forms could serve as immunogens in experimental animals even though their association with acute infectious diseases was doubtful [1-4]. The lack of apparent infectivity of these organisms and their susceptibility to the action of complement and normal serum components discouraged further investigation of their immunogenicity [5-7]. Reports indicating the possible intracellular parasitism and describing immunoregulatory activity for a number of membrane components suggest a renewed interest in the immunologic capability of protoplasts, spheroplasts, L-forms, and cell wall-defective microorganisms [8-14].

II. ANTIGENIC CHARACTERISTICS

A. Components in Common with Cell Walls

Dienes et al. [2] demonstrated with L-forms of two strains of proteus that the L-form shared antigenic determinants in common with the parent bacterial form. Adsorption of anti-L-form serum with the parent bacterial form removed all agglutinating antibodies to the L-form. Adsorption and antibacterial serum with the L-form lowered the agglutination titer of this serum with the bacterial form but did not remove all reactivity, indicating that some cell wall antigens were lacking in the L-phase organism. These authors [15] also reported that the L-form of *Salmonella typhi* shared common antigenic determinants with the bacterial form of *Salmonella typhimurium* as well as *S. typhi*. However, they did not react with antiserum to proteus. Tulasne [16] reported that the L-phase organism prepared from gram-negative bacteria, while losing some cell wall-unique antigens, retained the capacity to act as immunogens for the production of O and H antibodies. Minck and co-workers [17,18] reported that the stable L-form of *Proteus* 18 induced significantly lower levels of anti-O antibodies in rabbits when compared with the parent bacterial form. These investigators were able to demonstrate that the inhibitory antibody against L-form growth in the immune sera was not related to O or H antigenic specificity. In addition, they demonstrated that this growth-inhibitory activity was significantly greater than that produced following immunization of rabbits with the whole or disrupted parent bacterial form. Sharp and Dienes [19] reported that a glycoprotein antigen found in particularly high concentration in the cell wall preparations of *Proteus* 18 was also present in the stable L-form of this organism. Carey et al. [20] examined the capacity of several gram-negative protoplasts to agglutinate with somatic antisera prepared with the bacterial forms and reported that such protoplasts retained the capacity to agglutinate with these sera but at a significantly lower affinity. L-forms of gram-negative bacteria have been shown to retain endotoxic activity indicating a retention of the lipopolysaccharide moiety by these forms [21-26]. This lipopolysaccharide appeared less toxic in the L-form that the parent bacterial form [23]. Kotelko et al. [24] demonstrated that the endotoxin in the stable L-form of *Proteus mirabilis* could be extracted with the hot aqueous phenol method but not the trichloroacetic acid method, although active endotoxin could be extracted from the parent bacterial form by either method. These investigators concluded that the lipopolysaccharide was attached to a different moiety in the L-form. Gmeiner and Martin [25] reported that the stable L-form of *P. mirabilis* synthesized the same two types of lipopolysaccharide (types I and II) as the parent bacterial form but significantly lower amounts of the more hydrophilic form (type II). It has been reported that rabbits can be primed for the Shwartzman reaction utilizing the stable L-form of *P. mirabilis* and eliciting the reaction with *Escherichia coli* endotoxin [26]. The L-form elicited only a minimal area of reactivity in animals primed with the L-form, the parent bacterial form, or *E. coli* endotoxin.

Forsgren [27] demonstrated that the L-forms of *Staphylococcus aureus* retained small quantities of protein A, a significant component of the cell wall of this organism. A small quantity of protein A was also elaborated by this L-form.

Mirsky and co-workers [28] have demonstrated that antibodies to membrane adenosine triphosphatase caused agglutination of protoplasts or membrane preparations. Monteil and co-workers [29–32] have reported that the L-form of *P. mirabilis* yielded a Mg^{2+}-dependent ATPase that was immunogenic. These investigators postulated that the antibodies responsible for the growth inhibitory activity of anti-L-form serum were directed against this component.

Unstable L-forms, spheroplasts, and cell-wall-defective variants have been shown to retain varying amounts of residual cell wall materials which may be antigenic [33,34]. These variants could be used as effective immunogens for these selected cell wall components. By definition, protoplasts should be free of such antigens [35].

B. Components Unique to the Membrane

Dienes et al. [2] reported that antiserum produced to a stable L-form obtained from a type 52 *Proteus* reacted specifically with the L-form and not to the bacterial form when examined by the agglutination technique. In addition, the L-form did not react with antiserum prepared against the parent bacterial form. This suggests that immunogens were present in the L-form that were not available or masked in the parent bacterial form. Sharp et al. [36] found that some stable L-forms of Group A streptococci retained the capacity to produce M protein, although no evidence of the group-specific polysaccharide was detected. However, some L-forms do not react with typing sera, indicating the loss of this antigen also. Karakawa et al. [37] employed type-specific fluorescein-labeled antibody to demonstrate that L-forms of Group A streptococci retain significant amounts of specific M protein. They reported also that the M protein was released into the surrounding environment. Recently a comparison of a type 12 M protein obtained from L-forms and protoplasts and the parent bacterial form indicated a difference in molecular weight between that extracted from the coccal form and the M protein obtained from the L-form or protoplast [38]. The L-form antigen showed lines of partial identity in immunodiffusion with the

M protein extracted from the parent form when reacted against antiserum to the L-form M protein. The M proteins of the L-form and protoplast did not differ from that of the parent form in exhibiting antiphagocytic activity.

Crawford [39,40] reported that a complement-fixing antigen could be extracted from a stable L-form of Group A streptococcus that would react against sera from patients with streptococcal infections. Similar extraction methods did not result in such an antigen being obtained from the parent streptococcus. In addition, adsorption of the reacting sera with whole cells, cell wall preparations, or sonicated streptococci did not remove the reactivity of the sera for this complement fixing antigen. In our laboratory [41,42] rabbit antiserum against the stable L-form of Group A streptococci showed agglutination with soluble L-form antigens adsorbed to latex after adsorption of the serum with the parent bacterial form. The data suggested that immunogens masked in the parent coccal form were exposed in the L-form. Ultrasonically or mechanically disrupted streptococci were similar in antigenic reactivity with the L-form when reacted with anti-L-form serum [42]. James et al. [43] concluded that the envelope of the L-form was unique from either the cell wall or the protoplasmic membrane in a type 12 Group A streptococcus. The membrane of the L-form yielded lipoprotein with a greater concentration of lipid than the lipoprotein found in the protoplasmic membrane preparations. The L-form membrane showed significantly less mucopeptide than the cell wall preparations. Kanazawa and Wu [44] indicated that lipoprotein accumulated in the cytoplasmic membrane of a spheroplast of *E. coli*. The accumulation of such components as lipoprotein, glycolipids, and glycoproteins in cell wall-less variants could alter the immunogenicity associated with these membranes. It has been demonstrated that a low-molecular-weight glycoprotein in the type 12 streptococcal membrane shows antigenic similarity with a similar fraction of human glomeruli [45]. Stable L-forms of Group A streptococci of types 12, 14, and 19 were shown to share common antigens of a glycolipid nature with the membranes of the parent coccal form [46].

Lipoteichoic acid of the membrane of stable L-forms of Group A streptococci, while structurally different from that extracted from the parent bacterial form, was shown to be effective in preventing the attachment of the parent streptococcus as well as the L-form to mammalian cells [47]. It was reported that enzymes such as phospholipase A [48], *N*-acetylmuramyl-L-alanine amidase [49], and adenosine triphosphatase [29-32,50,51] have been shown to be present in membrane preparations of spheroplasts and L-forms of bacteria. Antibodies to the ATPase of *P. mirabilis* have been shown to inhibit the in vitro growth of the stable L-form prepared from this bacterium [29-32].

C. Components Elaborated by the L-Form

Experiments with the stable L-forms of Group A streptococci indicated that these organisms retain the property of releasing extracellular components into the medium. These L-forms were shown to elaborate hemolysin and M protein [52,53], hyaluronic acid, streptolysin O and S, streptokinase, deoxyribonuclease [54,55], and erythrogenic toxin [42], as well as streptococcin [56]. It has been noted that the L-phase organism may show increased production of such extracellular components [57,58]. Kalmanson et al. [59] reported that an L-form of *Streptococcus faecalis* produced a bacteriocin with a different spectrum of activity from that produced by the parent streptococcus.

Smith and Willis [60] noted that stable L-forms obtained from strains of *S. aureus* continued to elaborate such components as pigment, catalase, coagulase, deoxyribonuclease, gelatinase, and lipase as did the parent bacterial form. It was suggested that the medium components required for the growth of the L-form could have contributed to the lack of detection of such components as hemolysins and fibrinolysin. Simon and Yin [61] reported that L-forms of a penicillinase-producing *S. aureus* continued to show this activity but at a significantly reduced level. Urease production by stable L-forms of *P. mirabilis* have been shown to contribute to the production of bladder stones in rats [62]. It would be of interest to determine if L-forms of other species of *Proteus* which have been shown to produce ureases with different biochemical properties [63] could initiate the formation of such stones. It has been reported that L-forms of *Clostridia* continue to produce exotoxin similar to that of the parent bacteria [64-66].

III. IMMUNITY: HUMORAL RESPONSE

A. Serum Antibody

Numerous reports have been published indicating the development of serum antibodies to L-form components following inoculation of such organisms into laboratory animals. Such antibodies have been manifested by a variety of serologic techniques. Agglutination has been utilized for a number of the L-forms of gram-negative bacteria [1-4]. Soluble antigens have been utilized in the complement fixation, precipitation, and indirect agglutination [41,42]. Edward and Fitzgerald [67] demonstrated that antisera were capable of inhibiting the growth of stable L-forms of proteus. This activity was shown to be stable to heating at 56°C for 60 min. Similar growth inhibitory activity has been demonstrated with L-forms of streptococci [42]. The level of growth inhibitory activity did not appear to be correlated with the titers of antibody determined by precipitation and indirect agglutination.

B. Secretory Antibody

The reports of Agarwal and co-workers [68,69] indicated that antigenic preparations of L-forms of *Vibrio cholera* administered orally gave rise to corproantibodies as well as serum antibodies. Others [70] have indicated a correlation of corproantibodies with those of other secretory sites. The predominant immunoglobulin associated with these secretions was IgA. It was reported that human secretory IgA antibodies to cholera showed the properties of agglutination, toxin neutralization, and antiadherence [71]. Such antibodies were not vibriocidal. It would be interesting to examine the immune response to oral and/or intranasal inoculation with other stable L-forms.

IV. IMMUNITY: CELLULAR RESPONSE

A. Delayed Hypersensitivity

Kagan et al. [72] have reported that the intraperitoneal injection of stable L-forms of Group A streptococci into mice leads to the development of lesions characteristic of both immediate and delayed-type hypersensitivities. These conclusions were based primarily on histological examination. These authors and others [73] have noted that injection of L-forms of Group A streptococci lead to changes in the thymus-dependent areas of the lymph node and spleen. Ratnam and Chandrasekhar [74] were unable to induce tuberculin hypersensitivity in guinea pigs with spheroplasts of *Mycobacterium tuberculosis* even though these forms persisted for a considerable length of time in the animals. Agarwal and Sundararaj [75,76] reported the induction of cell-mediated immunity in rabbits with ribonucleic acid-protein fractions of L-forms of *V. cholerae*. Parameters of cell-mediated immunity examined included leukocyte migration inhibition, macrophage migration inhibition, macrophage aggregation, and delayed hypersensitivity skin test. The cell-mediated immunity was induced after either intramuscular or oral introduction of the immunogen.

B. Granulomatous Reactions

The appearance of reticuloendothelial cells such as giant cells, macrophages, histocytes, and epitheloid cells are characteristic of a granulomatous reaction [77]. Such reactions have been described as a manifestation of the immune response to substances that are poorly solubilized and/or persist locally in the host. Orr et al. [78] reported that injection of the L-form of *S. faecalis* into the wall of the terminal ileum of rabbits leads to the production of focal granulomatous lesions in the ileal submucosa. Similar injections with the parent bacterial form or L-form medium did not induce such lesions. The granuloma persisted in these animals for a period in excess of the 3 months' observation time. Recently, Beaman [79,80] reported that intraperitoneal or intravenous inoculation of mice with an L-form of *Nocardia caviae* led to the formation of a granulomatous reaction after 7-8 months which developed into a spreading mycetoma. The L-form but not the parent bacterial form could be isolated from the brain of these mice. Both forms were observed in the mycetoma (see Chap. 10).

V. L-FORMS AS AGENTS OF IMMUNE MODULATION

A. Mitogens

Takada et al. [81] reported that the cytoplasmic membrane of L-forms induced from *S. aureus* was a potent mitogen for spleen lymphocytes of mice and guinea pigs. They concluded that the active component was not protein A because of differing properties on silicic acid column chromatography. Protein A has been shown to be a polyclonal B-cell activator [82,83]. L-forms of *S. aureus* have been shown to retain this component at low concentrations [27]. Serological comparison of the mitogenic component reported by Takada et al. [81] with protein A should be carried out.

Lipoteichoic acid, which has been shown to be present in stable L-forms of streptococci, has been reported to be mitogenic for T lymphocytes [84-86]. Streptolysin S has been reported to have a heat-stable, nondialyzable mitogenic factor associated with it. The lack of antigenicity of this component hampers the elucidation of the relationship of the hemolytic and mitogenic factors [87,88]. The pyrogenic exotoxins of Group A streptococci have been shown to react both as specific immunogens and as mitogens for rabbit lymphocytes [89,90]. B-lymphocyte mitogenicity has been demonstrated with the lipopolysaccharide of gram-negative bacteria [91]. As indicated above, all of these components have been found in L-forms, although few studies have been reported pertaining to the mitogenicity of such components from L-forms or L-forms themselves.

B. Suppressors

It has been noted that L-forms of *Listeria* induced an atrophy of lymphoid tissue in rabbits and thus acted as a suppressor of the immune response [92]. Miller et al. [93] reported that streptococcal lipoteichoic acid suppressed both the primary and secondary humoral response in mice to a thymus-dependent immunogen. The same substance acted to enhance the antibody response to *E. coli* lipopolysaccharide. Bacterial endotoxins have been shown to act as immunosuppressive agents as well as B-cell mitogens and adjuvants [94]. The streptococcal pyrogenic exotoxin has been reported to suppress antibody response in rabbits to sheep red blood cells [95], but too few studies have been reported to evaluate the L-form properly as an immunosuppressor. Obviously more interest and research should be directed to these areas.

VI. CONCLUSIONS

The L-forms of bacteria have been shown to be immunogenic for a variety of hosts. The L-form may present immunogens to the host that are masked and/or suppressed by cell wall components in the parent bacterial form. Some of these membrane components have antigenic determinants in common with mammalian tissue.

Immunization with the L-form can lead to the development of both humoral and cell-mediated immunity. The products of such immunity could enhance the inflammatory response of the host and lead to autoallergic types of reaction. The persistence of the L-form, despite the lethal effects of host serum components, could lead to continuous low-level immunogenic stimulation.

Many of the cellular and extracellular components associated with the L-forms have been shown to possess immunoregulatory activity. The role of these variant microorganisms as agents of immunological disease deserves further investigation.

REFERENCES

1. Klieneberger-Nobel, E. (1962). *Pleuropneumonia-like Organisms (PPLO) Mycoplasmataceae*, Academic, New York.
2. Dienes, L., Weinberger, H. J., and Madoff, S. (1950). Serological reactions of L type cultures isolated from proteus. *Proc. Soc. Exp. Biol. Med. 75*: 409–412.
3. Freundt, E. A. (1956). Experimental investigations into the pathogenicity of the L-phase variant of *Streptobacillus moniliformis. Acta. Path. Microbiol. Scand.* 38:246–258.
4. Lynn, R. J. (1967). Immunology of mycoplasma and bacterial L-forms in *A Microbial Enigma: Mycoplasma and Bacterial L-Forms* (C. Panos, ed.), World Publishing, Cleveland, pp. 213–252.
5. Muschel, L. H. and Jackson, J. E. (1966). The reactivity of serum against protoplasts and spheroplasts. *J. Immunol.* 97:46–51.
6. Guze, L. B., Hubert, E. G., Montgomerie, J. Z., and Kalmanson, G. M. (1967). Observations on the killing of microbial protoplasts by serum. *Nature 214*:1343–1346.
7. McGee, Z. A., Ratner, H. B., Bryant, R. E., Rosenthal, A. S. and Koenig, M. G. (1972). An antibody-complement system in human serum lethal to L-phase variants of bacteria. *J. Infect. Dis.* 125:231–241.
8. Babudieri, B. (1972). Mycoplasma-like organisms, parasite of red blood cells of an amphibian, *Hydromantes italicus (Spelerpes fuscus). Infect. Immun.* 6:77–82.
9. Green, M. T., Heidger, Jr., P. M., and Domingue, G. (1974). Demonstration of the phenomena of microbial persistence and reversion with bacterial L-forms in human embryonic kidney cells. *Infect. Immun.* 10:889–914.

10. Pease, P. E. (1974). Identification of bacteria from blood and joint fluids of human subjects as *Bacillus licheniformis*. *Ann. Rheum. Dis. 33*:67–69.
11. Bourgeois, L. and Beaman, B. L. (1974). Probable L-forms of *Nocardia asteroides* induced in cultured mouse peritoneal macrophages. *Infect. Immun. 9*:576–590.
12. Butler, H. M. and Blakey, J. L. (1975). A review of bacteria in L-phase and their possible clinical significance. *Med. J. Aust. 2*:463–467.
13. Domingue, G. J., Schlegel, J. U., Heidger, Jr., P. M., and Ehrlich, M. (1977). Novel bacterial structures in human blood: Cultural isolation, ultrastructural and biochemical evaluation. Ed. INSERM, Paris, pp. 279–278.
14. Bisset, K. A. (1979). Origin of the diphtheroid bacteria, mycoplasma, etc. reported in association with autoimmune conditions. *Ann. Rheum. Dis. 38*:199.
15. Weinberger, H. J., Madoff, S., and Dienes, L. (1950). The properties of L-forms isolated from Salmonella and the isolation of L-forms from *Shigella. J. Bacteriol. 59*:765–775.
16. Tulasne, R. (1951). Les formes L des bacteries. *Revue d'Immunologic et de Therapic Antimicrobienne 15*:223–251.
17. Minck, R., Kirn, A., and Fleck, J. (1961). Etude de l'action inhibitrice specifique des antiserums sur les cultures L des bacteries. I. Exclusion du role des anticorps O et H dans le phenomene d'inhibition specifique des culture L. *Ann. Inst. Pasteur 101*:178–184.
18. Kirn, A., Fleck, J., and Minck, R. (1962). Etude de l'action inhibitrice specifique des antiserums sur les cultures L des bacteries. II. Presence d'agglutinines H dan les antiserums. *Ann. Inst. Pasteur 102*:113–117.
19. Sharp, J. T. and Dienes, L. (1959). Carbohydrate containing antigen from the bacterial and L-forms of proteus. *J. Bacteriol. 78*:343–351.
20. Carey, W. F., Muschel, L. H., and Baron, L. S. (1960). The formation of bacterial protoplasts *in vivo. J. Immunol. 84*:183–188.
21. Tulasne, R. and Lavillauriex, J. (1955). Mecanisme de l'action pathogene d'une forme L des bacteries d'origine vibrionnienne. *Comp. Rend. Soc. Biol. 149*:178–180.
22. Lavillaureix, J. (1957). Action de formes L pathogenes sur de cultures de cellules cancereuses. *Comp. Rend. Soc. Biol. 244*:1098–1101.
23. Dansinger, B. L. and Suter, E. (1962). Endotoxic activity of L-forms derived from *Salmonella paratyphii* B. *Proc. Soc. Exp. Biol. Med. 111*: 399–400.
24. Kotelko, K., Luderitz, O., and Westphal, O. (1965). Vergleichende untersuchungen an antigenen von *Proteus mirabilis* und einer stabilen L-form. *Biochem. Zeitschrift. 343*:227–242.
25. Gmeiner, J. and Martin, H. H. (1976). Phospholipid and lipopolysaccharide in *Proteus mirabilis* and its stable protoplast L-form. Difference in content and fatty acid composition. *Eur. J. Biochem. 67*:487–494.
26. Kalmanson, G. M., Kubota, M. Y., and Guze, L. B. (1968). Production of the Shwartzman reaction with microbial L-forms. *J. Bacteriol. 96*:646–651.

27. Forsgren, A. (1969). Protein A from *Staphylococcus aureus*. VIII. Production of protein A by bacterial and L-forms of *Staphylococcus aureus*. *Acta. Pathol. Microbiol. Scand. 75*:481-490.
28. Mirsky, R., Barlow, V., and Berman, P. (1974). Antibodies to purified membrane-bound ATPase from *Bacillus megaterium* KM and their reaction with protoplasts and cytoplasmic membranes. *Biochim. Biophys. Acta 345*: 55-61.
29. Monteil, H., Schoun, J., and Guinard, M. (1974). A Na^+K^+-activated Mg^{++}-dependent ATPase released from proteus L-form membrane. *Eur. J. Biochem. 41*:525-532.
30. Monteil, H., Roussel, G., and Boulouis, D. (1975). Membrane ATPase of proteus L-forms: solubilization and molecular properties. *Biochem. Biophys. Acta 382*:465-478.
31. Monteil, H. and Roussel, G. (1975). Immunogenic properties of membrane-bound ATPase from stable proteus P18 L-forms: a kinetic study of inhibition by specific antibodies. *Biochem. Biophys. Res. Commun. 63*: 313-322.
32. Monteil, H. (1977). L'ATPase membranaire des formes L stables de proteus P18: properties enzymatiques et neutralisation par les anticorps inhibant la croissance des formes L in *Spheroplasts, Protoplasts and L-forms of Bacteria* (J. Roux, ed.), Vol. 64, Ed. INSERM, Paris, pp. 149-162.
33. Chandler, H. M. and Hamilton, R. C. (1975). The protective antigenicity of protoplasts and sphaeroplasts of a highly protective strain of *Clostridium chauvoei*. *J. Gen. Microbiol. 88*:179-183.
34. Bertolani, R., Elberg, S. S., and Ralston, D. (1975). Variations in properties of L-forms of *Pseudomonas aeruginosa*. *Infect. Immunity 11*:180-192.
35. McGee, Z., Wittler, R., and Gooder, H. (1971). Wall defective microbial variants: Terminology and experimental design. *J. Infect. Dis. 123*:433-438.
36. Sharp, J. T., Hijmans, W., and Dienes, L. (1957). Examination of the L-forms of Group A streptococci for the group-specific polysaccharide and M protein. *J. Exp. Med. 105*:153-159.
37. Karakawa, W. W., Rotta, J., and Krause, R. M. (1965). Detection of M protein in colonies of streptococcal L-forms by immunofluorescence. *Proc. Soc. Exp. Biol. Med. 118*:198-210.
38. Van de Rijn, I. and Fischetti, V. A. (1981). Immunochemical analysis of intact M protein secreted by cell wall-less streptococci. *Infect. Immunity 32*:86-91.
39. Crawford, Y. E. (1960). Studies of a complement-fixing antigen from group A streptococcal L-forms. I. Preparation and preliminary tests in rabbits and man. *J. Immunol. 84*:86-92.
40. Crawford, Y. E. (1962). Studies of a complement fixing antigen from group A streptococcal L-forms. II. Antibody reactions of naval recruits in streptococcal outbreaks and acute rheumatic fever. *J. Immunol. 89*:698-708.
41. Lynn, R. J. and Mellenberg, M. B. (1965). Immunological properties of an L-form of a group A beta hemolytic streptococcus. *Antonie van Leeuwenhoek 31*:15-24.

42. Lynn, R. J. and Haller, G. J. (1968). Bacterial L-forms as immunogenic agents in *Microbial Protoplasts, Spheroplasts, and L-forms* (L. B. Guze, ed.), Williams & Wilkins, Baltimore, pp. 270–278.
43. James, A. M., Hill, M. J., and Maxted, W. R. (1965). A comparative study of the bacterial cell wall, protoplast membrane and L-form envelope of *Streptococcus pyogenes*. *Antonie van Leeuwenhoek 31*:423–432.
44. Kanazawa, H. and Wu, H. C. (1979). Lipoprotein synthesis in *Escherichia coli* spheroplasts: accumulation of lipoprotein in cytoplasmic membrane. *J. Bacteriol. 137*:818–823.
45. Markowitz, A. S. and Lange, Jr., C. F. (1964). Streptococcal related glomerulonephritis. I. Isolation, immunochemistry and comparative chemistry of soluble fractions from type 12 nephritogenic streptococci and human glomeruli. *J. Immunol. 92*:565–575.
46. Feinman, S. B., Prescott, B., and Cole, R. (1973). Serological reactions of glycolipids from streptococcal L-forms. *Infect. Immunity 8*:752–756.
47. DeVuono, J. and Panos, C. (1974). Effect of L-form, *Streptococcus pyogenes* and of lipoteichoic acid on human cells in tissue culture. *Infect. Immunity 22*:255–265.
48. Patriarca, P., Beckerdite, S., and Elsbach, P. (1972). Phospholipase and phospholipid turnover in *Escherichia coli* spheroplasts. *Biochim. Biophys. Acta 260*:593–600.
49. Forsberg, C. W. and Ward, J. B. (1972). N-acetylmuramyl-L-alanine amidase of *Bacillus licheniformis* and its L-form. *J. Bacteriol. 110*:878–888.
50. Fukui, Y., Nachbar, M. S., and Salton, M. R. J. (1971). Immunological properties of *Micrococcus lysodeikticus* membranes. *J. Bacteriol. 105*:86–92.
51. Whiteside, T. L. and Salton, M. R. J. (1970). Antibodies to adenosine triphosphatase from membranes of *Micrococcus lysodeikticus*. *Biochemistry 9*:3034–3040.
52. Freimer, E. H., Krause, R. M., and McCarty, M. (1957). Studies of L-forms and protoplasts of group A streptococci. I. Isolation, growth, and bacteriologic characteristics. *J. Exp. Med. 110*:853–874.
53. Haller, G. J. and Lynn, R. J. (1968). The response observed in rabbits following implantation of diffusion chambers containing L-forms of group A beta hemolytic streptococcus in *Microbial Protoplasts, Spheroplasts, and L-forms* (L. B. Guze, ed.), Williams & Wilkins, Baltimore, pp. 352–355.
54. Hryniewicz, W. (1977). Streptococcal L-forms and some of their properties in *Spheroplasts, Protoplasts, and L-forms of Bacteria* (J. Roux, ed.), Vol. 64, Ed. INSERM, Paris, pp. 39–56.
55. Akema, R., Okazaki, N., Ono, A., and Miyamoto, Y. (1977). Production of streptolysin S by L-form organisms induced from a strain of group A streptococcus. *Jpn. J. Med. Sci. Biol. 30*:46–47.
56. Hryniewicz, W. and Tagg, J. R. (1976). Bacteriocin production by group A streptococcal L-forms. *Antimicrob. Agents Chemother. 10*:912–914.

57. Fernandes, P. B. and Panos, C. (1976). Persistence, pathogenesis and morphology of an L-form of *Streptococcus pyogenes* adapted to physiological isotonic conditions when in immunosuppressed mice. *Infect. Immun. 14*: 1228-1240.
58. Maruyama, Y., Sugai, S., and Egami, R. (1959). Formation of streptolysin S by streptococcal protoplasts. *Nature 811*:832.
59. Kalmanson, G. M., Hubert, E. G., and Guze, L. B. (1970). Effect of bacteriocin from *Streptococcus faecalis* on microbial L-forms. *J. Infect. Dis. 121*: 311-315.
60. Smith, J. A. and Willis, A. T. (1967). Some physiological characters of L-forms of *Staphylococcus aureus*. *J. Path. Bact. 94*:359-365.
61. Simon, H. J. and Yin, E. J. (1970). Penicillinase studies on L-phase variants, G-phase variants and reverted strains of *Staphylococcus aureus*. *Infect. Immun. 2*:644-654.
62. Braude, A. I. and Siemienski, J. (1968). Production of bladder stones by L-forms. *Trans. Assoc. Amer. Phys. 81*:323-331.
63. Rosenstein, I. J., Hamilton-Miller, J. M., and Brumfitt, W. (1981). Role of urease in the formation of infection stones: Comparison of ureases from different sources. *Infect. Immun. 32*:32-37.
64. Scheibel, I. and Assandri, J. (1959). Isolation of toxigenic L-phase variants from *Cl. tetani*. *Acta. Pathol. Microbiol. Scand. 46*:333-338.
65. Mahony, D. E. (1977). Stable L-forms of *Clostridium perfringens*: growth, toxin production, and pathogenicity. *Infect. Immun. 15*:19-25.
66. Kanei, C., Uchida, T., and Yoneda, M. (1977). Toxin production by strain C7 (beta); its mutants and their L-phase variants of *Corynebacterium diphtheriae*. *Jpn. J. Med. Sci. Biol. 30*:39-40.
67. Edward, D. G. and Fitzgerald, W. A. (1954). Inhibition of growth of pleuropneumonia-like organisms by antibody. *J. Path. Bact. 68*:23-30.
68. Agarwal, S. C. and Ganguly, N. K. (1972). Experimental oral immunization with L-forms of *Vibrio cholerae*. *Infect. Immun. 5*:31-34.
69. Agarwal, S. C. and Ganguly, N. K. (1972). Oral immunization with L-forms of *Vibrio cholerae* in human volunteers. *Infect. Immun. 6*:17-20.
70. Majumdar, A. S., Dutta, P., Dutta, D., and Ghose, A. C. (1981). Antibacterial and antitoxin responses in serum and milk of cholera patients. *Infect. Immun. 32*:1-8.
71. Majumdar, A. S. and Ghose, A. C. (1981). Evaluation of the biological properties of different classes of human antibodies in relation to cholera. *Infect. Immun. 32*:9-14.
72. Kagan, G., Gusman, B., Vulfovitch, Yu., and Besouglova, T. (1977). Group A streptococcal L-forms as a trigger of immuno-morphological changes of the heart and immunogenic organs in *Spheroplasts, Protoplasts and L-forms of Bacteria* (J. Roux, ed.), Vol. 64, Ed. INSERM, Paris, pp. 259-264.
73. Mauss, H. and Schmitt-Slomska, J. (1977). Changes due to streptococcal L-forms in parathymic lymph nodes and in the spleen of the mouse in *Spheroplasts, Protoplasts, and L-forms of Bacteria* (J. Roux, ed.), Vol. 64, Ed. INSERM, Paris, pp. 345-354.

74. Ratnam, S. and Chandrasekhar, S. (1976). The pathogenicity of spheroplasts of *Mycobacterium tuberculosis*. *Am. Rev. Resp. Dis.* 114:549–554.
75. Agarwal, S. C. and Sundararaj, T. (1976). Cell-mediated immunity to *Vibrio cholerae* with ribonucleic acid-protein fractions of *V. cholerae* L-form lysates. *Infect. Immun.* 14:363–367.
76. Agarwal, S. C. and Sundararaj, T. (1977). Cell mediated immunity after oral immunization with ribonucleic acid-protein fractions of *Vibrio cholerae* L-form lysates. *Infect. Immun.* 16:527–530.
77. Adams, D. O. (1976). The granulomatous inflammatory response. *Am. J. Pathol.* 84:164–192.
78. Orr, M. M., Tamarind, D. L., Cook, J., Fincham, W. J., Hawley, P. R., Quilliam, J. P., and Irving, M. H. (1974). Preliminary studies on the response of rabbit bowel to intramural injections of L-form bacteria. *Br. J. Surg.* 61:921.
79. Beaman, B. L. (1981). L-forms of Nocardia pathogenic for mice. *Abstr. Ann. Meeting, Am. Soc. Microbiol. 1981*:76.
80. Beaman, B. L. (1980). Induction of L-phase variant of *Nocardia caviae* within intact murine lungs. *Infect. Immun.* 29:244–251.
81. Takada, H., Hirachi, Y., Hashizume, H., and Kontani, J. (1980). Mitogenic activity of cytoplasmic membranes isolated from L-forms of *Staphylococcus aureus*. *Microbiol. Immunol.* 24:1079–1090.
82. Forsgren, A., Svedjelund, A., and Wigzell, H. (1976). Lymphocyte stimulation by protein A of *Staphylococcus aureus*. *Eur. J. Immunol.* 6:207–213.
83. Ringden, O. and Rynnel-Dagoo, B. (1978). Activation of human B and T lymphocytes by protein A of *Staphylococcus aureus*. *Eur. J. Immunol.* 8:47–52.
84. Knox, K. W. and Wicken, A. J. (1973). Immunological properties of teichoic acids. *Bacteriol. Rev.* 37:215–257.
85. Beachey, E. H., Dale, J. B., Grebe, S., Ahmed, A., Simpson, W. A., and Ofek, I. (1979). Lymphocyte binding and T cell mitogenic properties of group A streptococcal lipoteichoic acid. *J. Immunol.* 122:189–195.
86. Miller, G. A. and Jackson, R. W. (1973). The effect of *Streptococcus pyogenes* teichoic acid on the immune response of mice. *J. Immunol.* 110:148–156.
87. Cook, J. and Fincham, W. J. (1969). The effect of streptococcal L-form cultures on lymphocytes. *Life Sci.* 8:357–361.
88. Taranta, A., Cuppari, G., and Quagliata, F. (1969). Dissociation of hemolytic and lymphocyte transforming activities of streptolysin S preparations. *J. Exp. Med.* 129:605–622.
89. Nauciel, C. (1973). Mitogenic activity of purified streptococcal erythrogenic toxin on lymphocytes. *Ann. Immunol.* 124:383–390.
90. Barsumian, E. L., Schlievert, P. M., and Watson, D. W. (1978). Nonspecific and specific immunological mitogenicity by group A streptococcal pyrogenic exotoxin. *Infect. Immun.* 22:681–688.
91. Peavy, D. L., Shands, J. W., Adler, Jr., W. H., and Smith, R. T. (1973). Mitogenicity of bacterial endotoxin: characterization of the mitogenic principle. *J. Immunol.* 111:352–357.

92. Prosorovsky, S., Kotljarova, J., Fedotova, I., and Bakulov, I. (1977). Pathogenicity of listerial L-forms in *Spheroplasts, Protoplasts, and L-forms of Bacteria* (J. Roux, ed.), Vol. 64, Ed. INSERM, Paris, pp. 265-272.
93. Miller, G. A., Urban, J., and Jackson, R. W. (1976). Effect of a streptococcal lipoteichoic acid on host responses in mice. *Infect. Immun. 13*: 1408-1417.
94. Finger, H., Fresenius, H., and Angerer, M. (1971). Bacterial endotoxins as immunosuppressive agents. *Experientia 27*:456-458.
95. Hanna, E. E. and Watson, D. W. (1968). Host parasite relationships among group A streptococci. IV. Suppression of antibody response by streptococcal pyrogenic exotoxin. *J. Bacteriol. 95*:14-21.

13
Interaction of Cell Wall-Defective Bacteria with Host Defenses

ZELL A. McGEE
Department of Medicine, Center for Infectious Diseases, University of Utah School of Medicine, Salt Lake City, Utah

I. Introduction	277
II. Osmotic Effects of Host Environments	278
III. Interaction with Serum Factors	279
IV. Interaction with Phagocytic Cells	281
V. Environments Theoretically Favorable to Cell Wall-Defective Variants	283
VI. Conclusions	284
References	284

I. INTRODUCTION

Most bacteria that are pathogenic for humans can be induced under appropriate conditions in vitro to undergo profound morphologic change and to multiply with defective cell walls [1–4]. These cell wall-defective bacteria (e.g., L-forms, L-phase variants [4]) are indifferent to the presence of cell wall-active antimicrobials such as penicillin, are undetectable by routine clinical microbiologic techniques, and are capable of reverting to the original bacterium when the inducing agent (e.g., an antimicrobial) is withdrawn. Because of these characteristics, basic microbiologists and clinicians have been intrigued for years with the concept that bacteria might undergo transition to cell wall-defective forms in animal or human hosts and play a role in a variety of relapsing infections and chronic inflammatory diseases. There is compelling evidence that cell wall-defective bacteria are involved in infectious processes of some experimental animals (e.g., mice [5,6]) and in occasional patients with a variety of diseases (e.g., pyelonephritis [7], endocarditis [8], meningitis [9]). To date, there is no consensus that cell wall-defective bacteria regularly play a role in any infectious disease (see Chap. 14).

The theoretical transition of a bacterium to a cell wall-defective form (by action of its own autolytic enzymes, in response to host factors or in response to treatment with a cell wall-active antimicrobial) has often been assumed to enhance the potential of the microbe for survival in the host. This is likely to be true, however, only if the cell wall-defective bacterium is less susceptible than its bacterial parent to the host's antibacterial defense mechanisms. An examination of the interaction of cell wall-defective bacteria with host defenses may help predict whether or not it is to the advantage of a bacterium to exist in a cell wall-defective form in vivo. The presence or absence of this advantage determines in large part the likelihood that cell wall-defective variants occur in vivo. In addition, knowledge of which cell wall-defective bacteria best avoid host defenses and which sites in the body have the least number of operative host defenses can help predict the most likely species of bacteria to produce cell wall-defective forms in vivo and where these variants are likely to be found. Such information should be of great value in designing experiments to examine the role of cell wall-defective bacteria in naturally occurring infections.

II. OSMOTIC EFFECTS OF HOST ENVIRONMENTS

The formation of cell wall-defective variants in vitro has usually required that the osmotic pressure of the medium balance or exceed the internal osmotic pressure of the bacterium. Theoretically, if these conditions are not met, water moves from the external environment across the cytoplasmic membrane to the intracellular space of the bacterium which, lacking a rigid cell wall, distends and ruptures. It has been assumed by some authors that only the environment of the renal medulla, which is quite hypertonic (approximately 500 to over 1000 mOsm/kg of water, depending on the state of hydration) would provide sufficiently high osmotic pressure to provide stability to cell wall-defective variants. This is almost certainly not true. The internal osmotic pressure of gram-negative bacteria is 300-400 mOsm/kg and that of gram-positive bacteria 900 mOsm/kg or greater [10]. Osmotic pressures similar to those found inside gram-negative bacteria occur in normal human serum and in purulent exudates. Further, cell wall-defective variants have been shown to survive at osmolalities lower than those of their internal environment if their cytoplasmic membranes are stabilized by divalent cations, polyamines, or a change to a higher proportion of saturated fatty acids in the membrane [11]. Thus, strictly from the point of view of their osmotic stability, cell wall-defective variants of gram-negative bacteria theoretically could survive almost anywhere in the body, including the internal environment of human cells. Cell wall-defective variants of gram-positive bacteria might survive in the kidney and, if their cytoplasmic membranes were stabilized, in areas of lower osmotic pressure.

III. INTERACTION WITH SERUM FACTORS

A first line of defense against cell wall-defective variants in vivo is likely to be killing of these variants by normal human serum. Such serum is lethal to the cell wall-defective variants of a variety of gram-negative and gram-positive human

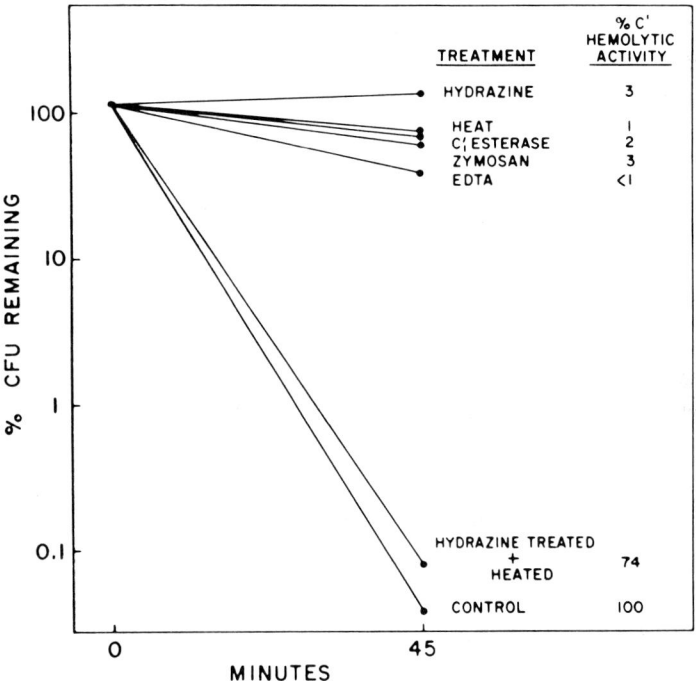

Figure 1 Effect of inactivation of complement by various treatments on the ability of normal human serum to kill L-phase variants of *Proteus mirabilis*. Hydrazine-treated serum (deficient in $C'4$) and heated serum (deficient in $C'1$ and $C'2$), though neither killed when used alone, had almost complete restoration of hemolytic complement activity and complete restoration of killing activity when mixed in proportions half those usually used in the incubation mixture. Untreated human serum was used as a control. The results of these experiments indicate that active complement is required for killing of L-phase variants by normal human serum. (From McGee et al. [12] by courtesy of the Journal of Infectious Diseases.)

pathogens which in their classical bacterial phase are not killed by serum [12]. These pathogens include *Salmonella typhi, Pseudomonas aeruginosa, Proteus mirabilis, Staphylococcus aureus, Streptococcus pyogenes,* and *Streptococcus faecalis* [13]. In a series of studies concerned with the mechanism of killing of cell wall-defective variants of bacteria by normal human serum under conditions in which the variants were osmotically stable, the killing was rapid and was accompanied by lysis and fragmentation of the cytoplasmic membrane [12]. Studies of the mechanism of killing indicated that serum deficient in lysozyme and β-lysin readily killed the variants. Thus, these factors were not essential to

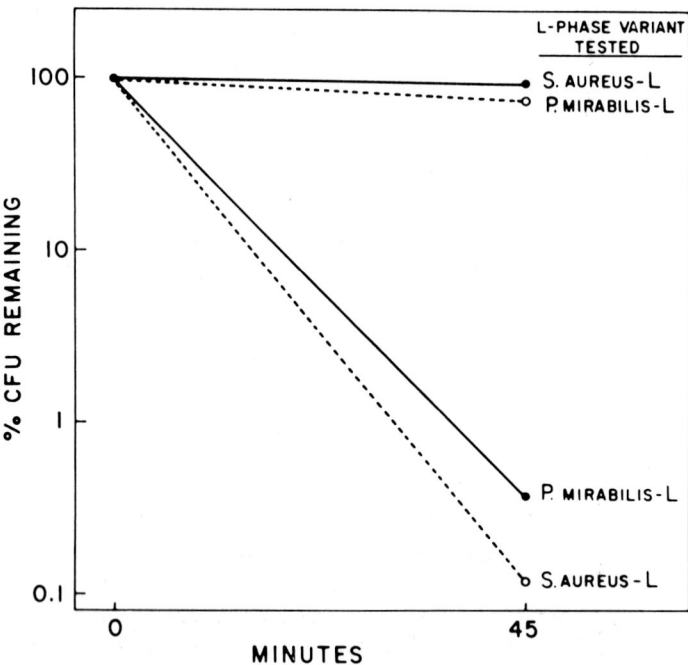

Figure 2 Effect of absorption with L-phase variants on the ability of normal human serum to kill variants of the same species or a species different from that used to absorb the serum. Serum absorbed with L-phase variants of *Proteus mirabilis* (o-----o); serum absorbed with L-phase variants of *Staphylococcus aureus* (●-----●). The sera were absorbed in a manner that maintained hemolytic complement activity. The results of these experiments indicate that an absorbable factor with at least some specificity, presumably specific antibody, is required in addition to complement activity, for killing of L-phase variants by normal human serum. (From McGee et al. [12] by courtesy of the Journal of Infectious Diseases.)

the lethal action of serum. In contrast, serum rendered free of hemolytic complement by a variety of methods did not kill cell wall-defective variants (Fig. 1). Serum absorbed with *P. mirabilis* L-phase variants under conditions that maintained complement activity failed to kill L-phase variants of *P. mirabilis* but did kill the L-phase variants of *S. aureus* (Fig. 2). Serum absorbed with *S. aureus* L-phase variants failed to kill L-phase variants of *S. aureus* but did kill the L-phase variants of *P. mirabilis*. This suggested that in addition to complement, specific antibody was required for killing. Indeed, combining specifically absorbed serum as a source of complement with IgM or IgG as sources of antibody (although none of these alone killed L-phase variants) restored killing activity comparable to that of normal human serum. Killing of *P. mirabilis* L-phase variants was greatest with complement plus IgM, and killing of *S. aureus* L-phase variants was greatest with complement plus IgG. Therefore the serum system lethal for cell wall-defective variants is comprised of the classical complement pathway plus primarily IgG, IgM, or both, depending on the species of the cell wall-defective variant [12].

The presence in normal human serum of antibodies to cell wall-defective variants does not necessarily mean that humans normally have contact with L-phase variants. Such antibodies could theoretically be elicited by the cytoplasmic membrane or other antigens held in common by L-phase variants and the classical bacterial phase of the organism.

Studies of the alternative complement pathway with L-phase variants of *S. aureus* and *S. faecalis* indicated that both were able to activate the pathway and consume C3 in C4-deficient guinea pig serum. Activation of the alternative pathway resulted in death of the L-phase variants [14]. Thus the alternative complement pathway, which is present in normal serum, may also be a host defense against cell wall-defective variants.

Animals immunized or infected with cell wall-defective variants develop antibodies that inhibit the growth of these organisms [15,16]. These growth-inhibiting antibodies, which may also be elicited by the classical bacterial phase, are not complement-requiring and appear to be directed at antigens in the cytoplasmic membrane. Neither the nature of these growth-inhibiting antibodies nor their mode of action is well characterized. Also, there is virtually no information regarding how often such antibodies are present in the serum of patients with chronic infections.

IV. INTERACTION WITH PHAGOCYTIC CELLS

The interaction of cell wall-defective variants with host cells in acute inflammatory exudates—polymorphonuclear (PMN) leukocytes—has only been studied in a limited way. In quantitative studies comparing results with parent bacteria and those with cell wall-defective variants, the parent bacteria more readily attracted

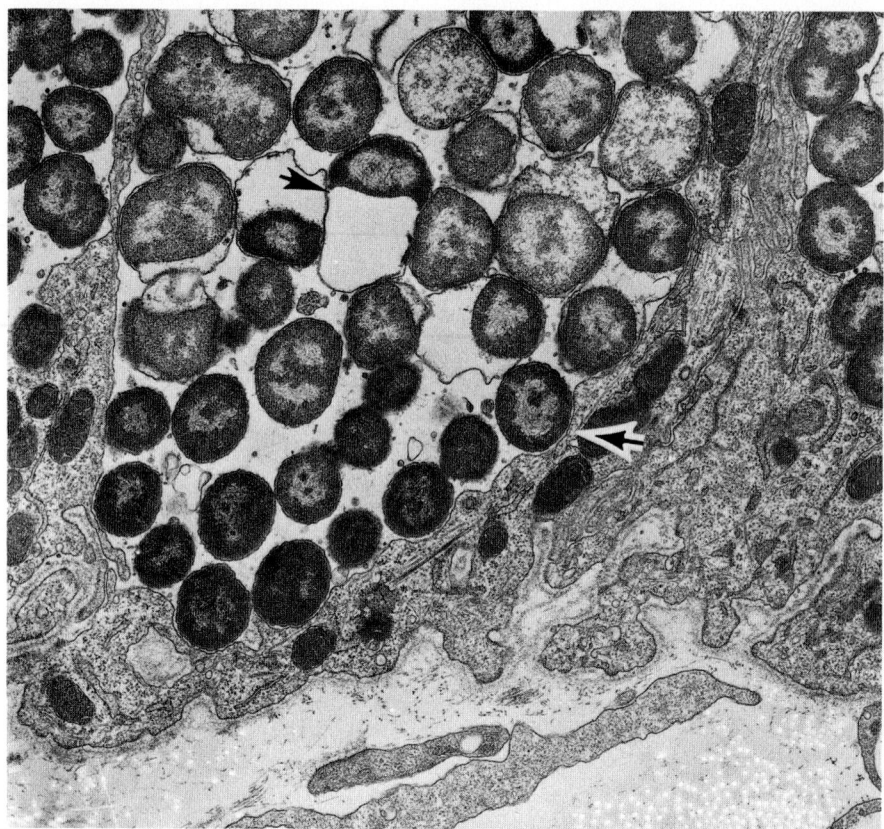

Figure 3 Transmission electron micrograph showing a phagocytic vacuole at the base of a nonciliated cell in the epithelium of human Fallopian tube mucosa in organ culture. The organ culture was infected 48 hr previously with a piliated, transparent colony type of *Neisseria gonorrhoeae*. The lamina propria and subepithelial tissues are in the lower quarter of the photo. The gonococci attach specifically to microvilli of nonciliated cells during the first 24 hr of the infection and are phagocytized during the second 24 hr of the infection. There is no apparent fusion of lysosomal granules to the vacuole and viable gonococci can be recovered from the tissues. Some gonococci in the vacuoles maintain normal morphology with intact cell walls (white-outlined arrow). A majority of the gonococci in the vacuoles have separation of the apparently still intact outer membrane from most of the circumference of the organism with disappearance of the peptidoglycan layer (black arrow). The ultrastructural appearance of the latter gonococci is identical to that of gonococcal L-phase variants induced on hypertonic medium by penicillin.

PMN leukocytes and were more readily phagocytized than were cell wall-defective variants [17]. PMN leukocytes appear capable of phagocytizing cell wall-defective variants in fluid systems as well as in systems favoring surface phagocytosis. However, the requirements for optimal phagocytosis and the fate of phagocytized cell wall-defective variants are not clear.

A number of authors have presented evidence that cell wall-defective variants can be formed within macrophages, monocytes, or other cells in tissue culture [11,18,19]. This suggests the possibility that cell wall-defective variants might be able to form and reside for prolonged periods in certain cells in vivo—possibly to emerge later as significant pathogens.

It is possible that cells other than professional phagocytes might provide an intracellular environment in which bacteria could undergo transition to cell wall-defective variants and be protected from humoral and cellular host defenses. For instance, recent studies of the interaction of *Neisseria gonorrhoeae* with nonciliated cells of human Fallopian tube mucosa suggest that such cells might provide the gonococci a protective environment. Gonococci have been shown to attach specifically to the luminal surface of nonciliated cells of human Fallopian tube mucosa in organ culture and to be transported, inside phagocytic vacuoles, to the base of the cells. They reside within the phagocytic vacuoles at the base of the cells for varying periods of time and some of the organisms appear to undergo multiplication [20]. A majority of the organisms within the vacuoles have an appearance similar to that of gonococcal L-phase variants induced in vitro—there is separation of the outer membrane from the cytoplasmic membrane with absence of a detectable peptidoglycan layer (Fig. 3). Although a number of lines of evidence indicate that at least some of the intracellular gonococci are viable, it is not certain that the cell wall-defective forms are viable. This phenomenon deserves further study.

V. ENVIRONMENTS THEORETICALLY FAVORABLE TO CELL WALL-DEFECTIVE VARIANTS

The presence in normal human serum of the antibody-complement system lethal to cell wall-defective variants of both gram-positive and gram-negative bacteria suggests that such cell wall-defective variants are most likely to form and be able to survive in areas to which this and other humoral host defenses (e.g., the alternative complement pathway) do not have access or in which they are inactivated. The environment of the renal medulla seems most likely to favor survival of cell wall-defective variants. This is not necessarily true because the hyperosmolality of the renal medulla provides them osmotic stability. Most renal pathogens do not need the hypertonic environment. Rather, the high salt content of the renal medulla inhibits complement and may protect cell wall-defective variants from the lethal antibody-complement system.

Bacteria—especially those that have high autolytic activity and those with relatively low internal osmotic pressure—may have a greater potential for forming and surviving as cell wall-defective variants within certain professional or nonprofessional phagocytic cells. Within these cells the cell wall-defective variants are likely to have their osmotic requirements met and would likely be protected from serum factors and destructive phagocytic cells. Thus, the wall-defective variants of bacteria such as gonococci and meningococci seem ideally suited for study of their potential role in human disease.

VI. CONCLUSIONS

Despite a plethora of information about the isolation of cell wall-defective variants from one type of infection or another, there are few systematic studies of the interaction of host defenses with these microorganisms. There are many excellent research opportunities in this area. The information currently available about host defenses against cell wall-defective variants allows predictions concerning which diseases and which disease sites are most likely to yield important information about the role of cell wall-defective variants in infectious processes.

REFERENCES

1. McGee, Z. A. (1977). Cell wall-deficient bacteria in *CRC Handbook Series in Clinical Laboratory Science*, Section E: *Clinical Microbiology*, vol. I, (A. von Graevenitz, ed.), CRC Press, Cleveland, pp. 367–375.
2. Madoff, S. and Pachas, W. N. (1970). Mycoplasma and the L-forms of bacteria in *Rapid Diagnostic Methods in Medical Microbiology* (C. D. Graber, ed.), Williams & Wilkins, Baltimore, pp. 195–217.
3. Clasener, H. (1972). Pathogenicity of the L-phase of bacteria. *Ann. Rev. Microbiol.* 26:55–84.
4. McGee, Z. A., Wittler, R. G., Gooder, H., and Charache, P. (1971). Wall-defective microbial variants: Terminology and experimental design. *J. Infect. Dis.* 123:433–438.
5. Mortimer, E. A., Jr. (1967). The production of L-forms of group A streptococci in mice in *Microbial Protoplasts, Spheroplasts and L-forms* (L. B. Guze, ed.), Williams & Wilkins, Baltimore, pp. 345–351.
6. Beaman, B. L. and Scates, S. M. (1981). Role of L-forms of *Nocardia caviae* in the development of chronic mycetomas in normal and immunodeficient murine models. *Infect. Immun.* 33:893–907.
7. Gutman, L. T., Shaller, J., and Wedgewood, R. J. (1967). Bacterial L-forms in relapsing urinary-tract infection. *Lancet* i:464–466.
8. Wittler, R. G., Malizia, W. F., Kramer, P. E., Tuckett, J. D., Pritchard, H. N., and Baber, H. J. (1960). Isolation of corynebacterium and its transitional forms from a case of subacute bacterial endocarditis treated with antibiotics. *J. Gen. Microbiol.* 23:315–333.

9. Louria, D. B., Kaminski, T., Grieco, M., and Singer, J. (1969). Aberrant forms of bacteria and fungi found in blood or cerebrospinal fluid. *Arch. Intern. Med. 124*:39–48.
10. Razin, S. and Argaman, M. (1963). Lysis of mycoplasma, bacterial protoplasts, spheroplasts and L-forms by various agents. *J. Gen. Microbiol. 30*: 155–172.
11. Leon, O. and Panos, C. (1976). Adaptation of an osmotically fragile L-form of *Streptococcus pyogenes* to physiological osmotic conditions and its ability to destroy human heart cells in tissue culture. *Infect. Immun. 13*: 252–262.
12. McGee, Z. A., Ratner, H. B., Bryant, R. E., Rosenthal, A. S., and Koenig, M. G. (1972). An antibody-complement system in human serum lethal to L-phase variants of bacteria. *J. Infect. Dis. 125*:231–242.
13. McGee, Z. A., Ratner, H. B., and Koenig, M. G. (1971). Media exchange method for demonstrating killing of L-phase variants in solid media by normal human serum. *Infect. Immun. 4*:237–239.
14. Saulsbury, F. T. and Winkelstein, J. A. (1979). Activation of the alternative complement pathway by L-phase variants of gram-positive bacteria. *Infect. Immun. 23*:711–716.
15. Kagan, G. Y. (1967). The results of some comparative experimental investigations of L-forms of bacteria and mycoplasma. *Ann. N.Y. Acad. Sci. 143*: 734–748.
16. Lynn, R. J. and Haller, G. J. (1967). Bacterial L-forms as immunogenic agents in *Microbial Protoplasts, Spheroplasts and L-forms* (L. B. Guze, ed.), Williams & Wilkins, Baltimore, pp. 270–278.
17. Harwick, H. J., Barajas, L., Montgomerie, J. Z., Kalmanson, G. M., and Guze, L. B. (1972). Phagocytoses of microbial L-forms. *Infect. Immun. 5*: 976–981.
18. Hatten, B. A. and Sulkin, S. E. (1966). Intracellular production of *Brucella* L forms. II. Induction and survival of *Brucella abortus* L forms in tissue culture. *J. Bacteriol. 91*:14–20.
19. Thacore, H. and Willett, H. P. (1966). The formation of spheroplasts of *Mycobacterium tuberculosis* in tissue culture cells. *Am. Rev. Resp. Dis. 93*: 786–796.
20. McGee, Z. A. and Horn, R. G. (1979). Phagocytosis of gonococci by nonprofessional phagocytic cells in *Microbiology–1979* (D. Schlessinger, ed.), American Society for Microbiology, Washington, pp. 158–161.

14

L-Forms and Bacterial Variants in Infectious Disease Processes

WILLIAM N. PACHAS
Department of Medicine, Spaulding Rehabilitation Hospital and Harvard Medical School, Boston, Massachusetts

I. Introduction	288
II. Experimental Evidence	289
A. L-Forms of Gram-Positive Bacteria	289
B. The Role of Streptococcal L-Forms in Experimental Infection	290
C. Listeria and *Erysipelothrix rhusiopathiae*	291
D. Experimental Infections with Staphylococcal L-Forms	293
E. L-Forms in Brucellosis	294
F. Experimental Studies with Gram-Negative Bacteria L-Forms	295
G. Experimental Urinary Tract Infections	295
H. Experimental Studies with Salmonella L-Forms	296
I. Other Studies on Mechanisms of L-Form Pathogenicity	297
III. L-Forms in Human Infections: The Clinical Evidence	299
A. Evidence for the Role of L-Forms in Urinary Tract Infections	300
B. L-Forms from Blood Isolates	301
C. L-Forms in Rheumatic Fever	305
IV. L-Form Infections in Other Sites	306
A. Staphylococcal Osteomyelitis	306
B. L-Forms in Central Nervous System Infections	307
C. L-Forms in Tuberculosis	307
D. L-Forms in Miscellaneous Conditions	308
E. Atypical Bacteria in Rheumatoid Arthritis	309
V. Summary and Conclusions	309
References	311

I. INTRODUCTION

Since the early studies by Louis Dienes [1-5], Kleineberger-Nobel [6,7], and others, the L-forms of bacteria have intrigued investigators because of their close resemblance to the mycoplasma and, since they are clearly derived from bacteria, many of them pathogens, their own potential for pathogenicity has been an important concern over the years. Historically, at one time or another, the L-forms of bacteria have either enjoyed acceptance as pathogens, or their etiologic role was promptly discarded when the experimental observations failed to reveal direct pathogenicity unless they first reverted to the parent bacterium. In all fairness, however, the arguments presented for or against their function as etiologic agents were limited by important difficulties in the study of cultures, and by the rather crude experimental approaches in which the L-forms were used as infecting agents. Previous reviews on the subject have pointed out some of the problems that the clinical investigator and the experimental pathologist must overcome, in order to interpret properly the clinical and histologic findings thought to be connected with the isolation of bacterial L-forms [4,8-15].

A brief discussion of the present concept of the biology of bacteria as it concerns the production of L-forms may provide some basis for understanding the state of the art in this interesting and important field.

Because of natural influences or laboratory manipulations, bacteria can be induced to lose their cell wall or a part of it, and may then survive with new biologic properties—at least during growth in artificial media. The reproductive process and growth characteristics of the L-forms of bacteria were originally described in the pioneering work by Dienes and Madoff [1,2,16].

Other forms of bacterial growth, different from that of the intact bacterium, have also been identified and given varied designations such as bacterial protoplasts, bacterial variants, spheroplasts, and cell wall-defective bacteria. These forms represent different stages of bacterial cell wall alteration brought about by cell wall-active antibiotics, by components of the culture media used for their isolation such as high osmolality, or by cell wall injury induced by host tissue factors such as lytic complement, antibody, lysozyme, and other humoral elements (Chap. 1). Eventually, these bacterial variants resume their typical morphology upon subcultivation. The term "protoplast" refers to the wall-less bacterium that is obtained by treating the bacteria with lysozyme in a hyperosmolar environment. The protoplasts thus obtained have the dual potential to either become L-forms or to revert to bacteria.

This wide range of biologic possibilities by bacteria are important at the same time that they are perplexing. Their ability to survive and reproduce, with cell wall modifications ranging from absence to all intermediate states of cell wall reconstruction, is remarkable and unique. Moreover, the possibility of stabilizing a bacterial variant at a certain state of cell wall reconstruction, or in a wall-less state, offers interesting opportunities to study their new physiologic state and their biologic potential as infectious agents.

Whether the L-forms represent a true phase in the life of the bacteria, or whether they are merely laboratory artifacts, remains an unsettled issue. It should be emphasized, however, that there are bacteria in nature such as the *Streptobacillus moniliformis*, capable of a spontaneous bidirectional life cycle going from bacteria to L-forms and vice-versa [1,4]. This property may also be seen in other bacteria when they are subject to environmental or immunologic injury that may threaten their survival [2]. In the process, the generation of these variant forms within a given host could lead to produce toxic or immunologic reactions of pathogenic significance. With this background, the existing evidence for the role of L-forms and bacterial variants in animal and human pathology will be reviewed briefly.

II. EXPERIMENTAL EVIDENCE

A. L-Forms of Gram-Positive Bacteria

Most organisms in this group require media of high osmolarity enriched with nutrients for the production of L-forms, together with the presence of an inducing agent such as a β-lactam antibiotic. The conditions for L-form induction and growth are thus fairly strict, and any adaptation to media of lower osmolarity or lesser nutrients usually requires a careful and stepwise manipulation of the cultures [4]. This adaptation process may fail however, resulting in the loss of viability of the L-forms.

These experimental facts in the laboratory may or may not have a parallel in clinical or experimental in vivo situations, and they need not follow the same process (although to my knowledge there is no information on the in vivo adaptation of L-forms). Some animal studies with L-forms of gram-positive bacteria cultivated in hyperosmolar media may have been unsuccessful because they did not take into account their need for slow adaptations. However, when pathogenicity was observed following the parenteral administration of L-forms, the pathology was most probably due to the revertant bacterial form and not to the L-form itself; there are exceptions to this concept, especially with some recent studies that clearly suggest a direct pathogenic role for the L-forms [17].

Given the possibility that live L-forms are successful in adapting to a host, they may then establish either a reproductive cycle resulting in immediate pathology or a latent state that, depending on opportunity, may exert a pathogenic role at a later time. If the L-form state could be maintained as such for appropriate periods of time, one could more objectively and specifically determine the role of L-forms in pathogenicity, albeit this is a difficult proposition; some recent experimental work notably that of Beaman et al. with *Nocardia caviae* [17], demonstrates the pathogenicity of the nocardia L-forms in mice as they transform from the vegetative form to the wall-less state at the height of the pneumonic process. This suggests that the pulmonic lesions were caused by the nocardia L-forms. This kind of evidence deserves further investigation in relation to the pathophysiology of the tissue injury.

B. The Role of Streptococcal L-Forms in Experimental Infection

The role of streptococcal L-forms in conditions such as rheumatic fever and glomerulonephritis has been pursued intensely over the years. Ginsburg has classified the types of tissue lesions that are elicited by streptococcal antigens, including the streptococcal L-forms, in a diversity of animal models [18]. The immune system has a primordial role in the production of histologic lesions because of the presence of cross-reactive streptococcal and human tissue antigens with specific anti-streptococcal antibodies that may cause the characteristic lesions of rheumatic fever in the heart and joints and of glomerulonephritis in the kidneys [18].

Earlier studies with tissue cultures failed to show pathogenicity of streptococcal L-forms by morphologic criteria, in spite of the fact that the L-forms could be recovered in viable state for as long as 270 days [18]. In the experiments by DeVuono and Panos [19] (see Panos, this volume) with a stable streptococcal L-form that had been adapted to growth in media of normal osmolarity, the L-forms demonstrated the ability to kill human embryonic kidney and liver tissue culture cells via the toxic effect of the lipid component of lipoteichoic acid that was secreted in the tissue culture medium. These authors also demonstrated constitutional modifications in the cell proteins that were induced by infection with the streptococcal L-forms. The organisms persisted in the tissue cultures while the pathologic changes were taking place. Iesmantaite et al. have shown that streptococcal L-forms adhere to the surface of human lymphocytes and to red blood cells of human and various animal species [20]. The attachment of L-forms to lymphocytes may bear some significance in relation to modulations or stimulations of the immune response of the activated lymphocytes.

The work of Kagan and collaborators [21,22] revealed the surprising mobility of the streptococcal L-forms and their antigens within the cytoplasm of "reactive" cells. The site of localization of the antigens changed from intracellular to extracellular in relation to the progression of the cardiac lesions and with the various degrees of disease activity that occurred over the length of the study. L-forms were actually detected within areas of the myocardium adjacent to collagen tissue, and reactive changes in the thymus and in the lymph nodes were also described.

Gusman recently showed progressive tissue changes in cardiac valves and membranes that were induced by the intraperitoneal injection of Group A β-hemolytic streptococcal L-forms in mice [23]. Streptococcal antigens were identified by immunofluorescence in the tissues up to 1 year. Recovery of live L-forms was apparently not successful, suggesting that streptococcal antigens per se may have induced the tissue changes. Moreover, the work of Matsunaga et al. further supports this view; in experiments using extracts of cytoplasmic membranes of streptococcal L-forms they were able to produce pericarditis and myocarditis in mice [24]. Iesmantaite et al. [25] elicited rheumatic fever-like lesions in the cardiac valves and in the myocardium of rabbits injected with hemolytic streptococcal L-forms placed in intraperitoneal chambers. L-forms were isolated from the blood and from the chambers for as long as 15 days, and a low-titer serum antibody response to the L-forms was detected throughout.

Crude extracts of Group A streptococcus induced rheumatic fever-like lesions in the myocardium of mice [26]. Similar extracts were found to adsorb to the sarcolemmal sheaths and to the glomerular basement membrane in vitro. Antisera prepared against the streptococcal cytoplasmic membranes had greater reactivity to the cardiac tissue-bound streptococcal products than antisera prepared against cell wall material [27].

These studies seem to point out the existence of an affinity of live and prepared streptococcal membrane antigens for cardiac tissues and their interplay with the immune system to elicit inflammatory tissue injury and reactive scarring in the cardiac valves, kidneys, and in other tissues such as the synovial membrane [28].

C. Listeria and *Erysipelothrix rhusiopathiae*

Early in vivo studies with *Listeria monocytogenes* L-forms failed to show any pathogenicity unless it was caused by the revertant bacteria. Prosorovsky et al. [29], working with listeria L-forms induced on high salt media with penicillin, demonstrated absence of pathogenicity in the chicken embryo and guinea pig. However, in rabbits and lambs, the L-forms produced a picture characterized by encephalomyelitis, liver disease, and peripheral monocytosis. In all respects, this illness resembled the parent bacterial disease, although bacteria were not recovered. Another interesting finding was the marked involution of the lymphoid tissue and of the bone marrow in animals that developed central nervous system disease induced by the L-forms. Studies in tissue cultures showed wide heterogeneity of cytopathic effect, indicating possible biological differences of the various L-form cultures. Listeria L-form-induced disease thus appears to show many facets of pathology in need of further clarification, such as the pathogenesis of tissue damage, effects on the immune system, and biological variability of the L-forms.

Erysipelothrix rhusiopathiae is the agent that causes swine erysipelas, a disease characterized by skin lesions and a progressive form of chronic arthritis that resembles rheumatoid arthritis in many respects. Characteristically, during the acute phase of the arthritis, the bacteria can be easily isolated from the synovial fluid and tissues; in the chronic stages (usually after the fourth month of the illness) the recovery of the organisms occurs less frequently. Experimentally, *E. rhusiopathiae* arthritis has been produced in rats and rabbits not only with live [30-32] and whole dead organisms, but also with cell-free extracts [33,34]. Regardless of the route of inoculation (e.g., intravenous, intraarticular, or subcutaneous), an inflammatory synovitis with many of the features of rheumatoid arthritis is produced. The fact that the reaction invariably occurred in the joints suggests the existence of a tropism for the localization of the bacteria or of their products in the synovial tissue. Once the infection develops, and in spite of the presence of an appropriate antibody response, the synovial inflammation and proliferative reaction persist uninhibited and the course then tends to be progressive. It is also known that preimmunized animals become protected by IgG antibody [35] and immune macrophages effectively destroy virulent bacteria [36]. On the other hand, prior immunization may sensitize the animals to challenge with live organisms and cause more severe disease [37].

These immunologic events are important because they may be responsible for some pathologic changes involved with the production of the chronic synovitis. Moreover, it has been found that the animals are capable of producing an autoimmune response by forming anti IgG antibodies similar to the rheumatoid factor. These rheumatoid factor-like antibodies are predominantly found in the fluid of diseased joints and cannot be detected in the synovial fluid of the unaffected joints [38].

Agglutinating antibodies against *E. rhusiopathiae* also appear in lesser concentration than would be expected in relationship to the total increase in the protein of the fluid [39]. The possibility then exists that, in spite of the presence of specific agglutinins, the organisms survive in sufficient numbers to localize successfully in the synovial tissue. Assuming that the immune mechanism, including macrophages, is activated by the infection with *E. rhusiopathiae*, the failure to eradicate the infection may be due in part to an insufficient immune response and in part due to the development of blocking antibodies which, like the rheumatoid factor, may inactivate IgG antibodies with useful agglutinating activity.

Other mechanisms of bacterial opsonization may be affected by autoantibodies, and the activation of complement may be altered. The failure to activate lytic complement may also favor the persistence of the bacteria in the synovial tissue. It is also possible that the partially opsonized bacteria may be stripped of the cell wall and rendered viable in the form of protoplasts that, under the proper conditions, may initiate L-form growth. Toshkov et al. have apparently been successful in demonstrating L-forms of *E. rhusiopathiae* for up to 15 months in experimental animals. The presence of L-forms was documented by electronmicroscopy [40].

When *E. rhusiopathiae* L-forms are induced in vitro with penicillin in hyperosmolar medium and then allowed to revert, some of the revertants are capable of spontaneously transforming to L-forms in the presence of 2% sodium chloride in the medium [41]. If a process of alternating L-form inductions and reversions is maintained, mutants develop with the ability to transform into L-forms spontaneously even without addition of salt to the medium (our unpublished data). This property of *E. rhusiopathiae* in vitro may have relevance to the experimental and natural disease in animals, where successful L-form production and reversion to bacteria may possibly occur.

The appearance of mutants or variants may further diversify the immunologic response and lead to ineffective control of infection, eventually developing into the chronic infectious state that results in chronic arthritis. This possibility may have a parallel in experimental infection of mice with *Nocardia caviae* in which a similar process of L-form production followed by bacterial reversions may be the mechanism responsible for the production of mycetomas [42] (see Chap. 10). Changes in the cell wall composition of the bacterial revertants of *Nocardia asteroides* have been reported by the same group of investigators [43]. With the information available on the experimental disease with *E. rhusiopathiae*, there should be enough incentive to study the role of L-forms and bacterial revertants in the pathogenesis of chronic arthritis.

Without question, any progress in this area will be welcome by workers engaged in the study of infectious experimental models of rheumatoid arthritis. The difficulty of isolating organisms from the joints of diseased animals, and during the late stages of the arthritis, is puzzling and lends support to the possibility that L-forms of *E. rhusiopathiae* may be involved in the perpetuation of this inflammation. The study by Toshkov is relevant to this possibility; however, this work needs further confirmation. In another investigation [44], a highly sensitive technique of RNA-DNA hybridization failed to demonstrate the presence of *E. rhusiopathiae* in the synovial tissue of pigs affected with chronic arthritis. In that study, however, the cultures for *E. rhusiopathiae* were also negative and L-forms were not investigated [44].

D. Experimental Infections with Staphylococcal L-Forms

Contrasting evidence for the role of staphylococcal L-forms exists in the literature. Some workers have reported induction of experimental meningitis with staphylococcal L-forms in rabbits [45,46]. On the other hand, attempts to produce pyelonephritis in properly conditioned animals (rabbits were made hydronephrotic by treatment with oxamide) were unsuccessful [47]. In another experiment, rabbits were subjected to cardiac valvular damage by appropriate traumatic injury. A strain of stable staphylococcal L-forms failed to colonize these areas of aseptic endocarditis [48]. These studies suggest that perhaps some staphylococcal L-forms may lack pathogenicity for certain tissues such as heart and kidney, whereas other L-form strains may be virulent for the meninges. As with other organisms, the staphylococci seem to lose or at least partially lose pathogenicity after reversion from the L-form [49].

Cytoplasmic membranes and cytoplasmic fractions of staphylococcal L-forms produce a mitogenic effect on human lymphocytes. This stimulatory effect is apparently blocked by human serum [50]. It would be of interest to study the effect of staphylococcal L-forms on the function of lymphocytes in in vivo experiments.

E. L-Forms in Brucellosis

Natural brucellosis in man and animals tends to have a chronic and recurrent course (see Hatten and Schmitt-Slomska, this volume). The possibility of bacterial transformation to L-forms during the course of the infection has been invoked from time to time by observations made on clinical specimens from which brucella L-forms apparently were isolated [8]. This view, however, has not been supported by experimental data or by the in vivo demonstration of L-forms in human or animal hosts.

A more direct look into the mechanisms of bacterial survival in the host, and whether or not there is a pathogenic role for the L-forms as the source of chronicity, was shown by studies with penicillin-treated mice prior to infection with brucella cells. These experiments showed the appearance of L-form growth when spleen sections were inoculated onto agar medium. Stabilized L-forms were reinoculated into mice and were easily recovered again from the spleens of these animals. Electronmicrographs from these in vivo-induced L-forms grown on agar showed typical L-forms and protoplasts surrounded by lamellar structures suggestive of cell wall material loosely assembled around the protoplasts [51]. These findings support earlier work demonstrating the spontaneous transformation of brucella cells into L-forms in tissue cultures, and the enhancement of the L-form yield when penicillin was added to the system [52].

Other studies present evidence for the role of immune mechanisms as L-form inducers. Mouse bone marrow cells obtained from animals immunized with brucella antigen were cultivated with live brucella cells; the immunologically active cell clones either killed the vegetative brucella forms or triggered their conversion to L-forms, probably by degrading the bacterial cell wall [53]. In experiments with guinea pigs, the L-forms persisted for periods of up to 90 days, and produced mild to moderate lymphoreticular proliferation with significant enlargement of the lymph nodes, liver, and spleen, as well as some general toxicity to the animals [54].

It seems clear from these experiments that the brucella cells, either spontaneously or by the action of mechanisms disturbing cell wall synthesis such as antibiotics or antibodies, may be converted into L-forms in vivo or in tissue culture systems. These wall-less organisms appear capable of stimulating a lymphoproliferative response of unknown significance. One would wonder whether such lymphoreticular hyperplasia may in time merely produce a hyperimmune state, or cause a more fundamental change such as cell transformations of the type induced by certain viruses that cause lymphomas or leukemias in animals.

F. Experimental Studies with Gram-Negative Bacteria L-Forms

The induction of L-forms from gram-negative organisms is usually less complicated than from gram-positive bacteria, especially if one is working with *Proteus* and *Salmonella* spp. *E. coli, Klebsiella*, and other enterobacteriaceae are more fastidious and rarely produce L-forms that can be maintained in culture indefinitely. Usually there is no requirement for osmolar protection, and the nutritional requirements may be less strict. A number of inducing agents can be selected from among the β-lactam antibiotics, and specific antibody and complement may act as L-form inducers, as noted with *Salmonella* spp. [5]. Penicillin, unless used in large quantities, may fail to induce L-forms from gram-negative bacteria due to resistance of the organisms to the antibiotic. Substitution with semisynthetic penicillins or cephalosporins may obviate the difficulty.

Proteus spp. and sometimes *Salmonella* spp. develop L-forms quite readily, often within hours of their initial interaction with the inducing agent. The L-form colonies that result are of two types: (1) B type, those that show an ability to maintain a certain amount of organized cell-wall; (2) A type, L-forms that lose cell wall entirely and are surrounded merely by protoplastic membrane. The latter may be indistinguishable from mycoplasma by ultrastructural analysis [3]. Proteus L-forms revert easily to bacteria when the inducing agent is withdrawn from the environment. Salmonella and *E. coli* tend to produce stable L-forms of the A-type, that is, without a cell wall. The property of *Salmonella* spp. to transform to L-forms in the presence of specific antibody and complement may have relevance for some of the in vivo experimental infections and possibly for certain clinical situations. Pertinent data on experimental models of infection with gram-negative bacterial L-forms is now briefly reviewed.

G. Experimental Urinary Tract Infections

The enthusiasm for a study of the pathogenicity of L-forms in the urinary tract has been quite limited for the past several years and little new information has emerged. Nevertheless, the classical studies with experimental urinary tract infections are worth mentioning. Braude et al. [55,56] called attention to the fact that normal human urine of high osmolarity could spontaneously induce protoplasts or spheroplasts in *Proteus* spp., and that the number of protoplasts could be greatly increased by the addition of penicillin. They also noted that as long as the organisms were kept in an osmolarly protective environment they remained viable, but they rapidly lysed if they were transferred to hypotonic urine. In pathologic urine specimens, these authors were able to demonstrate the presence of spheroplasts of varous gram-negative bacteria which apparently had developed spontaneously in vivo. These organisms displayed the morphologic changes noted during L-form induction with penicillin, including elongation of the bacteria and the appearance of dilatations in the body of the cells and large body formation. In the study, however, no attempt was made to recover L-forms after filtration of both the urine specimens or of the sucrose media used for the in vitro experiments.

The role of *E. coli* variants was tested experimentally in rats [57]. These organisms had morphologic and colonial characteristics of L-forms that had been induced with penicillin in hyperosmolar media. They failed to produce any significant pathology in the kidneys of the experimental animals, in spite of the fact that they had an improved survival in kidney tissue when compared with their survival in spleen or liver. Furthermore, it was found that the local tissue response to the L-form variants, the media, and killed variants was exactly the same, including mild fibrosis and round cell infiltration. The limited experimental data thus far have not produced definitive proof of the pathogenic properties of the L-forms. Many studies have been aimed at merely recovering intermediate or variant forms in media of high osmolarity. The development of histologic lesions as a result of the presence of these organisms in the tissues has always raised the question as to whether the tissue damage or reaction is due to a true pathogenetic effect, or simply due to the deposition of foreign material that then triggers a local response. The demonstration of viable organisms in the tissues, with some degree of reproducible virulence, is therefore fundamental to ascribing pathogenetic properties to the L-forms.

H. Experimental Studies with Salmonella L-Forms

Dienes et al. first studied the effect of specific antibody and complement in *Salmonella typhi* and quite elegantly showed that the immunologic injury caused in the bacteria led to a sequence of morphologic changes beginning with swelling of the bacilli and formation of large round bodies from which small granules started to grow into the agar; after 3 days of incubation, typical L-form colonies appeared on the surface of the culture medium. These changes occurred without osmolar protection [5]. This dramatic discovery has been the source of multiple attempts to demonstrate the possible role of salmonella L-forms induced by immunologic mechanisms in chronic salmonellosis, as well as in the carrier state.

Russian investigators have presented experimental evidence of the in vivo transformation of *S. typhi* into L-forms, by using diffusion chambers introduced into animals that had been previously immunized with the same organism [58].

In other experiments, they were able to produce a chronic carrier state in rabbits, with recovery of L-forms for as long as 18 months postinfection. Presumably the transformation had been mediated by an immune reaction [59]. It is unclear, however, where and how the transformation from bacillus to L-forms took place. Kawakami et al. [60] carried out experiments in mice injected intravenously with either *Salmonella enteritidis* or *Salmonella typhimurium*. These animals produced osmotically dependent bacterial forms that were recovered from liver homogenates that grew in media containing 0.35 M sucrose, but not in the media without sucrose. The yield of this osmotically sensitive form increased when the experiments were conducted in previously immunized mice. Electronmicrographs from the liver cells showed the bacteria to be incorporated, within a few minutes of injection, in phagosomes of the Kupffer cells, and the bacteria appeared intact and had a normal thickness cell wall. After 5-12 hr, the propagating bacteria showed significant thinning of the cell wall, which probably represented a disturbance in the cell physiology with the production of a defective cell wall requiring osmolar protection for growth in the culture medium. These abnormal bacteria presumably resulted from cell wall injury induced by antibodies in the immunized animals, or from enzymatic damage from lysosomal enzymes.

Morphologically, the resulting cell wall-defective variants showed the characteristics of the type B L-forms. Stable A-type L-forms were not isolated and no attempt was made to recover organisms. Pathogenicity of salmonella L-forms has been studied in chick embryos infected with *S. typhimurium* L-forms [61]. Hemorrhagic plaques of the chorioallantoic membrane were detected, but after three passages, the L-forms were not able to cause the death of the embryos, perhaps suggesting that the L-forms had lost their initial pathogenicity. One must bear in mind that these experiments were not performed with in vivo-induced L-forms. The existence of natural mechanisms favoring the transformation of salmonella into L-forms in vivo appears now to be well established. Their significance in regard to the epidemiology of both the chronic state and the carrier state in the animal and human host requires further elucidation.

I. Other Studies on Mechanisms of L-Form Pathogenicity

One of the important properties of the L-forms relates to their ability to reconstruct cell wall and to reproduce bacteria with properties similar to those of the parent bacterium. These phenomena have been the subject of intense research with bacterial protoplasts [10]. Studies with L-form revertants have shown interesting problems. When the pathogenicity of revertants of *Klebsiella pneumoniae* L-forms was tested in mice, it was shown that even after 40 consecutive passages in the mice, the L-form revertants remained totally avirulent. The organisms, however, preserved their antigenicity and elicited protective antibodies against the virulent parent bacterium [62]. This study again demonstrates the loss of virulence by some organisms once they have passed through the L-form state; in some cases the avirulent state appears to be irreversible, raising the possibility of genetic alterations occurring concomitant with the temporary loss of the cell wall.

In contrast, L-form revertants from meningococcus strains preserved their virulence even after many passages in the L-form state; however, as long as the organisms remained as L-forms they did not demonstrate any pathogenicity [63]. Truly pathogenic L-forms appear to derive from bacteria that secrete toxins, such as *Clostridium tetani* and *Vibrio cholera* [2]. In addition, *Clostridium botulinum* L-forms have been shown to share the same property [64]. There are no ultrastructural studies to indicate that these organisms totally lack cell wall. In these cases, however, it appears that toxin secretion is independent of cell wall reconstruction.

Spheroplasts of *Mycobacterium tuberculosis* injected into guinea pigs may persist in the animals for prolonged periods of time, without eliciting either tuberculin hypersensitivity or tissue damage; only when reversion to bacilli occurs do the typical changes of tuberculous infection develop [65]. In this case, the retention of some cell wall components by these spheroplasts precluded neither the loss of virulence nor the loss of the ability of inducing tuberculin hypersensitivity.

In the disease pseudotuberculosis in mice [66], a corynebacterium with modified cell wall that survives in resistant animals in an avirulent state may become virulent when the animals are treated with a single injection of hydrocortisone. The bacterium lacks an M protein-like factor (which is present in the cell wall of the virulent strain), is deficient in some metabolic activities, produces tiny translucent colonies on agar, and structurally resembles the tiny G variant of *Corynebacterium diphtheriae*.

Proteus spheroplasts induced with penicillin were effectively phagocytized by human macrophages and at a higher rate than the normal bacteria [67]. The possibility that spheroplasts (or B type L-forms) may induce greater chemotactic activity than the parent bacterium on the human macrophages may reflect important species differences in terms of the behavior of phagocytic cells and their reactivity to different antigens.

There may also be species differences. Another study, using mouse peritoneal macrophages that did not phagocytize Proteus L-forms and various mycoplasmas, induced lysis of these organisms by secreting hydrolytic enzymes and the C3a component of complement [68]. In this context, it is relevant that intact L-forms of *Staphylococcus aureus* and *Streptococcus faecalis*, as well as their isolated membranes, can activate the alternate complement pathway [69]. The effect of these complement fractions on L-forms or mycoplasma in in vivo conditions is presently unknown. Other phagocytic cells, such as human polymorphonuclear leukocytes, offered yet another variant of response to the wall-less bacteria. In experiments with L-forms of *S. faecalis, E. coli,* and *P. mirabilis,* the granulocytes displayed decreased chemotactic response to these L-forms while still showing strong chemotaxis for the respective parent bacteria [70]. When tested for chemotactic activity against *Mycoplasma pneumoniae* and *Mycoplasma hominis,* the white blood cells were entirely indifferent.

The apparent loss of chemotactic inducing activity by some L-forms is an important issue and relevant to the possibility of L-forms surviving in a given host. The potential for inhibition of chemotactic activity, rather than the lack of stimulation to chemotaxis, should be addressed in future experiments. It would also be important to know what is the role of certain bacterial components, especially those located in the cell wall that may be lost during the process of transformation to L-forms, such as the enterobacterial common antigen [71]. The absence of this antigen in the L-forms of proteus or other enterobacteria may preclude the expression of chemotaxis stimulating activity by these organisms. Significant also is the formation of L-forms under the effect of peritoneal macrophages in vitro as noted in experiments with *Nocardia asteroides* [72]. Much work is needed before any conclusion can be drawn regarding the response to phagocytic cells from various species and of their interaction with L-forms or mycoplasmas. In addition, standardization of the techniques used for this type of study seems highly desirable.

III. L-FORMS IN HUMAN INFECTIONS: THE CLINICAL EVIDENCE

The advances made in this field have been presented in a number of monographs and review articles [8-13,15,73]. Most contributions were made in the 1960s and early 1970s, the time when the pioneering work of earlier investigators generated interest on the possible role of L-forms in infectious processes. This flurry of enthusiasm did not meet with the expected clinical success, and by the mid-1970s, progressive decline had set in. Consequently, little new material has been produced, and the role of the L-forms in disease remains as obscure now as it was 20 years ago. Many important questions are still pressing for answers. For instance, do these organisms have the potential to produce infection, and if so, what is the pathogenesis of such infection? Is the resultant pathology the consequence of an infection or of a special interaction between the L-forms and the immune mechanism causing changes in the lymphoreticular system that are of such a nature as to produce an autoimmune disease like rheumatoid arthritis? Are the L-forms recovered in cultures truly viable in the host, or are they the product of a rescue operation carried out by the hyperosmolar culture medium and, therefore, lacking any role as pathogenic agents? Without further clinical data, it is not possible to answer any of these questions conclusively. On the other hand, some experimental work substantiates the possibility that the L-forms may have a pathogenic role: Hence sufficient argument can be made to pursue the demonstration of potentially pathogenetic mechanisms of these modified bacteria in certain clinical conditions.

A. Evidence for the Role of L-Forms in Urinary Tract Infections

Because the kidney provides a hyperosmolar environment for protoplasts or L-forms to develop and reproduce in situ, almost two decades ago several investigators studied the problem of recurrent and chronic urinary tract infections in relation to the possible existence of cell wall-defective bacteria as the etiologic agent [74-76]. Two general conclusions can be drawn. The first concerns the isolation of bacterial protoplasts in urine specimens of patients with urinary tract infections. Because these forms are insensitive to cell wall-acting antibiotics, they may be a cause for recurrent infection after the drug is withdrawn. The second point concerns the presence of L-forms in the kidney itself as a probable cause of pyelonephritis. Studies dealing with the first issue suggest that during the active infection both protoplasts and regular bacteria can be identified in the urine; but during the asymptomatic periods, only protoplasts are found. These data are difficult to interpret. One cannot establish with certainty whether these atypical bacteria are actually lodged as such in the kidney and then shed to the lower urinary tract and urine, or whether they result from changes caused by the urine itself, or from parental bacteria remaining in the bladder. It could be argued that factors such as hypertonicity of the urine or lysozymes secreted by inflammatory cells and macrophages could induce changes in the bacterial cell wall leading to protoplast formation.

Another possibility concerns the local specific antibody response that is generated in the kidney against invasive bacteria. This immunologic reaction can be recognized by demonstration with the immunofluorescent technique, the bacterial coating antibody [77]. Such antibody response is not seen in infections of the lower urinary tract. One would wonder as to the role of antibodies in the generation of protoplasts in these urine specimens. However, there has been no description of bacterial protoplasts coated with antibody during the course of urinary tract infections.

In experimental attempts to produce pathology in the kidney with L-forms or protoplasts, the results have been disappointing, even in situations where protoplasts were said to have persisted in the kidney for prolonged periods of time. The clinical data, on the other hand have produced rather surprising findings. In one study where kidney biopsies were obtained from 25 human subjects at the time of surgery, seven specimens produced protoplasts and not L-forms in hyperosmolar media, and in five specimens bacteria were isolated. Evidence of pyelonephritis did not necessarily correlate with the presence of either protoplasts or bacteria in the kidneys. The most striking finding in this study was the nature of the protoplast isolates, that when fully reverted to bacteria were identified as *Staphylococcus aureus*, α-hemolytic streptococcus, *Staphylococcus epidermidis*, non-Group A β-hemolytic streptococci, and in one case, *Streptococcus faecalis* [78]. Of these bacteria, only the latter is recognized as a common urinary pathogen, and occasionally *S. aureus*. This study poses fundamental and intriguing questions as to the role of such isolates in the kidneys of patients with chronic pyelonephritis. Indeed one would have expected to find L-forms or protoplasts of gram-negative enteric flora, rather than of dubious renal pathogens such as gram-positive bacteria. It is also important to note that in the laboratory gram-negative enterobacteria usually do not require osmolar protection to produce L-forms; furthermore, the formation of protoplasts in vitro does not necessarily lead to the production of reproductive elements unless the protoplasts are allowed to transform into L-forms or revert to bacteria. For all practical purposes, protoplasts probably have very little potential for survival unless they are carefully preserved and properly primed into bacteria or L-forms [79]. At present, the relevance of L-forms to urinary tract infectious needs further emphasis. The rapid increase in the elderly population, for example, has brought about special situations that have become the cause of significant morbidity and mortality, e.g., development of various bladder malfunctions, use of catheters, etc. In addition, new antibiotics are being introduced constantly, and the appearance of bacteria with multiple antibiotic resistant patterns is an everyday phenomenon. The treatments are therefore quite difficult and not without risk for the patient. In this context one has to reexamine the role of some of the new antibiotics as facilitators of recurrent urinary tract infections by inducing L-forms in vivo followed by reversion to bacteria once the antibiotic has been discontinued. It is obvious that there is a need for new experimental and clinical evidence to determine the role of L-forms in the recurrence and chronicity of these infections.

B. L-Forms from Blood Isolates

The isolation of L-forms from blood specimens has been reported sporadically in the literature [80-94]. The clinical conditions varied, but they were found most prominently in subacute bacterial endocarditis [80,81] and thrombophlebitis [93,94]. Of interest also are reports of blood isolates in chronic renal disease [88,89] and even in normal blood specimens [91]. Significant controversy exists regarding the pathogenic role of these isolates. The safest explanation is that the L-form probably represents a transient state of latent pathogenicity that will only become fully developed when the organisms return to the bacterial state. The case reported by Wittler and associates [80] many years ago illustrates this situation well. Their patient was a youngster with subacute bacterial endocarditis caused by a corynebacterium that was isolated from the blood during the active phase of the disease; the L-forms were isolated only after the patient had been treated with penicillin. It appeared that treatment with penicillin caused the in vivo transformation of the organisms to the L-form, hence the failure of penicillin treatment to eradicate infection. Neu and Goldmeyer [81] isolated protoplasts of enterococcus in high-osmolarity medium from a patient with culture-negative bacterial endocarditis. This patient had also received prior antibiotic treatment with penicillin and streptomycin, and enterococcus had been isolated initially; but the antibiotic treatment had failed to produce resolution of the infection. Because of persistent fever and borderline cardiac function, aortic valve replacement was performed. Enterococcus protoplasts were isolated from the valve specimen, but not from the blood, in the hyperosmolar medium. None of the routine cultures showed growth. The patient was treated with high doses of penicillin and streptomycin, and apparently did well in follow-up examinations. The authors concluded that the protoplasts probably represented a "dormant" form of the bacterium with no pathogenetic role except as a revertant.

Another case of bacterial endocarditis probably caused by cell wall-defective *Streptococcus viridans* was described. In this case, the clinical course was complicated by coronary embolism from the bacterial endocarditis and subsequently the patient was successfully treated by surgery. The organisms that grew out from the blood were isolated in hyperosmolar media and did not grow in regular media [82]. However, there were no descriptions of morphology or other cultural characteristics that could have allowed their identification as protoplasts or L-forms.

Kagan and Mikhailova [83] reported the largest series thus far of patients with endocarditis from whom L-forms of streptococci were isolated in hyperosmolar culture. Ten of the 14 patients had atypical bacteria in their cultures. Six were L-forms, one a transitional form, and three showed a mixed culture of L-forms and vegetative bacteria. Louria et al. [84] described atypical organisms in five of more than 300 patients suspected of having a septic process. All the patients had negative routine cultures. The organisms that grew out in the hyperosmolar media did not show typical L-form morphology. In four of the five cases, the bacteriologic findings were supported by serological tests. In another large series of febrile patients with negative routine cultures [85], 160 isolates from 41 patients were obtained from a variety of clinical conditions, including 21 patients with septicemia, of whom nine had subacute bacterial endocarditis. Seven patients had abscesses and other purulent conditions, such as septic arthritis, empyema, and one skin lesion. Most commonly the atypical organisms reverted to streptococci or *Staphylococcus* species, and less frequently to corynebacteria, gram-negative enterics, *Hemophilus influenzae*, or *Candida* species. The morphology of the isolated organism was examined by air-dried preparations for gram stain which clearly showed the granular appearance of the organisms, whereas the heat-dried preparations showed only debris. Another significant point in this study was the nature of the underlying disorder of these patients, the majority having conditions compromising their immune state. This actually is the only report that so far has emphasized this problem.

Since patients with immune defiency states are subject to frequent and multiple infections, a prospective study of patients who show predictable trend of infections, (e.g., fevers that follow discontinuation of antibiotic treatment) could be appropriate subjects for investigation of latent and overt infections caused by atypical bacteria. Mashkov studied streptococcal L-forms and their revertants recovered from children with sepsis. The revertants had the same antibiotic sensitivity as standard streptococci, but failed to produce hemolysin, a property that was also shared by the L-forms [86]. This anomaly has also been observed by other authors [87] and agrees with experimental data with other organisms in which the bacterial properties changed after organisms passed through the L-form stage [49].

Domingue et al. have isolated cell wall-deficient bacteria from filtrates of red cell lysates of patients with a variety of kidney disorders [88,89]. Some of the organisms eventually reverted to bacteria that were characterized as streptococcal species, whereas others could not be classified. The presence of these organisms in patients with chronic renal disease is difficult to explain, and their existence presumably within the red cells is most intriguing and requires further documentation. A pathogenetic mechanism for the glomerulopathies in relationship to these bacterial isolates could not be established. Moreover, since such bacterial forms can also be found in the blood of normal individuals, additional studies become critical for the proper assessments of these findings.

Tedeschi et al. [90] have found L-forms as well as vegetative forms of *Staphylococcus epidermidis* as inclusions within platelets of normal subjects, and Bisset and Bartlett have described L-forms and vegetative forms of a strain of *Bacillus licheniformis* in the erythrocytes of normal persons [91]. These isolates were the result of very prolonged incubation up to 25 months. Twenty-eight percent of these normal blood specimens grew out the bacillus. The authors described progressive morphologic changes from L-forms (initial state), to diphtheroid-like, and ultimately to the sporogenous bacillary forms.

Tedeschi et al. [92] presented electron microscopic evidence of diphtheroid-like organisms in human blood of patients with a multiplicity of conditions. The detection of these microorganisms was totally independent of their diagnosis, and their growth also developed over a long period of cultivation, in general between 4-8 weeks. These isolates and those cited above apparently belong in a different category whose exact relationship to a normal state or the pathologic condition is totally unclear. Future investigations should clarify their origin and their biologic significance.

Altemeier et al. [93,94] isolated L-forms of *Bacteroides* spp. from patients with acute and recurrent deep venous thrombosis. A possible role of the anticonceptive estrogens in the pathogenesis of the infectious thrombophlebitis was postulated by enhancing the growth of the L-form cultures, and also by enabling these L-forms to interfere with the anticoagulant effect of heparin. Unfortunately, no further work has been done in this important field of venous disease which yearly causes significant morbidity and mortality in hospitalized patients.

Another important problem that has not been properly addressed concerns the breakthrough phenomenon that occurs in patients with sepsis who are receiving appropriate antibiotic therapy. In these situations, organisms are recovered from body fluids or blood that contain inhibitory or bactericidal levels of the antibiotics. In some cases, organisms have been recovered exclusively in hyperosmolar media, thereby creating the idea that ineffectiveness of treatment was due to the presence of L-forms. When these L-forms were placed in routine culture media, they reverted to the parent bacterium. We have seen the breakthrough phenomenon in patients with *E. coli* sepsis treated with adequate doses of antibiotic. The organisms usually appear in the enriched hyperosmolar cultures after 2-3 days of cultivation and often present a pleomorphic morphology on gram stain. Unfortunately, it was not possible to determine whether these atypical forms had developed from L-forms or whether they were the result of deformation in the presence of antibiotic remaining in culture media of high osmolarity. These patients responded clinically to combined treatment with cephalosporins and aminoglycosides, and the cultures subsequently became negative (unpublished observations).

In the case described by Palmer [95], *Salmonella enteritidis* was isolated from the joint fluid on routine medium in the presence of inhibitory levels of the antibiotic. The isolate produced L-forms when placed in hyperosmolar media with penicillin. This "breakthrough" phenomenon was interpreted as being the result of L-form transformation in vivo, indeed a difficult fact to prove. On the other hand, modifications of the cell wall may yield variants such as the B type of *Proteus mirabilis*, occasionally seen also with *Salmonella*, that rapidly reverts to regular bacteria in media without inducing agent. The use of hyperosmolar media with gram-negative organisms such as *Proteus* and *Salmonella* may lead to erroneous conclusions. These bacteria may produce L-forms within a wide range of salt concentrations but often, as indicated before, there is no need for hyperosmolarity for L-form induction.

In a negative vein, a study by Gleckman et al. [96] of 33 patients with fever of unknown origin failed to reveal the presence of L-forms. In another article dealing with fever of unknown origin, there was no mention of any case in which L-forms were found [97]. From a patient with Hodgkin's disease studied by us L-forms of an unclassified streptococcus were isolated from the blood in media containing 2% sodium chloride (unpublished observation). The patient had a long febrile course and degenerative cysts in the liver, thought initially to be liver abscesses. Bloody material aspirated from the cyst was cultured in regular media and yielded no growth. Cultures of cyst fluid for L-forms were not done. The patient finally succumbed to her illness and the pathology showed hypocellular type Hodgkin's disease. The isolation of streptococcal L-forms in this case was most perplexing, but it is unlikely that the patient's illness would have responded to antibiotic treatment. The role of L-forms in situations with immunocompromised hosts may reflect an opportunistic invasion with otherwise low-grade bacterial pathogens, with the ability to transform to L-forms under special circumstances in vivo.

C. L-Forms in Rheumatic Fever

There is clear epidemiologic and clinical evidence that infections with Group A hemolytic streptococci are responsible for the occurrence of rheumatic fever. Experimental studies have further suggested the existence of a link between streptococcal products and the development of cardiac lesions that resemble rheumatic carditis [98,99]. (Also, see section on experimental studies.) It has also become evident that the streptococcal cell membranes provide an antigen with similar antigenicity to a component of the sarcolemma, the cytoplasmic membrane of the cardiac muscle cell, with the result that antistreptococcal cell membrane antibodies could react with the sarcolemmal antigen in immunofluorescent studies [98]. Similar antibody to sarcolemma is formed in the serum of patients with uncomplicated streptococcal infection, but this occurs in much higher titers in patients with rheumatic fever; the antibody formation also appears to have a longer course of production in these patients [98]. The experimental background appears to support the existence of a possible role for the L-forms of the Group A streptococcus in the pathogenesis of rheumatic fever. First, because the streptococcal L-forms are of the A type, the cell membrane, having similar antigenicity with the cardiac muscle, becomes subject to immune recognition and response with the dual capability of reacting to streptococcal and cardiac targets. Second, because the L-forms are known to produce bacterial products, they may also induce toxic damage and inflammatory changes in the target tissues. Russian investigators Kagan [73] and Klodnitskaia [100] have reported finding Group A streptococcal L-forms in the blood of patients with rheumatic fever. The latter recovered the L-forms frequently from the blood of these patients and, interestingly, independently of the state of activity of the disease.

Immune complexes to both streptococcal cell wall antigens and L-form antigens have been detected in higher quantities in the sera of rheumatic fever patients than in normal persons [101,102]. Whether or not these immune complexes reflect activity of viable streptococcal L-forms is unknown. Experimentally, L-forms have been identified in the myocardium in areas near the connective tissue [22,23]. The reason for this preferential location of the L-form is unclear, but recent studies stimulate some provocative thoughts [103]. First, rheumatic fever appears to have a genetic predisposition involving the presence of a certain B-cell lymphocyte HLA Ir gene called 883. Second, if indeed streptococcal antigens are deposited in areas near connective tissue, the possibility exists that the increase in plasma cells and lymphocytes also noted in the vicinity of collagen tissue in the heart valves may be a direct immunologic response to the presence of the streptococcal antigens. The resulting cross-reacting antibodies to streptococcal and sarcolemma antigens may then explain the local nature of tissue damage in the heart. Kagan et al. [104] have shown typical electrocardiographic changes in monkeys developing throat infections with streptococcal L-forms, and lesions of rheumatic carditis have been produced by the injection of the streptococcal membranes into rhesus monkeys [103]. These, undoubtedly, are big steps in the conquest of rheumatic fever. The ultimate task will then be to determine if the genetically predisposed individual with the Ir gene 883 handles streptococcal infections in a manner that allows the development of L-forms.

IV. L-FORM INFECTIONS IN OTHER SITES

A. Staphylococcal Osteomyelitis

Staphylococcus aureus has been implicated as the main cause of chronic osteomyelitis. The reasons for its persistence in bone tissues are unknown. We know of one patient who, in the course of 50 years, had three independent, well-documented bouts of suppurative staphylococcal osteomyelitis with fistula formation in the same site. All three infections responded to prolonged anti-infective regimens as they were available at the time. These included irrigation with bacteriostatic solutions for many months during the first attack, Aureomycin given for many weeks during the second bout, and one of the newly developed cephalosporins in the most recent infection. Following each healing of the fistula, the patient entered into prolonged remissions lasting many years (our unpublished observations). One could argue that if L-forms existed following the first infection, the recurrences were mediated by subsequent reversions to the bacterial form. Although there was no isolation of L-forms in this case, the situation is not unlike those reported in the literature [105].

Isolation of staphylococcal L-forms from cases of persistent or recurrent osteomyelitis have brought into focus the fact that these bacterial forms may persist in a viable state for many years, and that along with this they may also retain the potential for regenerating the cell wall. Staphylococcal L-forms have also been isolated from empyema fluids on a special L-form medium with high osmolarity. In the future, sequential serological studies against certain staphylococcal markers such as teichoic acids or L-form antigens will be most appropriate in determining the natural course of these infections. In addition to isolation in culture, L-forms or vegetative staphylococcal forms could be closely studied in the tissues by electronmicroscopy and by highly specific fluorescent antibody techniques.

B. L-Forms in Central Nervous System Infections

A number of investigators have presented evidence that L-forms of streptococci, *Staphylococcus epidermidis*, and corynebacteria [73,84,106] were isolated from the spinal fluid of patients with various infectious processes of the central nervous system, including meningitis, encephalitis, brain abscesses, and ventricular infections. An *H. influenzae* L-form has been detected by fluorescent antibody and by isolation in culture [87]. Other organisms such as gram-negative enterobacteria and pseudomonas have been cultivated in the L-form state and then reverted to the bacterial form upon subculture [106]. Because some of these patients had evidence of abnormalities in the spinal fluid as well as clinically, antibiotics that were considered to be effective against the L-forms were used for treatment. Indeed the clinical improvement that followed could be used as an argument to suggest that the L-forms were responsible for the clinical abnormalities and for the changes in the spinal fluid. However, the isolation of these organisms in culture is not sufficient proof that they actually existed as such in the central nervous system. Careful observation of the clinical course and adequate examination of fresh specimens for morphologic variants or L-forms are necessary for proper evaluation of the bacteriologic findings, especially in view of the fact that L-forms can develop in such a poor nutrient environment as spinal fluid which is also devoid of hypertonic properties.

C. L-Forms in Tuberculosis

The role of L-forms of *Mycobacterium tuberculosis* has been recently studied by Khomeno et al. [107]. In 115 patients undergoing treatment for pulmonary tuberculosis, it was noted that the bacterial forms were rapidly eliminated from the sputum whereas the L-forms persisted for much longer periods of time. In half of the patients, the L-forms and the bacteria coexisted prior to the treatment, but in other patients the L-form induction coincided with the onset of chemotherapy. A correlation between the severity of infection and the persistence of the L-forms in the sputum was emphasized as a prognostic factor. Other authors have made similar claims [108,109]. Mattman devised an immunological method for detection of *M. tuberculosis* L-forms in the sputum and in the body fluids by fluorescent antibody methods [87]. The L-forms apparently induced the production of specific antibodies in the immunized rabbits that allowed identification of the L-forms independently from the bacillus. With this technique the L-forms of *M. tuberculosis* were identified in the blood of a patient with disseminated tuberculosis. The role of the L-forms of *M. tuberculosis* in the persistence of tuberculous infection or in resistant states needs further exploration. Tuberculous infection is still a major problem in many parts of the world, including the United States.

D. L-Forms in Miscellaneous Conditions

Reports of unusual L-form isolates have sporadically been presented in the literature. It is difficult to ascribe any significance to these isolates in relation to a pathologic process. Nelson and Pickett [110] recovered "L-forms" of brucella from human blood cultures and thought that these organisms had a role in persistent infections. Shchegolev and Starshinova [111] isolated L-forms of *Salmonella typhi* from patients with active salmonellosis as well as from carriers, and also thought that the L-forms were involved in the chronicity as well as in the carrier state of salmonellosis. The adaptability of salmonella L-forms has been tested with the experiments in chick embryos which showed that the L-forms rapidly lost pathogenicity in serial subcultures [61]. It is possible then that in the human infection with salmonella, if factors such as immunologic reactions favor the development of salmonella L-forms, these organisms can remain in the body for long periods of time without causing any pathogenicity except at the time that they revert to bacterium. Since the organisms are excreted in the bile, a certain amount of reversion to bacteria may take place and continue on in the journey of the bacteria in the intestinal tract. After a few call divisions in the bowel, the bacteria may recover their full pathogenic potential and by the time they are eliminated, they are ready to be infective to a new host.

The possibility that L-forms may occur transiently during the healing phase of certain infections is illustrated by the report of Barile et al. [112] who studied cases of aphthous stomatitis produced by *Streptococcus sanguis*. During the active ulcerative phase of the disease, only streptococcal forms were isolated from the lesions, whereas when the disease entered into its healing phase, only L-forms could be isolated from these lesions. Since this infection tends to have a cyclic course, immunological studies in relation to the natural course of the disease are highly desirable.

Staphylococcal L-forms were isolated from a patient with conjunctivitis resistant to treatment [113], and Kagan studied the spontaneous occurrence of staphylococcal L-forms in patients with cystic fibrosis [114]. Although no particular role was ascribed to these organisms, they were frequently encountered in the sputum of cystic fibrosis patients. In the case of a young girl, the L-forms might have been responsible for a prolonged febrile course that did not respond to antibiotics. The isolate had typical L-form appearance and ultimately reverted to the parent bacterium. The patient was then treated with tetracycline, and apparently improved.

An interesting report by Fernandes and Panos appeared in the literature describing the isolation of a stable L-form from the kidney biopsy of a patient with diffuse acute proliferative glomerulonephritis [115]. The isolate was thought to be an L-form and not a mycoplasma because it required hyperosmolar medium (but mycoplasma species may grow in hyperosmolar media). Unfortunately serological studies were not done, and thus the role in the nephritis remains obscure. In one patient with sterile pyuria, *M. hominis* was isolated from the urine in abundance and repeatedly, in a medium containing 2% sodium chloride. The organism also grew out in normal osmolarity media (our unpublished data). Therefore, in isolates that are originally grown in hyperosmolar media, adaptation to medium of lower osmolarity together with proper identification for mycoplasma should be carried out.

E. Atypical Bacteria in Rheumatoid Arthritis

Rheumatoid arthritis has often been considered to be of an infectious nature. Indeed, many organisms have been isolated from joint fluids and from the blood of patients with this disease. The range is quite wide and involves the full spectrum of microbiological forms including viruses, mycoplasmas, L-forms, and bacteria. Some authors believe that the various bacterial forms described are different evolving stages of a bacterium classified as *Bacillus licheniformis*. Because 10% of normal individuals also carry these forms in their blood, the suggestion has been made that, perhaps through an altered immunity, the state of tolerance that may normally exist to these organisms may be lost [116-119]. Rheumatoid arthritis may then result from a reactive state to the infective agent if proper genetic and immunologic conditions are given. Experimental and properly controlled studies with *Bacillus licheniformis* or its L-form are sorely missing.

V. SUMMARY AND CONCLUSIONS

From the above review, it is clear that in spite of slow progress in the field, many interesting areas of bacterial biology relating to the function of the L-forms have surfaced in the scientific literature, mainly from European investigators. Among the gram-positive bacteria the streptococcus continues to offer interesting possibilities for the study of the L-forms and their relation to experimental and human pathology. Streptococcal L-forms have been shown to produce cardiac lesions in various animal models perhaps via their exposed cytoplasmic membranes that could readily elicit cross-reacting antibodies to the sarcolemmal membrane of the cardiac muscle. The presence of L-forms in cardiac tissue thus could become the appropriate stimulus for the production of continued immunologically mediated tissue damage. Definitive evidence for this possible pathogenetic mechanism in rheumatic fever is still lacking. The experimental model of listeria L-form infection resembles the bacterial disease, and it also causes involution of the lymphoid tissue of the bone marrow. This model offers possibilities to study the role of listeria L-forms as immune suppressive agents. *Erysipelothrix rhusiopathiae* infection has been extensively studied in pigs and other animals. The hallmark of the infection is the production of chronic destructive arthritis with much similarity to rheumatoid arthritis. Since in the chronic phase of the disease the bacteria can no longer be recovered, it is plausible that L-forms of *E. rhusiopathiae* may play a role. This is a highly speculative possibility but one that merits attention. Neither recovery of L-forms of *E. rhusiopathiae* from chronically infected tissues, nor experimental infection with L-forms have been attempted.

Staphylococcal L-forms are apparently incapable of producing pathologic changes in the endocardium and the renal pelvis of experimental animals, even under astringent conditions. They, however, can induce mitogenic activity on human lymphocytes. These experiments suggest issues relating to host and tissue specificities, but they are of little relevance to the problem of chronic staphylococcal infection in man, namely chronic osteomyelitis.

Nocardia L-forms have been shown to be pathogenic for mice. In fact the infection occurs only when the bacteria transforms to L-forms in vivo. This work, thus far, represents the only model of direct L-form pathogenicity where neither reversion to bacteria nor production of exotoxin are at work. Data on brucella infection in humans have not shown any role for the L-forms. Animal experiments have revealed the feasibility of inducing brucella L-forms in vivo, and a state of lymphoreticular reactivity. These are interesting models whose relevance to chronic brucellosis in humans remains to be shown.

In regard to the L-forms of gram-negative bacteria, no significant new contributions have appeared in the clinical literature. The old question of the role of L-forms or cell wall-defective bacteria as the source of recurrent infection via reversion to bacteria is still unsettled, especially in urinary tract infections. Past experiments with salmonella L-forms induced by specific antibody still offer possibilities for future studies, such as the production of chronic or latent infections in animals and their relationship to similar human conditions.

Sporadic reports on the isolation of L-forms from clinical material have been anecdotal and difficult to interpret. The presence of L-forms in human tuberculosis are worth noting as they appear to have prognostic significance. Further work is needed in this important area of human infection. The existence of L-forms of gram-positive organisms in human red cells and platelets from diseased and normal individuals is puzzling and needs confirmation by others. The suggestive role of these organisms in diseases such as rheumatoid arthritis remains speculative.

In the last decade, progress on the biology and clinical significance of the L-forms has produced little new information; on the other hand, some strong new data such as the work with nocardia L-forms have clearly shown their pathogenic potential. This and other evidence hopefully will maintain and increase the scientific interest in the field, and some of the issues raised previously may find the proper solution.

REFERENCES

1. Dienes, L. (1946). Complex reproductive processes in bacteria. *Cold Spring Harbor Symp. Quant. Biol. 11*:51-59.
2. Dienes, L. (1968). Morphology and reproductive processes of bacteria with defective cell wall in *Microbial Protoplasts, Spheroplasts and L-Forms* (L. B. Guze, ed.), Williams & Wilkins, Baltimore, Maryland, pp. 74-93.
3. Dienes, L. and Bullivant, S. (1967). Comparison of the morphology of PPLO and L-forms of bacteria with light and electron microscopy. *Ann. N.Y. Acad. Sci. 143*:719-733.
4. Dienes, L. and Weinberger, H. J. (1951). The L-forms of bacteria. *Bact. Rev. 15*:245-288.
5. Dienes, L., Weinberger, H. J., and Madoff, S. (1950). The transformation of typhoid bacilli into L-forms under various conditions. *J. Bacteriol. 59*: 755-764.
6. Klieneberger, E. (1935). The natural occurrence of pleuropneumonia-like organisms in apparent symbiosis with *Streptobacillus moniliformis* and other bacteria. *J. Path. Bact. 40*:93-105.
7. Klieneberger-Nobel, E. (1949). Origin, development and significance of L-forms in bacterial cultures. *J. Gen. Microbiol. 3*:434-443.
8. Clasener, H. (1972). Pathogenicity of the L-phase of bacteria. *Ann. Rev. Microbiol. 26*:55-84.
9. Feingold, D. S. (1969). Biology and pathogenicity of microbial spheroplasts and L-forms. *N. Engl. J. Med. 281*:1159-1170.
10. Guze, L. B. (1968). *Microbial Protoplasts, Spheroplasts and L-Forms*, Williams & Wilkins, Baltimore, Maryland.
11. Hijmans, W., Van Boven, C. P. A., and Clasener, H. A. L. (1969). Fundamental biology of the L-phase of bacteria in *The Mycoplasmatales and the L-phase of Bacteria* (L. Hayflick, ed.), Appleton-Century-Crofts, New York, pp. 67-143.

12. Kenny, J. F. (1978). Role of cell-wall defective microbial variants in human infections. *Southern Med. J. 71*:180-190.
13. Louria, D. B. (1971). L-forms, spheroplasts and aberrant forms in chronic sepsis. *Adv. Intern. Med. 17*:125-142.
14. Roux, J. (1977). *Spheroplasts, Protoplasts and L-Forms of Bacteria*, Ed. INSERM, vol. 64, Paris.
15. Sharp, J. T. (1971). Mycoplasmas and bacterial L-forms: Clinical considerations in *Mycoplasma and the L-Forms of Bacteria* (S. Madoff, ed.), Gordon and Breach Science Publishers, New York, pp. 85-94.
16. Madoff, S., Burke, M. E., Dienes, L. (1967). Induction and Identification of L-Forms of Bacteria. *Ann. N.Y. Acad. Sci. 143*:755-759.
17. Beaman, B. L. (1980). Induction of L-phase variants of *Nocardia caviae* within intact murine lungs. *Infect. Immun. 29*:244-251.
18. Ginsburg, I. (1972). Mechanisms of cell and tissue injury induced by Group A streptococci. Relation to post streptococcal sequelae. *J. Infect. Dis. 126*: 419-456.
19. DeVuono, J. and Panos, C. (1978). Effect of L-form *Streptococcus pyogenes* and of lipoteichoic acid on human cells in tissue culture. *Infect. Immun. 22*:255-265.
20. Iesmantaite, N. A., Rimkunas, A. J., Panaviene, D. P., Januleviciute, N. A., and Preiskeliene, I. J. (1981). Interactions of red blood cells and lymphocytes with streptococcal L-forms. *Zh. Mikrobiol. Epidemiol. Immunobiol.* 6:74-76.
21. Kagan, G., Gusman, B., Vulfovitch, Y., and Besouglova, T. (1977). Group A streptococcal L-forms as a trigger of immuno-morphological changes of the heart and immunogenic organs in *Spheroplasts, Protoplasts, and L-Forms of Bacteria* (J. Roux, ed.), Ed. INSERM, Vol. 64, Paris, pp. 259-264.
22. Kagan, G., Vulfovitch, B., Gusman, B., and Raskova, T. (1977). Persistence and pathological effect of streptococcal L-forms in vivo in *Spheroplasts, Protoplasts and L-Forms of Bacteria* (J. Roux, ed.), Ed. INSERM, vol. 64, Paris, pp. 247-258.
23. Gusman, B. S. (1980). Morphogenesis of the heart lesion in experimental infection with streptococcal L-forms. *Arkh Patol. 42*:26-32.
24. Matsunaga, K., Katoh, K., Takahashi, T., et al. (1982). The experimental myocarditis of mice immunized with Group A streptococcal cytoplasmic membrane fraction extracted from L-forms. *Jpn. J. Exp. Med. 52*:267-270.
25. Iesmantaite, N. A., Ptasekas, R. S., Astrauskatis, I. I., Austraskas, V. I., and Rimkunas, A. I. (1975). Eksperimental'noe Izuchenie Roli L-Form Gemoliticheskogo Streptokokka V Infektsionnoi Patologii. *Zh. Mikrobiol. Epidemiol. Immunobiol. 2*:62-64.
26. Cromartie, W. J. and Craddock, J. G. (1966). Rheumatic-like cardiac lesions in mice. *Science 154*:285-287.
27. Stinson, M. W. and Bergley, E. J. (1982). Isolation of a heart- and kidney-binding protein from Group A streptococci. *Infect. Immuno. 35*:335-342.
28. Cook, J., Fincham, W. J., and Lack, G. H. (1969). Chronic arthritis produced by streptococcal L-forms. *J. Pathol. 99*:283-297.

29. Prosorovsky, S., Kotliarova, J., Fedotova, I., and Bakulov, I. (1977). Pathogenicity of listeria L-forms in *Spheroplasts, Protoplasts and L-Forms of Bacteria* (J. Roux, ed.), Ed. INSERM, vol. 64, Paris, pp. 265-272.
30. Ajmal, M. (1969). *Erysipelothrix rhusiopathiae* and spontaneous arthritis in pigs. *Res. Vet. Sci. 10*:579-582.
31. Ajmal, M. (1970). Experimental *Erysipelothrix rhusiopathiae*. Infection in white rats. *Res. Vet. Sci. 11*:279-282.
32. Ajmal, M. (1971). Experimental *Erysipelothrix* arthritis. II. Observations on rabbits following systemic administration of live *E. rhusiopathiae* or an intra-articular injection of non-living substances including inactivated organisms. *Res. Vet. Sci. 12*:412-419.
33. White, T. G. and Puls, J. L. (1969). Induction of experimental chronic arthritis in rabbits by cell-free fragments of erysipelothrix. *J. Bacteriol. 98*: 403-406.
34. White, T. G., Puls, J. L., and Mirikitani, F. K. (1971). Rabbit arthritis induced by cell-free extracts of erysipelothrix. *Infect. Immun. 3*:715-722.
35. Yokomizo, Y. and Isayama, Y. (1972). Antibody activities of IgM and IgG fractions from rabbit anti-*Erysipelothrix rhusiopathiae*. *Sera. Res. Vet. Sci. 13*:294-296.
36. Timoney, J. (1969). The inactivation of *Erysipelothrix rhusiopathiae* in macrophages from normal and immune mice. *Res. Vet. Sci. 10*:301-302.
37. Timoney, J. (1971). Antibody and rheumatoid factors in synovia of pigs with erysipelothrix polyarthritis. *J. Comp. Pathol. 81*:243-248.
38. Timoney, J. F. and Berman, D. T. (1970). Erysipelothrix arthritis in swine. Bacteriologic and immunopathologic aspects. *Am. J. Vet. Res. 31*:1411-1421.
39. Timoney, J. F. and Berman, D. T. (1970). Erysipelothrix arthritis in swine: Serum-synovial fluid gradients for antibody and serum proteins in normal and arthritic joints. *Am. J. Vet. Res. 31*:1405-1409.
40. Toshkov, A., Mihnilova, L., Cherepova, N., and Gulubov, S. (1975). Persistence and isolation of L-cycle forms of *Erysipelothrix rhusiopathiae* in experimental infection. *Zentralbl. Bakteriol. Orig. 233*:370-375.
41. Pachas, W. N. and Currid, V. R. (1974). L-form induction, morphology, and development in two related strains of *Erysipelothrix rhusiopathiae*. *J. Bacteriol. 119*:576-582.
42. Beaman, B. L. and Scates, S. M. (1981). Role of L-forms of *Nocardia caviae* in the development of chronic mycetomas in normal and immunodeficient murine models. *Infect. Immun. 33*:893-907.
43. Beaman, B. L., Bourgeois, A. L., and Moring, S. E. (1981). Cell-wall modification resulting from in-vitro induction of L-phase variants of *Nocardia asteroides*. *J. Bacteriol. 148*:600-609.
44. Steinman, C. R. and Hsu, K. (1976). Specific detection and semiquantitation of microorganisms in tissue by nucleic acid hybridization. II. Investigation of synovia from pigs with chronic erysipelothrix arthritis. *Arthritis Rheum. 19*:38-42.

45. Koptelova, E. I., Pokrouskii, V. I., and Gorshkova, E. P. (1965). Model of experimental meningitis in rabbits evoked by streptococcal and staphylococcal L-forms. *Vestn. Akad. Med. Nauk. SSSR. 20*:60–64.
46. Povroskii, V. I., Ryzhkov, E. V., and Koptelova, E. I. (1969). Pathomorphologic aspects of experimental meningitis in rabbits caused by L-forms of streptococcus, staphylococcus and typhoid bacillus. *Vestn. Akad. Med. Nauk. SSSR. 24*:95–96.
47. Watanakunakorn, C. and Bakie, C. (1974). Pathogenicity of stable L-phase variants of *Staphylococcus aureus*. Failure to colonize normal and oxamide-induced hydronoephrotic renal medulla of rats. *Infect. Immun. 9*:766–768.
48. Linnemann, C. C., Jr., Watanakunakorn, C., and Bakie, C. (1973). Pathogenicity of stable L-phase variants of *Staphylococcus aureus*: Failure to colonize experimental endocarditis in rabbits. *Infect. Immun. 7*:725–730.
49. Wieckiewicz, J. (1979). Loss of virulence of revertants from *Staphylococcus aureus* L-phase variants in comparison with the parent strain. *J. Hyg. Epidemiol. Microbiol. Immunol. 23*:326–331.
50. Takada, H., Hirachi, Y., Hashizume, H., and Kotani, S. (1981). Mitogenic effect of cytoplasmic membranes and a cytoplasmic fraction of *Staphylococcus aureus* L-forms on human peripheral blood lymphocytes. *Microbiol. Immunol. 25*:381–326.
51. Schmitt-Slomska, J., Caravano, R., Anoal, M., Gay, B., and Roux, J. (1981). Isolation of L-forms from the spleens of *Brucella suis*-infected, penicillin-treated mice. *Ann. Microbiol. (Inst. Pasteur) 132A*:253–265.
52. Hatten, B. A. and Sulkin, S. E. (1963). Possible role of *Brucella* L-forms in the pathogenesis of brucellosis in *Microbial Protoplasts, Spheroplasts and L-Forms* (L. B. Guze, ed.), Williams & Wilkins, Baltimore, Maryland, pp. 457–471.
53. Elberg, S. S. and Ralston, D. J. (1980). Enhancement of murine bone marrow colony formation and L-transformation by *Brucella* antigen. *Can. J. Comp. Med. 44*:320–327.
54. Grekova, N. A., Tolmacheva, T. A., and Vershilova, P. A. (1979). On the pathogenicity of non-stable *Brucella* L-forms and their revertants. *J. Hyg. Epidemiol. Microbiol. Immunol. 23*:129–134.
55. Braude, A. I., Siemienski, J. and Jacobs, I. (1961). Protoplast formation in human urine. *Trans. Ass. Amer. Phys. 74*:234–245.
56. Braude, A. I., Siemienski, J., and Lee, K. (1968). Spheroplasts in human urine in *Microbial Protoplasts, Spheroplasts and L-Forms* (L. B. Guze, ed.), Williams & Wilkins, Baltimore, Maryland, pp. 361–405.
57. Gutman, L. T., Winterbauer, R. H., Turck, M., Wedgwood, R. J., and Petersdorf, R. G. (1968). The role of bacterial variants in experimental pyelonephritis in *Microbial Protoplasts, Spheroplasts and L-Forms* (L. B. Guze, ed.), Williams & Wilkins, Baltimore, Maryland, pp. 391–395.
58. Levina, G., Yagud, S. L., Grutman, M. I., and Prozorovsky, S. V. (1981). *Salmonella typhi* L-transformation process in *in vivo* experiments using diffusion chambers. *Zh. Mikrobiol. Epidemiol. Immunobiol. 6*:36–39.

59. Levina, G. A., Prozorovsky, S. V., Yagud, S. L., Grutman, M. I., and Gorelov, A. L. (1981). Formation and persistence of L-variants of *Salmonella typhi* in experimental typhoid and in carriers. *Zh. Mikrobiol. Epidemiol. Immunobiol.* 7:27–30.
60. Kawakami, M., Ishibashi, H., Mitsuhashi, S., Sakaino, K., and Fukai, K. (1970). Experimental Salmonellosis. Unstable L-forms in liver of infected mice. *Jpn. J. Microbiol. 14*:143–153.
61. Carre, L., Roux, J., and Mandin, J. (1955). Culture des organismes L sur membrane chorio-allantoide d'embryon de poulet. *Montpellier Med. 47*: 438–445.
62. Guze, L. B., Harwick, H. J., and Kalmanson, G. M. (1976). Klebsiella L-forms: Effect of growth as L-form on virulence of reverted *Klebsiella-pneumoniae*. *J. Infect. Dis. 133*:245–252.
63. Bohnhoff, M. and Page, M. I. (1968). Experimental infection with parent and L-phase variants of *Neisseria meningitidis*. *J. Bacteriol. 95*:2070–2077.
64. Brown, Jr., G. W., King, G., Sugiyama, H. (1979). Penicillin-lysozyme conversion of *Clostridium botulinum* types A and E into protoplasts and their stabilization as L-form cultures. *J. Bacteriol. 104*:1325–1331.
65. Ratnam, S. and Chandrasekhar, S. (1976). The pathogenicity of sphero-plasts of *Mycobacterium tuberculosis*. *Am. Rev. Resp. Dis. 114*:549–554.
66. Fauve, R. M., Pierce-Chase, C. H., and Dubos, R. (1964). Corynebacterial pseudotuberculosis in mice II. Activation of natural and experimental latent infections. *J. Exp. Med. 120*:283–304.
67. Koller, H., Adam, D., and Daschner, F. (1975). Phagocytosis of cell-wall defective bacteria by human macrophages. *Med. Microbiol. Immunol. (Berlin) 161*:107–112.
68. Taylor-Robinson, D., Schorlemmer, H. U., Furr, P. M., and Allison, A. C. (1978). Macrophage secretion and the complement cleavage product C3a in the pathogenesis of infections by mycoplasmas and L-forms of bacteria and in immunity to these organisms. *Clin. Exp. Immunol. 33*:486–494.
69. Saulsbury, F. T. and Winkelstein, J. A. (1979). Activation of the alternative complement pathway by L-phase variants of gram positive bacteria. *Infect. Immun. 23*:711–716.
70. Harwick, H. J., Kalmanson, G. M., and Guze, L. B. (1977). Chemotactic activity of L-forms and mycoplasma. *Aust. J. Exp. Biol. Med. Sci. (pt. 4)*: 431–434.
71. Rinno, J., Gmeiner, J., Golecki, J. R., and Mayer, H. (1980). Localization of enterobacterial common antigen: *Proteus mirabilis* and its various L-forms. *J. Bacteriol. 141*:822–827.
72. Bourgeois, L. and Beaman, B. L. (1974). Probable L-forms of *Nocardia asteroides* induced in cultured mouse peritoneal macrophages. *Infect. Immun. 9*:576–590.
73. Kagan, G. Y. (1968). Some aspects of investigations of the pathogenic potentialities of L-forms of bacteria in *Microbial Protoplasts, Spheroplasts and L-Forms* (L. B. Guze, ed.), Williams & Wilkins, Baltimore, Maryland, pp. 422–443.

74. Conner, J. F., Coleman, S. E., Davis, J. L., and McGaughey, F. S. (1969). Bacterial L-forms: Urinary tract infections in a veterans hospital population. *J. Am. Geriatr. Soc. 16*:893-900.
75. Rhodes, D., Brosman, S., Kalmanson, G., and Guze, L. B. (1973). L-forms and urinary tract infections. *Urology 1*:114-116.
76. Turck, M., Gutman, L., Wedgwood, R. J., and Petersdorf, R. G. (1968). Significance of bacterial variants in urinary tract infections in *Microbial Protoplasts, Spheroplasts and L-Forms* (L. B. Guze, ed.), Williams & Wilkins, Baltimore, Maryland, pp. 415-421.
77. Thomas, V., Shelokov, A., and Forland, M. (1974). Antibody-coated bacteria in urine and site of urinary tract infection. *N. Engl. J. Med. 290*: 588-590.
78. Kalmanson, G. M. and Guze, L. B. (1968). Pyelonephritis: Isolation of protoplasts from human kidney tissue in *Microbial Protoplasts, Spheroplasts and L-Forms* (L. B. Guze, ed.), Williams & Wilkins, Baltimore, Maryland, pp. 406-414.
79. Fass, R. J. and Barnishan, J. (1977). Detection and significance of cell-wall defective bacteria in the urine of bacteriuric patients in *Spheroplasts, Protoplasts and L-Forms of Bacteria* (J. Roux, ed.), Ed. INSERM, vol. 64, Paris, pp. 317-326.
80. Wittler, R. and Malizia, W. F., et al. (1960). Isolation of a corynebacterium and its transitional forms from a case of subacute bacterial endocarditis treated with antibiotics. *J. Gen. Microbiol. 23*:315-333.
81. Neu, H. C. and Goldmeyer, B. (1968). Isolation of protoplasts in a case of enterococcal endocarditis. *Am. J. Med. 45*:784-788.
82. Licht, A., Yeivin, R., and Levy, M. (1973). Successful resuscitation in coronary embolism occurring as a complication of bacterial endocarditis caused by cell-wall defective *Streptococcus viridans. Isr. J. Med. Sci. 9*: 1009-1013.
83. Kagan, G. Y. and Mikhailova, V. S. (1963). Isolation of L-forms of streptococci from the blood of patients with rheumatism and endocarditis. *J. Hyg. Epidemiol. Microbiol. Immunol. 7*:327-343.
84. Louria, D. B., Kaminski, T., Grieco, M., and Singer, J. (1969). Aberrant forms of bacteria and fungi found in blood or cerebrospinal fluid. *Arch. Int. Med. 124*:39-48.
85. Charache, P. (1978). Atypical bacterial forms in human disease in *Microbial Protoplasts, Spheroplasts and L-Forms* (L. B. Guze, ed.), Williams & Wilkins, Baltimore, Maryland, pp. 484-494.
86. Mashkov, A. V. (1974). A study of the properties of L-forms of isolated bacteria from children. *Zh. Mikrobiol. Epidemiol. Immunobiol. 12*:62-65.
87. Mattman, L. H. (1968). L-forms isolated from infections in *Microbial Protoplasts, Spheroplasts and L-Forms* (L. B. Guze, ed.), Williams & Wilkins, Baltimore, Maryland, pp. 472-483.
88. Domingue, G. J., Schlegel, J. U., Heidger, P. J., and Ehrlich, M. (1977). Novel bacterial structures in human blood in *Spheroplasts, Protoplasts and L-Forms of Bacteria* (J. Roux, ed.), Ed. INSERM, vol. 64, Paris, pp. 279-298.

89. Domingue, G. J., Turner, B., and Schlegel, J. U. (1974). Cell-wall deficient bacterial variants in kidney tissue. Detection by immunofluorescence. *Urology* 3:288-292.
90. Tedeschi, G. G. and Santarelli, I. (1977). Electron microscopical evidence of the presence of unstable L-forms of *Staphylococcus epidermidis* in human platelets in *Spheroplasts, Protoplasts and L-Forms of Bacteria* (J. Roux, ed.), Ed. INSERM, vol. 64, Paris, pp. 341-344.
91. Bissett, K. A. and Bartlett, R. (1978). The isolation and characters of L-forms and reversions of *Bacillus licheniformis* va. *Endoparasiticus* (Benedek) associated with the erythrocytes of clinically normal persons. *J. Gen. Microbiol.* 2:335-349.
92. Tedeschi, G. G., Bondi, A., Paparelli, M., and Sprovieri, G. (1977). Electron microscopical evidence of the evolution of corynebacteria-like microorganisms within human erythrocytes. *Experientia* 34:458-460.
93. Altemeier, W. A., Hill, E. O., and Fullen, W. D. (1969). Acute and recurrent thromboembolic disease. *Am. Surg.* 170:547-558.
94. Altemeier, W. A., Hummel, R. P., Hill, E. O., and Lewis, S. (1973). Changing patterns in surgical infections. *Ann. Surg.* 178:436-445.
95. Palmer, D. W. (1979). Inadequate response to "adequate" treatment of bacterial infection: L-forms and bacteroidal antibiotic activity. *J. Infect. Dis.* 139:725-727.
96. Gleckman, R., Esposito, A., and Madoff, S. (1977). Fever of unknown origin: Attempts to isolate L-forms and other aberrant bacterial forms. *J. Clin. Microbiol.* 5:225-226.
97. Musher, D. M. (1982). Fever of unknown origin: Diagnostic principles. *Hosp. Practice* 17:89-95.
98. Freimer, E. H. and Zabriskie, J. B. (1968). An immunological relationship between the protoplast membrane of Group A Streptococci and the sarcolemma, the cell membrane of cardiac muscle in *Microbial Protoplasts, Spheroplasts and L-Forms* (L. B. Guze, ed.), Williams & Wilkins, Baltimore, Maryland, pp. 356-371.
99. Van deRijn, I., Zabriskie, J. B., and McCarty, M. (1977). Streptococcal antigens cross reactive with myocardium. Purification of heart reactive antibody and isolation and characterization of the streptococcal antigen. *J. Exp. Med.* 146:579-599.
100. Klodnitskaia, S. N., Stepanov, P. N., and Adamchuck, V. D. (1977). L-forms of Streptococcus in the cultures of blood from patients with rheumatic fever in the active and inactive phases. *Zh. Microbiol. Epidemiol. Immunobiol.* 9:127-131.
101. Heymer, B., Schleifer, K. K., Read, S., Zabriskie, J. B., and Krause, R. M. (1976). Detection of antibodies to bacterial cell-wall peptidoglycan in human sera. *J. Immunol.* 117:23-26.
102. Gorina, L. G., Zheverzheeva, I. V., Chumachenko, N. V., Goncharova, S. A., and Labinskaya, A. S. (1981). Detection of an antigen of the L-forms of Group A hemolytic Streptococci in the sera of rheumatic patients following immune complex separation. *Zh. Mikrobiol. Epidemiol. Immunobiol. Jul.* 7:42-45.

103. Williams, R. C. (1982). Host factors in rheumatic fever and heart disease. *Hosp. Pract.* 17:125-138.
104. Kagan, G. Y., Prozorovsky, S. V., and Koptelova, E. I., et al. (1969). L'angine experimentale du singe provoquee par les formes L des streptocoques du groupe A. *Ann. Inst. Pasteur* 116:733-749.
105. Gordon, S. L., Greer, R. B., and Craig, C. P. (1971). Recurrent osteomyelitis. Report of four cases culturing L-form variants of staphylococci. *J. Bone Joint Surg. (Am.)* 53:1150-1156.
106. Kenny, J. F. (1973). Bacterial variants in central nervous system infections in infants and children. *J. Pediatr.* 83:531-542.
107. Khomeno, A. G., Karachunsky, M. A., Dorozhkova, I. R., Chukanov, V. I., and Balta, Yu. E. (1980). L transformation and the mycobacterial population during treatment of patients with newly identified destructive tuberculosis of the lungs. *Probl. Tuberk* 2:18-23.
108. Boqush, L. K. (1981). L-forms of *Mycobacterium tuberculosis* in chronic pleural empyema in tuberculosis patients. *Probl. Tuberk Dec.* 12:19-23.
109. Karachunskii, M. A. (1980). Clinical characteristics of newly detected destructive pulmonary tuberculosis in patients excreting mycobacterial L-forms. *Probl. Tuberk* 8:15-20.
110. Nelson, E. L. and Pickett, M. J. (1951). The recovery of L-forms of *Brucella* and their relation to Brucella phage. *J. Infect. Dis.* 89:226-232.
111. Shchegolev, A. C. and Starshinova, V. S. (1964). Isolation of L-form bacteria from typhoid patients and carriers. *Zh. Mikrobiol.* 41:15-20.
112. Barile, M. F., Francis, T. C., and Graykowski, E. A. (1968). *Streptococcus sanguis* in the pathogenesis of recurrent aphthous stomatitis in *Microbial Protoplasts, Spheroplasts and L-Forms* (L. B. Guze, ed.), Williams & Wilkins, Baltimore, Maryland, pp. 444-456.
113. Bakir, M. (1978). L-forms of *Staphylococcus aureus* as a cause of resistant conjunctivitis. *Bull. Ophthalmol. Soc. Egypt* 71:237-245.
114. Kagan, B. M. (1968). Role of L-forms in staphylococcal infections in *Microbial Protoplasts, Spheroplasts and L-Forms* (L. B. Guze, ed.), Williams & Wilkins, Baltimore, Maryland, pp. 372-378.
115. Fernandes, P. B. and Panos, C. (1977). Wall-less microbial isolates from a human renal biopsy. *J. Clin. Microbiol.* 5:106-107.
116. Pease, P. (1969). Bacterial L-forms in the blood and joint fluid of arthritic subjects. *Ann. Rheum. Dis.* 28:270-274.
117. Pease, P. (1970). Morphological appearances of a bacterial L-form growing in association with the erythrocytes of arthritic subjects. *Ann. Rheum. Dis.* 29:439-444.
118. Pease, P. (1974). Identification of bacteria from blood and joint fluids of human subjects as *Bacillus licheniformis*. *Ann. Rheum. Dis.* 33:67-69.
119. Duthie, J. J. R., Stewart, S. M., and McBride, W. H. (1976). Do diphtheroids cause rheumatoid arthritis? in *Infection and Immunology in the Rheumatic Disease* (D. C. Dumonde, ed.), Oxford, Blackwell Scientific, pp. 171-175.

Index

A

Acholeplasma
  DNA base composition, 23
  genome size, 32, 33
  lactate dehydrogenases, 23, 28
  relation to lactobacilli, 30
  relation to streptococci, 29-31
  ribonucleic acids, 31-35
  A. laidlawii, 13, 29, 33, 74, 80
Adhesion sites, 131, 134, 154
Antibiotic activities (see also specific organism), 229-255
  of aminoglycosides, 231, 245-247
  on cytoplasmic membrane, 235-238
  of macrolides, 231, 245
  of polyene macrolides, 237, 238
  on nucleic acid synthesis, 244
  of penicillins, 233, 234
  of polymyxins, 231, 235-243
  of tetracyclines, 231, 244-249
Antibiotics
  actinomycin, 103, 231, 244
  bacitracin, 104, 109, 231
  β-lactams, 28, 100, 134-158, 230, 233, 234
  carbenicillin, 189, 195, 196
  chloramphenicol, 103, 231
  cloxacillin, 104
  cycloserine, 100, 103, 104, 189, 234
  methicillin, 100
  novobiocin, 109, 191
  penicillin, 100, 189, 231, 233, 234

[Antibiotics]
  polymixin B, 198, 231
  puromycin, 103
  tetracycline, 188, 231, 244-249
  vancomycin, 104, 231, 234, 235
Antibiotics, resistance to, 245-252
  plasmid-mediated, 247, 251
Antibiotics, susceptibility to, 231-252
Antibody
  antibody-complement system, 55, 279-281
  growth-inhibiting, 280, 281
  IgG, 281
  IgM, 281
  secretory, 268
  serum, 267-268
Antigens (see also specific organism), 263-270
  cell wall, in common with L-forms, 264, 265, 269
  complement fixing, 265
  lipopolysaccharide, 265-267, 269
  membrane, 265, 266, 269
  protein, 265
ATPase
  antibodies to, 265-266
Autolytic activity, 101, 102, 284

B

Bacillus, 99-121
  cell division, 105-107, 118, 119

[*Bacillus*]
  induction, 7, 100–102
  morphology and replication, 104–107
  reversion and revertants, 100–104
  stable L-form, 100, 102, 111, 114, 118
  ultrastructure, 110–113
  unstable L-form, 103, 109
  B. licheniformis, 99–103
  B. megaterium, 99–103, 108
  B. pumilus, 99, 100, 104
  B. subtilis, 9, 12, 13, 99–121
  B. subtilis Sal-1, 100, 101, 105, 108, 114, 118, 119
  B. subtilis Sig-1, 106–113, 115–117
  B. subtilis Sig-2 and Sig-3, 108, 109
Bacillus, genetics, 117–121
  auxotrophic markers, 117–119
  DNA, plasmid, 118–120
  DNA, recombinant, 117–119
  transfection, 119–121
  transformation, DNA-mediated, 117–120
Bacillus, membrane
  diaminopimelic acid, 101, 105
  lipid, 104
  lipoteichoic acid, 109, 111, 120
  osmotic stability, 100
  peptidoglycan, 102–104, 111
  protein, 108, 111, 112, 116, 120
  SDS-PAGE, 111, 112, 116
  UDP nucleotide, 104
Bacteria, cell-wall defective (L-forms), 3, 215, 277–284, 287–311
  host defenses in, 277–284
Bacterial L-forms (see also specific organism)
  antibody-complement system, 55, 279–281
  A-type, 8, 215–217
  of *Brucella*, 163–181

[Bacterial L-forms]
  B-type, 8, 215–217
  in cell culture, 54, 55, 82–91, 169, 170
  cell division in, 105–107
  chemotaxis, 299
  clinical significance, 90–91, 309–311
  cytotoxicity, 81–91
  definition, 2, 3, 5, 24, 25, 128
  in evolution, 13, 14, 24, 25
  genetics, 12, 13, 50, 117–121
  of Group D *Streptococcus*, 43–55
  host defenses, 220, 277–284
  identification, 9–12, 50, 51
  immunology, 263–270
  induction, 5–8, 46, 47, 185–192, 195
  interaction with phagocytes, 281–283
  in vivo isolation, 189–192
  "large bodies," 8–11
  latent infection, 81–84
  morphology and replication, 6–11, 45–49, 104–107, 195–196
  of *Neisseria*, 185–192
  of *Nocardia*, 203–223
  nutrition, 47, 48
  parentage, 2, 24, 50, 51, 54, 55
  pathogenicity, 14, 15, 54, 55, 189–192, 201, 287–311
  physical environment, 47, 49
  of *Proteus*, 127–158
  of *Pseudomonas*, 195–201
  resistance to antibiotics, 88, 89, 195, 245–252
  reversion and revertants, 9, 11, 12, 45, 47, 49, 50, 51, 100–104, 217, 219
  sensitivity to antibiotics, 88, 89, 195, 231–252
  stable, 8, 12, 102, 103, 114, 118, 171, 175–179, 230
  stable protoplast, 151–156
  stable spheroplast, 143–151

INDEX

[Bacterial L-forms]
  of *Streptococcus pyogenes*, 59–91
  toxin production, 14, 298
  unstable, 8, 103, 109
  unstable spheroplast, 143–151
  ultrastructure, 6, 8, 9, 45, 46, 144, 145, 152, 153, 172–175, 197, 211, 216, 218, 238–243, 253
Bacterial revertants (see also specific organism)
  definition, 3, 5
  identification of, 3, 5, 8–12, 50, 51
Bacterial variants, 2, 3, 277–284
Bacteriocin, 267
Bacteriophage, 2, 119
Brucella, 163–187
  antigenic properties, 171–181
  in blood cultures, 163, 164
  brucellaphage, 164, 165, 175
  in cell culture, 169, 170
  in culture media, 170, 171, 181
  electron microscopy, 172–175
  macrophage inhibition factor (MIF), 177
  mitogenic activity, 180, 181
  protective immunity, 178
  spheroplasts, 169, 170, 171
  "stable" L-forms, 171, 175, 176–179
  "unstable" L-forms, 170, 171
  B. abortus, 165, 169, 170, 172, 174, 180
  B. suis, 165, 169, 171, 175, 180, 232

C

Cell wall (see also specific organism)
  antigens, 264, 265, 269
  diaminopimelic acid, 100, 104
  enzyme activity, 60–65
  glucosamine, 100, 105

[Cell wall]
  group substance, 52
  inhibition of, 60–65
  lipid, 72, 73, 74
  mucopeptide, 51, 52
  muramic acid, 100, 104
  nucleotide precursors, 60, 61
  peptidoglycan, 60–63, 102, 103, 204, 205
  physical structure, 205, 206
  M protein, 88, 265
Cell wall-deficient (-defective) bacteria, 3, 265, 277–284, 287, 309
Clostridia, 14, 30, 35, 298
Collagen, defective biosynthesis of, 89–91
Complement
  bacteriocidal activity of, 279, 280
  pathway, 281
Corynebacterium diphtheriae, 14, 298
Culture medium
  gelatin, 9, 50, 100
  minimal salts, 100, 102
  sodium chloride, 2, 6, 46, 47, 100–102
  sucrose, 2, 6, 46–47, 185–187, 191, 192
Cyanelles, genome size, 26
Cyanobacteria, genome size, 26
Cytochrome, in evolution, 26, 27, 28

D

Defined media, 6, 105–107
Dienes, Louis, 2, 4, 8, 100, 185, 288
Dienes stain, 4, 6, 44
DNA (deoxyribonucleic acid)
  chromosomal, 13, 32, 247
  extrachromosomal, 247, 248, 250–252
  inhibitors, 52, 53
  plasmid DNA, 118–120, 247, 251

[DNA (deoxyribonucleic acid)]
  plasmid DNA, in antibiotic
      resistance, 247–251
  recombinant, 117–119
  replication, 53, 54
  sequence losses, 31–35
  transfection, 119–121
  transformation, 117–120
DNA base composition (% G + C
      content), 12, 23, 28
  in *Acholeplasma*, 23
  in *Mycoplasma*, 23, 28
  in *Spiroplasma*, 23
  in *Ureaplasma*, 23

E

Electron microscopy (see also
      Ultrastructure)
  freeze fracture, 205–207, 241–243
  of *Bacillus*, 109–113
  of Group D *Streptococcus*, 45, 46
  of *Nocardia*, 2–5, 207
  of *Proteus*, 144–145, 152–153,
      238–243, 253
  of *Pseudomonas*, 197
  scanning, 144, 145, 152
Electron spin resonance spectroscopy,
      (*S. pyogenes*), 78, 79
Enzymes, 2, 46, 47, 66, 69, 100–102, 267
  amidase, 101, 102
  autolysin, 101, 102
  lysozyme, 46, 47, 100
  muralytic, 2, 46, 47
Erysipelothrix rhusiopathiae, 12,
      291–293
Escherichia coli, 6, 8, 129, 134–
      140, 142, 157, 232, 236–
      237, 266, 269
  cell envelope, 129
  endotoxin, 265
  spheroplast, 266
Evolution and origins
  of mycoplasmas, 31–35
  of wall-less prokaryotes, 21–35

F

Fatty acids (in *S. pyogenes*)
  analysis, 76, 77, 78
  composition, 77, 78
  monoenoic, 74–78
  oleic, 74–78
  spin label probes, 78, 79
Freeze-fracture replica
  of *Nocardia*, 205, 206, 207
  of *P. mirabilis*, 241–243

G

G + C (%) DNA composition of
      mycoplasmas, 23, 28
Genetics
  of *B. subtilis*, 117–121
  of resistance to antibiotics, 247–
      252
Genome size
  Chlamydia, 24, 26
  cyanelles, 26
  Mycoplasma, 23, 24, 32
  rickettsiae, 24
  streptococci, 25, 31, 32
Glomerulonephritis, 90, 91

H

Hemophilus influenzae, 8, 9–12, 24,
      220, 277, 284, 307
  induction and reversion,
      10–12
Host defenses, 220, 277–284
  antibody-complement system,
      280, 281
  interaction with phagocytes
      (*N. gonorrhoeae*), 281–
      284
  osmotic effects, 278, 279
  phagocytosis, 281, 283
  serum bactericidal activities, 279–
      281

I

Identification, laboratory (see also specific organisms)
 of L-forms, 3–12, 50–51
 of revertants, 9, 12, 50, 51
 of "stable" nonreverting L-forms, 9, 12, 50, 51
Immune deficiency states, 83, 84, 303, 305
Immune modulation, 269–270
 mitogens in, 269
 suppressors in, 269–270
Immunity, cellular
 granulomatous, 268–269
 hypersensitivity in, 268
Immunity, humoral
 secretory antibody, 268
 serum antibody, 267, 268
Immunogen, 263, 265
Immunology, 263–270
Induction (of L-forms) (see also specific organism)
 amino acids, 5
 β-lactams, 5, 134–158
 carbenicillin, 195, 196
 cycloserine, 5, 100
 in liquid medium, 101
 lysozyme, 5, 46, 99–101, 196
 methicillin, 100, 102
 muralytic enzymes, 5–7, 99–101
 penicillin, 2–6, 46, 99, 100, 101, 185
 polyvinylpyrrolidone in, 6, 186
 sodium chloride in, 6, 100, 185
 sodium succinate in, 100
 sucrose in, 6, 46, 47, 185
Infections, experimental (L-forms), 289–297
 Brucella, 294–295
 endocarditis, 301–304
 Erysipelothrix rhusiopathiae, 291–293
 gram-negative bacteria, 295–297
 Listeria monocytogenes, 291
 Nocardia, 293

[Infections, experimental (L-forms)]
 streptococci, 290–291
 in urinary tract, 295–296
Infections, human (bacterial variants, L-forms), 299–311
 aphthous stomatitis, 308
 osteomyelitis, 306, 307
 rheumatic fever, 305–306
 tuberculosis, 307, 308
 of urinary tract, 300–301

K

Klebsiella pneumoniae, 295, 297, 298
Klieneberger, Emmy, 1, 288
"Koch's postulates," 222

L

L-colonies
 conversion yield in streptococcus, 46–47
L-forms (see Bacterial L-forms)
Lactate dehydrogenase
 absence in *Ureaplasma*, 23
 in acholeplasmas, 23, 28
 in streptococci, 28
Listeria monocytogenes, 232, 291
Lysozyme
 effect of serum deficient in, 280
 in L-form induction, 5, 46, 99–101

M

Membrane (see also specific organism)
 antigens, 264–266
 of *B. subtilis*, 108–117
 basement, 90
 glycolipids, 268
 phospholipase, 268

[Membrane]
　　N-acetylmuramyl-L-alanine
　　　　amidase, 266
　　of *S. pyogenes*, 71–74, 78–80
Mitochondria, 25, 27
Morphology (see also specific
　　organism), 6–9, 100–105,
　　187–188, 205–209
Muralytic enzyme, L-form induced
　　by, 2, 6, 46, 47
Muramic acids, 129, 130, 140, 141, 148
　　N-acetyl, 129, 130
　　O-acetyl, 129, 130, 140, 141, 148
　　1,6-anhydro-N-acetyl, 130
Mycobacterium tuberculosis, 212,
　　307, 308
Mycolic acid, 204, 205, 219
Mycoplasma
　　DNA base composition, 23, 28
　　evolution and origins, 14, 21–35
　　fermentative, 28
　　M. capricolum, 33
　　M. mycoides, 2, 33
Mycoplasmatales, 22–26, 31, 32,
　　128, 156
　　genome sizes, 22–26, 31, 32

N

Neisseria gonorrhoeae, 4, 6, 185–
　　190, 192, 232
　　antibiotics, effect of, 188, 189
　　and cAMP (cyclic adenosine
　　　　monophosphate), 187–189
　　induction in vitro, 185–188, 192
　　interaction with phagocytic cells,
　　　　280–284
　　isolation in vivo, 189–190, 192
　　and PVP (polyvinylpyrrolidone),
　　　　186–187
　　reversion, 185–188
Neisseria meningitidis, 24, 190–192
　　induction and growth, 190–192
　　isolation in vivo, 191, 192
　　and PVP, 191

Neisseria perflava, 12
Nocardia, 8, 9, 203–223, 289, 290, 293
　　antibiotic sensitivities, 221, 222
　　chemical and physiological
　　　　properties, 214–217
　　freeze-fracture replicas, 206, 207
　　host defense mechanisms, 220
　　induction and growth, 207–215
　　"Koch's postulates," 222
　　morphology and ultrastructure,
　　　　205–209
　　mutation, 217–219, 223
　　reversion and revertants, 217–219,
　　　　222–223
　　role in disease, 220–223
　　Type A L-forms, 215, 217
　　Type B L-forms, 215, 217
　　N. asteroides, 204–223, 293
　　N. brasiliensis, 213
　　N. caviae, 212–214, 220–223,
　　　　259, 290, 293
　　N. corallina, 208
　　N. rubra, 207
Nocardia cell wall
　　chemical composition, 204, 205
　　physical structure, 205, 206

O

Origins
　　of mycoplasmas, 27–35
　　of wall-less prokaryotes, 21–35
Osmotic effects of host
　　　　environments, 278, 279
Osmotic pressure
　　of cell wall-defective bacteria,
　　　　278–280
　　of renal medulla, 278, 279
Osmotic stabilizer
　　polyvinylpyrrolidone (PVP), 6,
　　　　185–187, 189, 191, 196
　　sodium chloride, 2, 6, 100–102
　　sodium succinate, 6, 100
　　spermine, 6, 47
　　sucrose, 2, 6, 46, 47, 185–187,
　　　　190, 191, 192

P

Pathogenicity (L-forms, bacterial variants), 297–311
Penicillin(s) (see also specific organism)
   effect on cell wall synthesis, 143–154, 230, 233, 234
   induction of L-forms, 2–5, 134–158
Penicillin-binding proteins
   absence of, in mycoplasmas, 32
   in *Chlamydia*, 26
   in *Proteus*, 12, 52, 136, 138–140, 142, 143
Phagocytosis, 280–284
Plasmids, role in antibiotic resistance, 247, 248, 249, 250, 251
Prokaryotes, origins, 21–42
   wall-less prokaryotes, evolution of, 21–42
Proteus, 127–158
   antibiotic effects, 236–243, 248
   and β-lactam antibiotics, 128, 134–158
   β-lactamases in, 127, 142, 156, 157
   muramic acids, 129, 130, 140, 141, 148
   penicillin-binding proteins in, 12, 126, 138–140, 142, 143, 148–150, 155–158
   DD-peptidases, 134–139, 142
   LD-peptidases, 134, 136, 147
   peptidoglycan, 128–134, 140, 141, 147, 148, 156–158
   plasma membranes, 129, 131, 134, 146, 153, 154, 158
Proteus mirabilis, 62, 142, 146–158, 204, 232, 238–243, 264, 266, 267, 295, 299
   antibodies to, 266, 267
   antigenic determinants, 264
   endotoxin in, 204
   urease production, 267

Proteus outer membrane, 130–133, 141, 142, 147, 154–157
   lipopolysaccharide, 130–133, 141, 142, 147, 154–157
   lipoprotein, 130–133, 141, 142, 154
   phospholipids, 130–133, 155
   porins, 131, 147, 157
Proteus vulgaris, 151–153, 232
Pseudomonas aeruginosa, 9, 195–201, 280, 283
   antibiotic sensitivities, 198, 199
   biochemical reactions, 198, 199
   immunology of, 198, 199
   induction and growth, 195, 196
   morphology, 197, 198
   pathogenicity, 199, 201
   studies in animals, 200, 201
Protoplasts (see also specific organisms), 3, 6, 45–47, 100–102, 104, 108, 143–158, 212, 213, 265

R

Reproduction and growth (see also specific organism), 6–9
Reversion, mechanisms of, 8–12, 45, 47, 49, 102–104
   agar, 9, 103
   gelatin, 9, 103
   primer, 12, 103
RNA (ribonucleic acids), 31–53
   rRNA, 32–35
   16S RNA, 30–33
   23S RNA, 32–33
   5S rRNA, 27, 31–35
   16S rRNA, 30, 32, 33
RNA gene sequences, 31–35
RNA gene sets, 32–35
   in *Acholeplasma*, 32, 33
   in *B. subtilis*, 34, 35
   in *E. coli*, 33, 35
   in mycoplasmas, 32–35
   in streptococci, 32–35

S

Salmonella typhi, 264, 280, 296, 308
Salmonella typhimurium, 232, 264, 298
Serological tests
  agglutination, 267
  complement fixation, 267
  precipitation, 267
Serum
  anti-L-form, 264, 267
  hyperimmune, 2
  killing effect of, 279-281
Sodium chloride, in L-form medium, 2, 6, 100-102
Spheroplast L-forms, 3, 143-151
Spheroplast(s), 3, 47, 143-151, 212, 213, 265
Spin label probes, 79
Stable L-forms (see specific organism)
Staphylococcus aureus, 8, 14, 60, 66, 140, 232, 245, 248, 252, 254, 265, 269, 298, 301
Streptobacillus moniliformis, 2, 289
Streptococci, Group A, 2, 6, 59, 66, 91, 232, 247, 248, 265-267, 291
  antigenicity, 265-267, 269
Streptococci, Group B, 232, 247, 248, 249
Streptococci, Group D, 43-55, 66
  biochemical characterization, 51-53
  cell wall components, 51-52
  DNA inhibitors, 53
  DNA replication, 53, 54
  genetic relatedness, 50, 51
  induction, 46, 47
  morphology, 44, 46
  nucleic acid homology, 50, 51
  physical environment, 47, 49
  protein patterns, by PAGE, 50, 51
  reversion and revertants, 47, 51
  in tissue culture, 54, 55

Streptococcus
  aldolase(s), 30
  antigenic characteristics of, 265-267
  gene sequences in, 32, 33
  genome size, 31
  lactate dehydrogenase, 28
  relation to acholeplasmas, 28, 31
  S. cremoris, 32, 33
  S. faecalis, 9, 45, 47, 50, 51, 73, 268, 280, 289, 298, 299, 301
  S. faecium, 9, 12, 45, 55
  S. lactis, 33
  S. liquefaciens, 46
  S. pneumoniae, 157, 232
Streptococcus pyogenes, 4, 12-14, 59-91, 280
  cell wall nucleotide precursors, 60-65
  collagen biosynthesis, 89-91
  cytotoxicity, 59-89
  effect on host cells, 88-89
  enzyme activities, 61-71
  in immunosuppressed mice, 82-86, 91
  isotonic L-form, 74-83
  macromolecular synthesis, 60-74
  membrane D-alanine incorporation, 69-70
  osmotic fragility, 74-81
  peptidoglycan, 60-64
  teichoic and lipoteichoic acid, 65-74

T

Tissue culture
  Brucella, 169, 170
  N. gonorrhoeae, 281-283
  S. pyogenes
    human heart cells, 83-87
    human embryonic kidney cells, 85-87
    human liver cells, 85-87

INDEX

Thermoplasma, in evolution, 24, 33
Toxin production
   Clostridium botulinum, 14, 298
   Clostridium tetani, 14, 298
   Corynebacterium diphtheriae, 14
   Vibrio cholerae, 14, 298

U, V

Ultrastructure (see also Electron microscopy), 6, 8, 9, 45, 46, 109, 113, 197, 238–243, 253
Unstable L-forms (see specific organism)
Vibrio cholerae, 14, 298